Abstracts

XXIIIrd CONGRESS of the International Society of Blood Transfusion

Amsterdam 1994

CONTENTS PAGE

0002

MOLECULAR BASIS OF THE LACK OF EXPRESSION OF SOME Rh EPITOPES IN D CATEGORY PHENOTYPES.

C. Rouillac[1], I. Mouro[1], M. Beolet[2], J.P. Cartron[1], C. Le Van Kim[1], Y. Colin[1]
[1]INSERM U76, INTS 6, rue Alexandre Cabanel, 75015 PARIS
[2]CRTS, 19-21, rue Camille Guérin, 59012 Lille Cédex

The Rh D, Cc and Ee antigens are carried by at least three unglycosylated membrane proteins of the human erythrocytes encoded by two highly related genes, *D* and *CE*. The major antigen, D, is a mosaic composed of at least nine determinants (epD1 to epD9). The lack of expression of some of these D epitopes at the surface of variant red cells defines the so-called D category phenotypes.
In a first attempt to delineate the different D epitopes, we analysed the RH locus and the transcripts from D category red cells (D^{IVa}, D^{IVb}, D^{Va} and D^{VI}). Out of 10 D^{VI} genomes investigated, 8 exhibited a segmental DNA replacement between the D fragment encompassing exons 4, 5 and 6 and the equivalent region of the *CE* gene. In the 2 other variants, these 3 exons were deleted. Our results indicated also that D^{VI}Ce and D^{VI}cE haplotypes are associated with 2 types of genomic rearrangement: gene conversion and deletion respectively. Analysis of D^{IVa}, D^{IVb} and D^{Va} transcripts showed that the lack of expression of different D epitopes is always associated with substitutions of amino acids specific of the RhD protein by those encoded at the equivalent position in the *CE* gene.
This study points out the importance of some polymorphic positions between D and Cc/Ee proteins in D antigenicity. The related *D* and *CE* genes are involved in recombination or gene conversion events which could be one of the basis of the extreme polymorphism of the RH blood group system.

0003

RhE-GENOTYPING BY POLYMERASE CHAIN REACTION AMPLIFICATIONS WITH SEQUENCE-SPECIFIC PRIMERS (PCR-SSP)

B.H.W. Faas[1], S. Simsek[1], P.M.M. Bleeker[1], M.A.M. Overbeeke[1], H.Th.M. Cuijpers[1], C.E. van der Schoot[1,2], A.E.G. Kr. von dem Borne[1,2]
1 Central Laboratory of the Dutch Red Cross Blood Transfusion Service, 2 Academic Medical Centre, Amsterdam.

It has been demonstrated that the Rhesus (Rh) blood group antigens are encoded by two homologous genes: the RhD-gene and the RhCcEe-gene. In this study we made use of the polymerase chain reaction with sequence-specific primers (PCR-SSP) to determine the RhE-genotype of 134 donors (including rare haplotypes) on genomic DNA. With a set of primers, of which one primer had a 3′ end-nucleotide specific for nucleotide (nt) 676 of the proposed RhCcEx-gene but not to nt676 of the RhD- and RhCcee-gene, we obtained only a product in DNA-samples of all donors (n=37) which were serologically typed as being E-positive. So we can conclude that we have developed a simple and reliable technique to determine the RhE genotype. This can be very useful in recently transfused patients in which anti-E is detected, and in prenatal diagnostics. We also confirm the proposed association between the cytosine at position 676 and the E-phenotype in this large series of donors.

0004

RFLP analysis identifies Rh D gene fragments in two donors with the RhD negative CCee phenotype

C.A. Hyland[1], L.C. Wolter[1], A. Saul[2].
1 Red Cross Blood Bank, 2 Queensland Institute of Medical Research, Brisbane, Australia.

AIM: To determine whether the Rh D gene is invariably absent in Rh D negative individuals.
METHOD: Blood donors with Rh phenotypes ccee (n=25), CCee (n=3) ccEE (n=2) were studied. Genomic DNA was cut with *MSP I*, and a Southern blot performed after electrophoresis on 1% agarose gel. Blots were hybridized to a genomic and a cDNA probe which spanned, respectively, the upstream and exon 1 region (5′probe) and exons 8 to 10 (3′probe) of the Rh CcEe gene and the closely related D gene.
RESULTS: The 5′probe identifies 2.6, 2.5, and 1.1 gene fragments from the Rh CcEe gene and 2.45 and 2.2 Kb bands from the D gene. The 3′ probe identifies Rh CcEe bands of 2.8, 1.1 Kb and a 2.0 Kb fragments from the D gene. All Rh D gene fragments were absent in all Rh ccee and ccEE types and in one of the 3 CCee types. One CCee type showed the 2.45 and 2.2 Kb D bands were present but the 2.0 Kb band was absent. The other exhibited all D gene fragments from both the 5′ and 3′ regions.
CONCLUSION: The absence of D gene fragments in the Rh ccee phenotypes is consistent with the report that the Rh D negative trait arises from the complete absence of the D gene[1]. However, the presence of D gene fragments in two donors with the rarer CCee phenotype suggests that alternative mechanisms can also generate the D negative trait.

1. Colin Y, Cherif-Zahar B, Le Van Kim C, Raynal V, Van Huffel V, Cartron JP: Blood 78:2747, 1991.

0005

Lutheran blood group glycoprotein is a new member of the immunoglobulin superfamily of proteins

Parsons SF, Mawby WJ*, Anstee DJ
International Blood Group Reference Laboratory, Bristol, UK
*Dept. of Biochemistry, University of Bristol, UK

The Mr 85,000 and Mr 78,000 Lutheran glycoproteins[1] were isolated from human erythrocyte membranes by immunoaffinity chromatography using monoclonal antibody BRIC 221. Amino acid sequence analysis allowed the design of short (24mer), redundant oligonucleotides for use in PCR amplification. PCR using plasmid DNA from a human placental cDNA library (Invitrogen, San Diego, CA, USA) as template yielded a 459 base pair product which was subcloned, sequenced and used to screen cDNA libraries. A cDNA clone of 2,417 base pairs was isolated from a human placental, λgt11library (Clontech, La Jolla, CA, USA), sequenced and the deduced amino acid sequence studied.

The predicted mature protein has 597 amino acids. There are five disulphide bonded, extracellular, immunoglobulin superfamily domains, a single hydrophobic, membrane spanning domain and a cytoplasmic domain of some 60 amino acids. The predicted structure is consistent with immunochemical analysis data.

1 Parsons SF *et al* 1987 Transfusion **27**:61-63

0007

THE IMPACT OF A NOVEL DECISION AIDE ON RED BLOOD CELL TRANSFUSION.

B. Littenberg, H.L. Corwin, A. Gettinger, J.P. AuBuchon. Dartmouth-Hitchcock Medical Center, Lebanon, New Hampshire, USA.

We incorporated a point-of-decision educational intervention into the transfusion ordering process of a multidisciplinary intensive care unit (ICU) and studied its effect on physician behavior. In a 3-mo. control period of baseline data accumulation, the transfusion audit criterion was a hemoglobin (Hb) of 100 g/L. In Phase 2 (3 mo.), clinicians ordered on a form that suggested "triggers" of 86 g/L, hemorrhage or anemic morbidity (*eg*, acute ischemia, impaired O_2 transport). In Phase 3 (3-mo.), the form required a trigger of 70 g/L in asymptomatic patients (pts). For 529 transfusion events in 295 ICU pts, mean Hb at transfusion decreased from 85 to 83 to 81 g/L ($p < .008$). Single-unit transfusions decreased, but the proportion of pts transfused and the number of units transfused (per pt or per pt-day) did not change. The reduction in Hb trigger value was not associated with an increase in length of hospital stay or mortality. By multivariate analysis, total blood usage was associated with length of ICU stay and with hematocrit and illness severity (APACHE II score) on admission to ICU ($p < .001$). Thus the educational interventions were associated with transfusions being given at lower Hb levels but did not reduce total red cell usage. However, the interventions were not associated with increased mortality. Point-of-decision interventions can alter clinical practice but, in this setting, did not reduce red cell usage.

0008

INFLUENCE OF HEMOGLOBIN AND BLOOD LOSS ON MORTALITY IN ELECTIVE SURGERY IN THE JEHOVAH'S WITNESS

RK Spence, C Curry, RC Camishion, MJ Pello, JB Alexander, U Atabek, F Koniges. Cooper Hospital/ UMC, Robert Wood Johnson Medical School, Camden, New Jersey, USA

The Jehovah's Witness (JW) presents a unique challenge because of this group's refusal to accept transfusion. We analyzed the effect of preoperative Hgb (PreH), and estimated blood loss (EBL) on mortality in 206 consecutive JW patients who underwent elective, non-cardiac surgery for which transfusion was anticipated between 1982 and 1993. Mortality was 9/206 (4.4%). PreH was: mean=9.5 g/d (3.5-16.5); EBL was: mean 1139 ml (0-7000). Regression analysis for PreH, EBL, sex, race, and preexisting disease showed only PreH ($p=.025$) and EBL ($p=.003$) to be predictors of mortality. PreH correlated with outcome at $<$ 10 g/d (N=53; $p=.03$) but not for PreH $>$ 10 g/d (N=153). 4 of the 9 deaths occurred in patients with PreH $>$ 10 g/d with EBL averaging 2300 ml. Elective surgery can be done safely in the majority of JW patients if blood loss is kept to a minimum. Anemic JW patients may benefit from restoration of red cell mass prior to elective surgery.

0009

CURRENT BLOOD TRANSFUSION PRACTICE IN AORTIC ANEURYSM SURGERY IN SCOTLAND

A A Milne[1] and W G Murphy[2,3] (on behalf of the Scottish Vascular Audit Group).

[1]Department of Vascular Surgery, Royal Infirmary, Edinburgh.
[2]South East Scotland Blood Transfusion Service, Edinburgh.
[3]Department of Medicine, University of Edinburgh.

Thirty-one surgeons practising vascular surgery in Scotland provided details of blood ordering policies for elective and emergency aortic aneurysm repairs. A blood ordering schedule was operated by 29 surgeons for elective operations and by 26 surgeons for emergency operations. The number of units of red cell concentrate ordered for elective operations ranged from 3 to 8 units (mode = 4) and for emergency operations from 6 to 12 units (mode = 6). The average time required to obtain red cell concentrates in the operating theatre in emergencies was estimated to be 38 minutes (range 15-90 mins) for a first time request and 9 minutes (range 2-30 mins) to obtain further blood in a patient already crossmatched. Blood conservation techniques in use included the use of low porosity or sealed grafts (27 surgeons), auto-transfusion (6 surgeons, but only regularly by 3), pre-deposit autologous transfusion preoperative haemodilution (1 surgeon). Intravenous heparin was used by 90% of surgeons during elective operations and by 16% of surgeons during emergency operations. Most surgeons used a standard dose of 5,000 units of heparin. These observations demonstrate considerable variations in practice and indicate the need for formulating a consensus on the use of blood transfusion in aortic aneurysm surgery.

0010

CANCER RECURRENCE AND OVERALL SURVIVAL AFTER BLOOD TRANSFUSION IN COLORECTAL CANCER PATIENTS, "THE *CRAB* CLINICAL TRIAL"

JGA Houbiers[1,2], LMG van de Watering[1], J Hermans[3], CJH van de Velde[2] & A Brand[1]
[1]Immunohaematology & Blood Bank, [2]Surgery, University Hospital Leiden, the Netherlands, tel. 31-71-264007, [3]Medical Statistics, Leiden University

In a multicentre randomized controlled trial (CRAB) we investigated the putative detrimental effect of blood transfusion (BT) on the prognosis of colorectal cancer. Leukocyte depleted ("filtered") blood products have been shown not to induce immunosuppressive effects in organ-transplant settings.

Patients were randomized to receive either packed cells without buffy coat (PC) or leukocyte depleted blood (LD). From 1987 till 1991 1108 patients have been randomized by 16 participating hospitals and according to the inclusion criteria 871 appeared eligible for analysis of whom 697 had been operated upon with curative intent. No differences in prognosis between PC and LD patients were observed. Even if the comparison was limited to patients who had received more than 3 units of blood no significant differences between leukocyte depleted and standard packed cells were observed: 64% and 68% 3 yr survival. Transfused patients (LD or PC) showed a 12% lower 3 year survival rate than non-transfused patients ($p < 0.01$), colorectal cancer recurrence rates, however, were similar ($p = 0.22$).

0013

BLOOD DONATION AND RED CELL VOLUME (RCV) REGENERATION IN DONORS OF DIFFERENT WEIGHTS.

A. Heaton, S. Holme. Irwin Memorial Blood Centers, San Francisco, CA; American Red Cross, Norfolk, VA, USA.

Studies to quantify red cell volume regeneration post donation were performed in eight females and four males who donated 475 $\pm$ 24 mL whole blood on two occasions >56 days apart. ^{99m}Tc RCV was measured on days 1, 7, and 42. All donor hematocrits were > 38% for females and > 41% for males.

N=11, Mean $\pm$ SE:

	^{99m}Tc RCV(mL)	Δ RCV(mL)	Correlation
Day 7	1566 $\pm$ 102		
		168 $\pm$ 45	.952
Day 42	1734 $\pm$ 129		
		221 $\pm$ 38	.963
Day 1	1513 $\pm$ 116		

Although the differences between RCV 7 and 42, and RCV 1 and 42 were significant (p <.001), the difference between RCV 1 and 7 was small, 54 $\pm$ 38 mL (p = 0.184).

91 additional ^{99m}Tc RCV studies were performed on paired 440 mL whole blood donations >56 days apart. Mean ($\pm$ SE) RCV difference averaged 30 $\pm$ 12 mL which were significantly different (p=0.014), the standard error of prediction averaged 7% and the values correlated closely (r = 0.97). Only females exhibited a significant (p <.001) reduction in red cell volume (63 $\pm$ 12 mL) when the donors' RCVs were analyzed by gender.

An inverse relationship was found between the two-donation RCV difference and the RCV on the first donation, suggesting that female donors should have RCV >1350 mL to avoid a greater than 5% reduction in RCV as a result of donation.

0014

F.G. Korse, H. Dikken
Central Laboratory of the Netherlands Red Cross Blood Transfusion Service, Amsterdam, The Netherlands

STERILITY TESTING OF WHOLE BLOOD DONATIONS

Bacterial contamination of donor blood continues to be an important risk factor for the quality and safety of blood and blood products. The sterility test methods as described in pharmacopeias require incubation periods of one or two weeks. Recently alternative methods such as BacT/Alert ® [Organon Teknika, AKZO] (B.A.) have been introduced which use automated incubation and detection, allowing results to be obtained faster.

We have tested 1990 random units of whole blood from voluntary non-paid donors for sterility. All tests were performed by using both B.A. and european pharmacopeial methods. The sensitivity of both methods was not significantly different. In 4 units (0,2%) of whole blood we detected bacterial contamination by both methods. In 20 units we detected bacterial contamination discordantly positive, i.e. either positive in B.A./negative in pharmacopeial method or negative in B.A./positive in pharmacopeial method.

All non-sterile samples were followed up by: testing sterility of the corresponding units of red blood cel concentrates (RBC) and microbial identification.

In 8 units RBC derived from the initially positive 24 whole blood donations bacterial contamination was detected. Incubation of these sterility-test samples started at 5-8 days postdonation. The identification results demonstrated that a large number of the bacteria is part of the normal skin-flora.

Since all contaminated units RBC showed positive results in B.A.-testing on whole blood we conclude that the B.A. method is at least equivalent to the pharmacopeial method.

0016

AN ANTENATAL SCREENING PROGRAMME TO DETECT PREGNANCIES AT RISK OF NEONATAL ALLOIMMUNE THROMBOCYTOPENIA DUE TO ANTI-HPA-1A

Williamson LM[1], Hadfield R[1], Maciver C[1], Ouwehand WH[1,2].
[1]Division of Transfusion Medicine, University of Cambridge, [2]NIBSC, Potters Bar, UK.

Objectives: (1) To establish the relationship between feto-maternal alloimmunisation to HPA-1a as detected by population screening, cord platelet count and perinatal morbidity.
(2) To determine the logistics and cost-effectiveness of such a screening programme.
Study design: Routine antenatal samples from 25,000 women over 1 year (from Sept 1993) are typed for HPA-1a using a modified MAIPA technique (monoclonal anti-glycoprotein IIb/IIIa followed by polyclonal anti-HPA1a). HLA-DR52a typing is performed on HPA1a neg women by PCR followed by sequence-specific oligonucleotide probing. Women are screened either once (if HLA-DR52a neg) or 3 times (if HLA-DR52a pos) for anti-HPA1a in an ELISA assay with GPIIb/IIIa coated plates. HPA1a negative platelets are available at delivery if antibodies are found. Cord platelet counts and cerebral ultrasound scanning are performed on high risk infants.
Results: Of 9,000 women so far screened (Jan 1994), 2.2% are HPA1a negative, of whom 37% are HLA-DR52a positive. Antibody screening and follow up are ongoing.
Conclusion: Antenatal screening for the major cause of NAITP is feasible on a large scale.

0017

Antenatal Management of Alloimmune Thrombocytopenia (AITP)

Kanhai H.H.H.[1], Brand A.[2], R.H. Meerman[1], H. Viëtor[2], D.Oepkes[1], J.Bennebroek Gravenhorst[1]
[1] Department of Obstetrics and [2] Blood Bank, University Hospital Leiden, The Netherlands.

Although the pathophysiology of AITP is thought to be analogous to Rhesus disease, little is known about antenatal management. Between 1989 and 1993 we treated 20 pregnancies on basis of a protocol. The timing of the first cordocentesis was individualized and based on the obstetric history. In order to prevent bleeding complications due to the cordocentesis, maternal platelets were infused to obtain a fetal platelet count of $>100\times10^9$/l. IVIG was administered to the mother (1.0 g/kg/wk), in cases of low platelet count. All the siblings had platelet counts $<40\times10^9$/l at birth. Platelet antibodies involved were anti HPA-1a (16), HPA-5a (2), HPA-3a (1) and a private antibody in one woman. Nine women received IVIG from 28 weeks onwards.
Results: A total of 46 cordocentesis were performed, 37 were followed by platelet transfusions. There were no bleeding complications. In only 2 cases there was response to IVIG. Mean gest. age at birth was 37 wks (range 34-41) and mean birthweight 2825 g (range 2180-3850). The mean platelet count at birth was 140×10^9/l (range 36-210). One infant died perinataly due to asphyxia. Haemorrhage in the infants was not observed.
Conclusions: With the use of this protocol serious bleeding complications in AITP can be prevented.

0018

ANTENATAL MANAGEMENT OF SEVERE FETO-MATERNAL ALLOIMMUNE THROMBOCYTOPENIA (FMAIT): REPORT OF THE MANAGEMENT OF 13 AFFECTED PREGNANCIES.

M.F.Murphy[1], A.H.Waters[1], H.A.Doughty[1], H.Hambley[2], R.S.Mibashan[2], C.H.Rodeck[3], K.Nicolaides[3]. [1]Department of Haematology, St.Bartholomew's Hospital and [2]Department of Haematology and [3]Harris Birthright Fetal Medicine Research Centre, King's College Hospital, U.K.

The most serious complication of FMAIT is intracranial haemorrhage (ICH) which causes death or long-term neurological morbidity in up to 25% of cases. The recognition that spontaneous ICH may occur in utero led us to attempt to prevent this in women with previously affected pregnancies due to anti-HPA-1a. The therapeutic options included fetal platelet transfusions and maternal steroids and/or IVIgG. In the first affected pregnancy, ICH occurred between 32 and 35 weeks' gestation before any treatment had been given, emphasising the need for earlier intervention. Our experience with 12 further pregnancies is reported.

4 severely affected cases (initial platelet count <20 x 10^9/l) were managed successfully with weekly fetal platelet transfusions started between 18 and 29 weeks to maintain the fetal platelet count above 30 x 10^9/l until delivery at 33-35 weeks. 1 severely affected case was referred late and was managed successfully with one transfusion at 36 weeks. 4 cases were mildly affected (initial platelet count >80 x 10^9/l) and the platelet counts were maintained in 1 case with steroids and in 2 with IVIgG without the need for repeated transfusions but in the fourth the fetal platelet count fell despite steroids and IVIgG and transfusions were required. 3 pregnancies resulted in fetal death; 1 due to ICH soon after starting steroids and IVIgG, 1 despite the successful initiation of fetal transfusions after the mother had a severe fall and 1 due to a cord haematoma.

The management of severe FMAIT to prevent antenatal ICH is still evolving. Steroids and IVIgG may be effective in some mildly affected cases but serial fetal platelet transfusions are the preferred therapy for those who are severely affected.

0019

INEFFICACY OF INTRAVENOUS IMMUNOGLOBULIN TREATMENT FOR FETAL ALLOIMMUNE THROMBOCYTOPENIA

H. Kroll[1)], G. Giers[2)], R. Bald[3)], V. Kiefel[1)], C. Breitfeld[1)], J. Hoch[2)], P. Hanfland[2)], M. Hansmann[3)], C. Mueller-Eckhardt[1)]
[1)]Institute for Clinical Immunology and Transfusion Medicine, Justus Liebig University, Giessen, [2)]Institute for Experimental Hematology and Transfusion Medicine, University of Bonn, [3)]Dept. for Prenatal Diagnostic and Therapy, University of Bonn, Germany

Fetal alloimmune thrombocytopenia (FAIT) is caused by transplacental transfer of maternal platelet antibodies, mostly directed against the Zw^a antigen. Since the fetus is threatened by low platelet counts (pc) and consecutive intracranial hemorrhage (ICH), prenatal monitoring and treatment are essential. However, the appropriate approach is still under discussion.

We report here on prenatal management of 12 affected fetuses. All 11 mothers were multiparous women who previously had thrombocytopenic newborns due to Zw^a incompatibility. First umbilical blood sampling (UBS) was performed at 24.5 (mean, range: 18-33) weeks of gestation (wg). Subsequently maternal intravenous immunoglobulin (ivlg) treatment was started over a mean period of 7.1 weeks (range: 3-13 weeks) at a dose of 1g/kg body weight per week. The fetal pc was monitored by UBS (mean frequency: 5.8, range: 2-13) which was always followed by intraumbilical transfusion of maternal or compatible donor platelets. In one fetus the baseline pc minimally rose (10G/l to 35G/l), in 5 fetuses the baseline pc remained unchanged at a low level and in 6 cases it progressively declined. One fetus suffered from ICH and was subsequently treated by platelet transfusions. In another case maternal ivlg treatment was discontinued at a pc of 25G/l and ivlg administered directly to the fetus who was delivered 4 weeks later after a minor rise of pc to 46G/l.

We conclude that the application of ivlg to the mother has no relevant therapeutic effect on FAIT. Additional intrauterine ivlg administration to the fetus in one case was also ineffective but this approach needs further evaluation. At present, only compatible platelet transfusions to the fetus are sufficient to manage severely affected cases.

0021

MAX[a], A NEW LOW-FREQUENCY PLATELET-SPECIFIC ANTIGEN LOCALIZED ON GLYCOPROTEIN (GP) IIb

P.Noris[1], A.E.G. Kr. von dem Borne[2,3], S. Simsek[2],
1 IRCCS San Matteo, Pavia, Italy;2 Central Laboratory of the Netherlands Red Cross Blood Transfusion Service, Amsterdam, the Netherlands; 3 Academic Medical Centre, Amsterdam, the Netherlands.

A new platelet-specific antigen, Max^a, was identified in a newborn infant with typical signs of NAITP. In the monoclonal antibody-specific immobilization of platelet antigens (MAIPA)-assay, the new antigen was localized on GP IIb. A panel of monoclonal antibodies, directed against GPIIb/IIIa, GPIIb and GPIIIa was used for this purpose. The GPIIb location was confirmed in immunoprecipitation and western-blotting experiments. To unravel the molecular basis of the Max^a antigen, platelet RNA from the Max^{a+} father was isolated and reversely transcribed into cDNA. The entire coding region of the GPIIb cDNA was amplified by the polymerase chain reaction. Nucleotide sequence analysis is currently performed. Until now 3 out of 497 unrelated donors were found to be positive for the Max^a antigen. Therefore it must be considered as a low-frequency antigen and must be taken into account in transfusion reactions.

0022

HPA-3 GENOTYPING BY PCR AMPLIFICATION WITH SEQUENCE-SPECIFIC PRIMERS (PCR-SSP)

P Metcalfe* and W H Ouwehand*#, *Division of Haematology, NIBSC, Potters Bar, UK, #University of Cambridge, UK.

All of the human platelet-specific alloantigen (HPA) systems so far described are determined by a single base-pair substitution which leads to a single amino acid difference in the relevant glycoprotein. This report describes a method using the polymerase chain reaction with sequence-specific primers (PCR-SSP) to determine the HPA-3a/3b genotype of donors in a simple and rapid one stage technique.

Two allele-specific primers were designed. In each the 3' nucleotide was complementary to one form of the DNA sequence at the HPA-3 polymorphic site. An additional mis-match near the 3' end of the primers and selected PCR conditions (denaturation 25s at 97°, annealing 30s at 64° and extension 30s at 72°) were used to ensure allele-specific amplification.

DNA from 20 donors was typed for HPA-3a/3b by PCR-SSP. All the results were in exact concordance with the genotypes derived by allele-specific restriction enzyme analysis (ASRA) using the enzyme Fok 1.

PCR-SSP is simpler and cheaper than restriction enzyme analysis and is therefore more suitable for large-scale genotyping of platelet donors. It will be used to maintain the UK National Platelet Panel.

0023

DNA-RFLP TYPING OF HUMAN PLATELET ALLOANTIGENS ZW, KO, BAK, BR (HPA-1, -2, -3, -5)

V. Kiefel, K. Unkelbach, S. Santoso, R. Kalb, C. Breitfeld, H. Kroll, C. Mueller-Eckhardt

Institute for Clinical Immunology and Transfusion Medicine, Justus-Liebig-University, Giessen, Germany.

After elucidation of the genetic basis underlying platelet alloantigen systems HPA-1 to 4, and recently HPA-5 (1, 2), DNA based typing has become an attractive alternative to serological techniques with sera containing platelet specific alloantibodies. Reliability of DNA typing by restriction fragment length (RFL) anylsis for HPA-1, -2, -3, -5 was compared to serological typing (MAIPA, platelet agglutination) in 98 donors. As recently proposed, restriction enzyme Mnl I was used for RFL HPA-5 typing (2). Typing results were concordant with serological antigen determination by MAIPA.
HPA-1 typing by digestion of PCR-products with endonuclease Msp I revealed an additional restriction site near the base coding for HPA-1b in one donor. In the meantime, the underlying base exchange ($T^{217}G$) was found in 3 of 261 donors. A new configuration for HPA-1 RFL analysis using a larger PCR product and endonuclease ScrF I with the advantage of an "internal control" for completeness of digestion, was evaluated in a further sample of 40 donors.

(1) S. Santoso et al., J. Clin. Invest., 1993, 92: 2427; (2) R. Kalb et al., in press

0024

HPA-4b (Yuk[b]) NEONATAL ALLOIMMUNE THROMBOCYTOPENIA (NAIT) IN A CAUCASIAN FAMILY: ALLELE CHARACTERIZATION

D. Gallardo[1], M. Pérez[2], N. Puig[3], P. Pérez[1], A. Boronat[2], A. Ribera[1]
1 Banc de Sang de l'ICS, Barcelona; 2 Facultat de Bioquímica, Universitat de Barcelona; 3 Centro de Transfusión de la Comunidad Valenciana, Spain.

Since the HPA-4 system was first described in orientals, a great number of caucasian individuals had been screened for the presence of the HPA-4b antigen with no positive results. Recently, two cases of NAIT caused by HPA-4b antibodies have been reported in two unrelated caucasian families with no known ancestor from Asia on either side. Both reports are based on serological studies and, since antibodies may recognize the overall configuration of the antigen rather than its specific chemical structures, we investigated the exact molecular event leading to one of the caucasian HPA-4b phenotypes mentioned above.
Two of the five HPA-4b positive siblings, including the father of the affected newborn, were chosen for allelic characterization. Specific primers were designed for genomic amplification of exon number 3 of the GPIIIa gene and PCR products were cloned and sequenced. In both cases two different sequences were obtained: one corresponding to the HPA-4a allele and the other one showing a single G to A substitution leading to an Arg to Gln change at residue 143 of the GPIIIa. This mutation is the same as the one defined for the HPA-4b allele in orientals and this finding may suggest that HPA-4 dimorfism took place before ethnic differentiation.

0028

THE VALUE OF THE E2 AND NS5 ANTIGEN FOR DETECTION OF HEPATITIS C VIRUS INFECTION.

H.Zaaijer[1], D.Vallari[2], M.Cunningham[2], R.Lesniewski[2], H.Reesink[1], P.Lelie[1].
1 Central Lab Netherlands Red Cross Bloodtransfusion Service, Amsterdam, Netherlands.
2 Abbott Laboratories, Hepatitis/Aids R&D, N.Chicago, USA.

Aim: To study the value of the hepatitis C virus (HCV) non-structural-5 (NS5) and envelope-2 (E2) antigen for detection of HCV infection.

Method: We studied 3 panels of donor and patient samples:
panel A: Riba-2=indeterminate, HCV-RNA=positive, n=33 donors.
panel B: Riba-2=indeterminate, HCV-RNA=negative, n=39 donors.
panel C: Seroconversion series from 9 post-transfusion hepatitis C patients, drawn at close intervals (average=17 days) during 6 months or longer.
We tested all samples using an experimental version of the Matrix immunoblot assay, containing HCV core, NS3, NS4 and yeast expressed recombinant NS5 antigen; and an experimental ELISA employing recombinant E2 antigen, expressed in Chinese Hamster ovary cells.

Results: Specific antibody reactivity against:	**E2**	**NS5**
in panel A (n=33, PCR pos.):	88%	36
in panel B (n=39, PCR neg.):	5%	10%

In the 9 seroconversion series, E2 and NS5 reactivity did not appear earlier than HCV core, NS3 or NS4 antibodies. Eventually, antibodies against E2 and core appeared in all 9 patients; but NS3, NS4 and NS5 antibodies were not detectable in respectively 1, 2 and 3 patients.

Conclusion: In panel A and B presence and absence of E2 reactivity correlated best with presence and absence of HCV-RNA. E2, but not NS5, was reactive in all patients in panel C.From this limited study we conclude that the recombinant E2 antigen appears to be a promising candidate for new HCV-antibody screening assays.

0029

SIGNIFICANCE OF PERSISTING ISOLATED ANTIBODIES TO THE NON-STRUCTURAL REGION 5 (NS5) OF THE HEPATITIS C-VIRUS (HCV) IN GERMAN BLOOD DONORS.

B. Knoedler, P. Kuehnl, J. Hiller, C. Darda. Dept. of Transfusion Medicine, University Hospital Hamburg, FRG

In order to determine the prevalence and significance of isolated antibodies to the NS5 region (replicase) of the HCV genome in prescreened anti-HCV-negative blood donors, we tested 8,560 of our regular donors with a '3rd generation' anti-HCV ELISA (Wellcozyme anti-HCV, Murex Diagnostics). This test includes a non-structural component from the NS5 region adjacent to the 3' end of the HCV genome, as well as antigens from the putative core (C, structural) and protease/ helicase (NS3, non-structural) regions already used in the 2nd generation anti-HCV-EIAs.

A total of 50/8,560 (0.58%) samples were repeatedly reactive, the s/co-values ranging from 1.0 to 3.8. NS5-monoreactivity was confirmed by the Chiron RIBA HCV test system SIA 3.0 in 8/50 samples and by the Wellcozyme HCV Western Blot in 21/34 samples. All NS5-reactive samples were tested by PCR. One sample was PCR positive, two follow-up samples of this donor however were negative.

By testing stored frozen samples, we could show, that in most cases these antibodies had been persisting for at least three years. Follow-up samples showed no seroconversion to other HCV-antigens and no elevated ALT in any of the cases. We conclude that blood donors with persisting isolated NS5-antibodies are not infective.

0030

REPLACEMENT OF RIBA-2 BY RIBA-3 IMPROVES CONFIRMATION OF HCV-INFECTION.

N. Lelie, T. Cuypers, H. Zaaijer, H. Reesink. Central Lab. Blood Transfusion Service Amsterdam, the Netherlands

Objective: Comparison of RIBA-2 and RIBA-3
Method: A statiscal analysis of the HCV confirmatory test results of our diagnostic service to bloodbanks and hospitals enabled us to compare the previously used RIBA-2 with the currently applied RIBA-3. The sensitivity and non-specific reactivity of both assays were determined on samples of 739 HCV-RNA PCR positive patients/donors and 1437 HCV-RNA PCR negative blooddonors. Specificity could not be calculated since many of the donors were preselected for PCR-testing because of RIBA-reactivity.

Results: Sensitivity (of antigens) in RIBA-2 and RIBA-3 as measured among HCV-RNA positive subjects

	n	C22	C33c	C100	5-1-1	NS-5	Positive.
RIBA-2	595	95%	94%	63%	55%		93%
RIBA-3	144	98%	94%	89%		71%	99%

The number of indeterminates among HCV-RNA positive subjects decreased significantly (p=0.007) from 6.7 % in RIBA-2 to 0.7% in RIBA-3. The frequency of indeterminate testresults in HCV-RNA negative donors, probably caused by non-specific reactivities, is significantly lower in RIBA-3 than it was in RIBA-2 (86/214;40% versus 730/1224;60%, P<0.001).
Conclusion: The sensitivity of the new RIBA-3 is close to 100%. The significant decrease in the number of non-specific reactivities in RIBA-3 can be attributed to the replacement of the C22 and C100 recombinant antigens by synthetic peptides. However we noticed a slight, but significant increase in the number of C33c indeterminates. Isolated C100 and NS-5 reactions in RIBA were often observed but never among HCV-RNA positive subjects. Should these antigens be removed from the screening tests?

0031

CAPACITY OF ANTI-HCV ELISA TO DETECT HCV-INFECTED PATIENTS WITH NO ANTI-CORE ANTIBODY.

A.M. COUROUCE, N. LE MARREC, A. GIRAULT, F. BOUCHARDEAU. INTS - Paris - FRANCE

Sequential samples from subjects with chronic and acute Hepatitis C, anti-c22 negative by RIBA-3, were tested with the 5 anti-HCV ELISA commercialized in France at the end of 1993.
There were 6 chronic carriers HCV-RNA positive by PCR (4 with antibody to c33c and NS5 and 2 with antibody to c33c alone) and 11 seroconverters anti-c22 negative and anti-c33c positive in the first HCV positive specimens.

Anti-HCV ELISA	6 chronic carriers	11 seroconverters	
	No missed	Late detection No	Duration months
Abbott 2.0	1	2	1 to 2
Murex 47/48	2	6	1 to 30
Ortho 3.0	0	0	———
S.D. Pasteur	3	5	2 to 12
U.B.I. 2.1	5	7	1 to 48

Conclusion : Large differences in the anti-NS3 sensitivity were observed between ELISA while anti-core sensitivity was similar. UBI test which does not contain NS3 antigens and HCV tests which include them can miss HCV-infected individuals.

0033

HLA-CLASS I ELUTED PLATELETS; AN ALTERNATIVE FOR HLA COMPATIBLE PLATELETS IN PATIENTS WITH MULTIPLE HLA ANTIBODIES.

V.M.J. Novotny[1], R.van Doorn[1], T.W.J. Huizinga[3], E.Briët[2], A.Brand[1,2].
[1] Red Cross Bloodbank Foundation Leiden, [2] Dept. of Haematology, [3] Dept. of Immunohaematology, University Hospital Leiden, the Netherlands.

Allo-immunnized thrombocytopenic patients refractory to random donor platelet (plts) transfusions, often require HLA compatible plts. In an alloimmunized patient with multiple HLA antibodies and no compatible donors because of a rare HLA type, we used random plts and eluted the HLA antigens by incubation with citric acid (pH 3,0) 10 min. at 0°C. Using flowcytometry and monoclonal antibodies directed against platelet specific glycoproteins and HLA class I, expression of the antigens before and after elution was measured. Gp expression (IIbIIIa,IbIX) remained stable, HLA expression decreased from 75 to 15%. Using multiple random donor plts no transfusion increments could be obtained. After transfusion with acid-treated plt transfusion increments to a level of 30 x 10^9/L were obtained and a profuse gastrointestinal bleeding stopped while multiple skin haemorrhages resolved. No side effects were observed. We conclude that acid treated random donor plts can be used as an alternative for HLA-matched plts.

0034

FUNCTIONAL CAPACITY AND CORRECTED COUNT INCREMENT OF TRANSFUSED PLATELETS. COMPARISON BETWEEN PLATELET CONCENTRATES DERIVED FROM POOLED BUFFY COATS AND APHERESIS.

L. Eriksson[1], J.Kristensen[2], K.Olsson[2], C.Högman[1]
Departments of 1Transfusion Medicine and 2Hematology,University Hospital,Uppsala,Sweden

Platelet concentrates (PCs) were prepared from pools of 4 buffy coats stored over night (BC-PC) (Transfus.Sci 1993;14:35-39) and with apheresis (A-PC) using CS-3000. The PCs were leuco-depleted by filtration and stored in 1000 ml PL-732 bags. PCs transfused within 2 days of preparation were considered as fresh, 3-5 days as stored. To evaluate the functional capacity of the transfused platelets we determined the in vitro bleeding time (IVBT) using a Thrombostat 4000/2, before, 10 min and 24 h after Tx together with corrected count increment (CCI) (Eur.J Haematol 1993;51:152-155). 100 PCs were transfused to 36 thrombocytopenic patients . The mean pre-Tx IVBT was 449±67s, in 72 % of the patients >480s

	Fresh		Stored	
	BCPC	A-PC	BCPC	A-PC
IVBT 10 min	235±104	257±89	321±132	287±122
IVBT 24 h	316±102	380±113	376±110	377±119
CCI 10 min	18±10	18±7	15±5	15±7
CCI 24 h	6±7	5±6	4±5	3±8

Conclusion: No statistical difference in the functional capacity of the BC-PC versus A-PC was found.

0035

EVALUATION OF PLATELET ADDITIVE SOLUTION "PAS 2" FOR THE STORAGE OF PLATELET CONCENTRATES OBTAINED FROM 0.5 CPD ANTICOAGULATED POOLED BUFFY COATS.

D.J. van Rhenen[1][2], J. Vermeij[1], M. Kappers-Klunne[2], J.M. Payrat[3].
[1]Red Cross Bloodbank Rotterdam, [2]Department of Haematology, University Hospital Rotterdam, The Netherlands, [3]Baxter R & D Europe, Nivelles, Belgium.

A new formulation identified as PAS 2 (citrate-acetate-NaCl) was developed to prepare platelet concentrates (PC) from pooled 0.5 CPD anticoagulated buffy coats (BC). A Study was undertaken to evaluate PAS 2 against a commercially available solution (Plasmalyte-[R]A) in vitro and in vivo.
In a paired in vitro study a comparison was made of platelet and leukocyte concentration; blood gases and bicarbonate; glucose and lactate concentration; total intracellular concentration of adenine nucleotides and ß-thromboglobulin release. Results show that PAS 2 and Plasmalyte-[R]A allow adequate storage conditions for platelets obtained from 0.5 CPD BC. Because of a higher ß-thromboglobulin release with Plasmalyte-[R]A (p <0.0001) 0.5 CPD was changed to full CPD in the clinical study with Plasmalyte-[R]A.
In a clinical evaluation of 9 patients with bone marrow failure, all patients received PC with both PAS 2 and Plasmalyte-[R]A that had a shelf life of at least 4 days.
Corrected Count Increments (CCI) were as follows:

	0.5 CPD PAS 2	CPD Plasmalyte-[R]A
CCI (1 - 4 h)	22.9 ± 10.4	24.1 ± 14.7
CCI (12 - 24 h)	11.8 ± 11.6	14.2 ± 8.1
CCI (36 - 48 h)	4.6 ± 5.6	8.5 ± 9.4

Platelet additive solutions PAS 2 and Plasmalyte-[R]A are important contributions to platelet transfusion quality improvement and give an excellent CCI even after 4 days of storage.

0036

PLATELET SELECTION FOR REFRATORY PATIENTS BY CROSS-MATCHING RANDOM PLATELETS FROZEN IN PLATES

F. Marangoni, L. Porretti, G. Rossi, A. Floris M. Colombo, P.Mancuso, D. Riccardi, M. Marconi, G. Rossini, P. Rebulla, G. Sirchia. Centro Trasfusionale e di Immunologia dei Trapianti, Ospedale Maggiore, Milano, Italy.

We set up a system for selecting compatible donors for hematologic patients refractory to random donor platelets. The system is based on a flow cytometric cross-match (XM), performed by PSIFT (von dem Borne,1978) with frozen platelet plates (6% DMSO), followed by platelet apheresis of XM-negative donors. In this study we evaluated the efficacy of 55 platelet transfusions given during Jan 1992-Aug 1993 by 45 XM-negative donors selected in a panel of 544 frozen samples to 18 refractory patients (RP), in comparision with that previously observed in the same 18 RP when transfused with random platelets. No transfusion was excluded for the presence of non-immune factors capable of shortening platelet survival. Efficacy is reported in the table as corrected count increment (CCI) at 1 h and at 24 h.

	XM-negative	**random**
Median 1h CCI(range)	10155(0-40820)	905(0-10958)
Median 24h CCI(range)	9324(0-26000)	0(0-8840)

Notwithstanding the good median efficacy, 16 of the 55 XM-negative units (30%), although compatible in vitro, showed CCI values < 7500/µL.
This study shows that this simple approach to platelet XM is effective in approximately 2/3 of RP. To overcome ineffectiveness in the remaining cases we are currently investigating a strategy based on cross-matching HLA selected platelets.

0038

APPLICATIONS OF THE MAIGA-ASSAY IN GRANULOCYTE SEROLOGY

J. Bux, G. Behrens,, C. Mueller-Eckhardt, Institute for Clinical Immunology and Transfusion Medicine, Justus-Liebig University Giessen, Germany

The recently described "antigen capture"-assay MAIGA (1) was used 1. to determine the NA-specificity of alloantibodies 2. to define the NA-phenotype of granulocytes and 3. to identify the glycoprotein specificity of autoantibodies. 15 out of 18 maternal sera containing alloantibodies with determined NA-specificity by granulocyte immunofluorescence test [GIFT] could be also detected by MAIGA using one of the mabs BW209/2 or 3G8. The NA-phenotyping of 41 granulocyte donors in GIFT resulted in 6 NA1,-, 11 NA2,- and 24 NA1,NA2 positive donors. 8 results of the heterozygous classified cells were doubtful and should be retyped. Using the same typing sera in MAIGA all cells could be clearly typed: 10 NA1,-, 15 NA2,- and 16 NA1,NA2. The MAIGA results were confirmed by genotyping. 117 sera with GIFT pos. antibodies causing autoimmune neutropenia were investigated for binding to the following glycoproteins: Fc-gamma-R III (3G8, BW209/2), Leu CAMb (Bear 1, BL5), complement receptor 1 (J3D3) and decay-accelerating factor [DAF] (GI 21)
Results of 119 sera with autoimmune neutropenia:

	FcRIII	Leu CAMb	CR1	DAF
monospecific sera	12	5	4	0
total positive sera	33	26	15	10

23 sera showed binding to more than one glycoprotein and 76 sera did not react in MAIGA with any glycoprotein tested.

(1) Bux et al., Transfusion Medicine 3:157-162, 1993

0039

DETECTION OF ANTI-HUMAN GRANULOCYTE ANTIBODY BY THE MIXED PASSIVE HEMAGGLUTINATION (MPHA) TEST.

M.Miyamoto and Y.Shibata
The Department of Tranfusion Medicine and Immunohematology, University of Tokyo, Tokyo, Japan

The post transfusional complications due to the anti-granulocyte antibodies are of clinical relevance. Although the detection of these antibodies is of great importance, there is no adequate method for this purpose. We utilized the mixed passive hemagglutination (MPHA) test, a method largely used for the detection of anti-human platelet antibodies, for the detection of these antibodies. The results were strictly concordant with that obtained with the micro-agglutination test. This technique was found to be highly useful, being easily performed, with high reproducibility, and needing smaller volume of the sample than the micro-agglutination test or the fluorescein method. Moreover, the long-term preservation of the granulocytes fixed on microplates is now feasible.

0040

HLA DR4 SUBTYPYNG WITH PCR-SSP METHOD. A FURTHER CONTRIBUTION FOR A BETTER HLA TYPING

M.Testi, R.Rosati, M.Mariani e M.Purpura - Immunoem. Lab.
CNTS-CRI Rome (Italy).

The polymorphism of the HLA class II region plays an important role in the control of immunoreactivity in allogeneic transplantation and in the predisposition to characterized autoimmune disease. Recent studies of DRB1 sequence polymorphism revealed the existence of 14 different DR4 alleles, variants of the serologically defined specificity HLA DR4 which are often preferentially found in different populations. Studies of HLA disease associations have also shown HLA DR4 variants to be associated with a number of autoimmune disease. Therefore, it is important that HLA DR4 variants can be defined precisely in disease and population groups. We have investigated the molecular diversity of HLA DR4 in a group of Caucasoids living in Rome (n=50) who was previously been typed as HLA DR4 positive by serology and DRB1 "low resolution" PCR-SSP typing. High molecular weight DNA was isolated from frozen blood by phenol/chloroform extractions or by salting-out in mini-scale.
DRB1*04 PCR-SSP subtypings were performed as previously described by Olerup and Zetterquist, that involved PCR amplification with sequence specific primers (SSP) and assignment of alleles based on presence or absence of amplified product following agarose gel electrophoresis. Simultaneously HLA-DQA1 and DQB1 by the PCR-SSP technique were carried out. Seven of the fourteen known DRB1*04 alleles were detected. DRB1*0403 was encontered in 14 haplotypes, been the most common allele. The distribution of DR4 alleles on haplotypes from our population is different from that reported in the 11th IHWS.Errors introduced by the small sample size may also account for the failure to detect certain alleles and for different frequencies that our data show. All DR4 splits were associated with DQA1*0301-DQB1*0301 or with DQA1*0301-DQB1*0302.
The A.A. consider that the introduction of a new technique as DRB1*04 PCR-SSP typing method to define allelic variants of HLA DR4 and the development of new evaluation strategies can be usefull to predict the outcome of MLC for HLA- DR4 positive patients requiring bone marrow transplantation and to investigate the polymorphism of HLA DR4 and disease associations.

0041

A SIMPLE DNA TYPING METHOD FOR HLA-DRB1 USING ENZYMATICALLY AMPLIFIED DNA AND IMMOBILIZED PROBES ON MICROTITER PLATE.

K. Tokunaga[1], S. Kawai[2], M. Miyamoto[1], S. Moriyama[1], T. Akaza[1], K. Tadokoro[1], A. Yamane[2], T. Juji[1]
1Japanese Red Cross Central Blood Center, Tokyo, Japan
2Wakunaga Pharmaceutical Co. Ltd., Hiroshima, Japan

A new simple and economical method for HLA-DRB1 DNA typing, polymerase chain reaction-microtiter plate hybridization(PCR-MPH), was developed. This method is composed of a similar format to an enzyme-linked immunosorbent assay(ELISA). In brief, PCR amplified-fragments with biotin-labeled primers were hybridized with probes immobilized on a microtiter well, and the bound PCR products were detected by streptavidin-conjugated enzymes followed by color development. The entire procedure can be completed within 2 hrs after PCR. A system for HLA-DRB1 generic typing using microtiter wells coated with twelve different SSOs have been established. HLA-DRB types classified by this method agreed well with those by the serological or PCR-SSO typing. Probes for subtyping of DRB1 groups have also been prepared. This PCR-MPH method can be a useful DNA typing method for HLA class II genes because of the advantages of a short assay time, an easy processing of large numbers of samples, and the possibility of automated typing.

0043

IDENTIFICATION OF P ANTIGEN-NEGATIVE RED CELLS USING PARVOVIRUS B19 CAPSIDS. R.J. Davey, J.L. Procter, K.E. Brown. National Institutes of Health, Bethesda, MD, USA.

The human parvovirus B19 causes the common childhood illness, fifth disease, and less common disorders of erythropoiesis at all ages. Non-infectious, empty B19 viral capsids can be produced by a genetically-engineered cell line. These capsids bind specifically to the P red cell antigen (globoside). We investigated whether B19 capsids are useful for identifying the rare P-negative red cell phenotypes, p and P_1^k. Selected red cells were typed for the P antigen with conventional reagents and with B19 capsids.

RBC ϕtype	n	Conventional Typing	B19 Capsid Typing
P pos	20	17+/3±	20+
P neg	10	10-	10-

Conventional reagents yielded equivocal (±) typings with 3 of 20 P-positive cells. However, all 20 P-positive cells were clearly positive by the capsid method. The conventional reagents and the B19 capsids correctly identified the 10 P-negative samples. Parvovirus B19 capsids permit accurate, simple and economical identification of individuals with rare, P-negative phenotypes and may be useful for screening large populations.

0044

MONITORING OF CHIMERISM AFTER ALLOGENEIC BONE MARROW TRANSPLANTATION USING AMPLIFICATION FRAGMENT LENGTH POLYMORPHISM (AMPFLP)-TYPING OF MICROSATELLITE LOCI

D.W.M.Schwartz, E.M.Jungl, O.R.Krenek, W.R.Mayr

Clinical Institute for Blood Group Serology and Transfusion Medicine, University of Vienna, Austria

Polymorphic DNA-microsatellites (Variable Number of Tandem Repeat-Loci, VNTR) represent a powerful set of markers for genetic linkage mapping, disease association studies and individual identification or paternity testing in forensic haemogenetics. With the event of the Polymerase Chain Reaction (PCR) easy and powerful techniques have become available for the reliable typing of these markers. Since monitoring of engraftment and relapse is crucial for optimal managment of patients after allogeneic Bone Marrow Transplantation (BMT), the use of sensitive PCR-based VNTR-typing may provide a more sensitive technique to test for mixed chimerism in these patients.
We have established the typing for the unlinked polymorphic VNTR-loci D1S80 (pMCT118), ApoB, COL2A1, YNZ22 (D17S30), SE33 (ACTBP2) and TC11 (HUMTH01) by polyacrylamide gel electrophoresis after PCR-amplification of genomic DNA (Amplification Fragment Length Polymorphism, AMPFLP). Due to the enormous polymorphism in this systems (as a measure, the combined mean exclusion chance for paternity cases of >0.999 can be computed), informative constellations to discriminate between two genetically different individuals exist in virtually all BMT-donor-recipient combinations.
In order to assess the sensitivity of the method, we have tested artificial mixtures of peripheral blood samples with known erythrocyte and VNTR-markers by haemagglutination and VNTR-AMPFLP. As expected, VNTR-AMPFLP was able to detect far lower amounts of a second cell population than haemagglutination. However, the sensitivity was dependent on the locus as well as the phenotypes of the samples.
These results suggest that typing for VNTR-Loci by the AMPFLP-technique provides a more sensitive way to monitor for chimerism and therefore can help to select the optimal therapy in BMT-patients.

0045

COMPARISON OF COLUMN, SOLID-PHASE AND TUBE AGGLUTINATION FOR THE DETECTION OF IRREGULAR RED CELL ANTIBODIES

F. Morelati, N. Revelli, P. Vaccarino, F. Drago, R. Mistò, A. Parravicini, A. Villa, P. Rebulla, G. Sirchia. Centro Trasfusionale e di Immunologia dei Trapianti, Ospedale Maggiore, Milano (Italy)

We compared column (CAT, Ortho BioVue™ System) and solid-phase (SPAG, Capture-R™ Immucor) agglutination techniques to our polyethylene glycol tube test (PEG, Gamma) for red cell antibody screening. Assays were carried out following manufacturers' instructions, with a 3-cell antibody screen panel (TRIO™ Gamma). We tested 100 samples non reactive by PEG (NR), 39 with clinically significant antibodies (CSA) and 13 with clinically insignificant antibodies (CIA) detected by PEG. In addition, we tested 18 samples (7 CSA and 11 CIA) from patients with antibodies undetectable by PEG at the time of this study, but previously reactive with this technique. Results:

		No. POS detected by		
Type of Sample	*Number*	*PEG*	*CAT*	*SPAG*
NR	100	0	0	0
CSA	39	39	36	38
CIA	13	13	7	3
Previous CSA	7	0	2	3
Previous CIA	11	0	1	1

CAT missed 1 anti-c, 2 anti-E and 6 of 13 CIA; SPAG missed 1 anti-E and 10 of 13 CIA. In regard to previous antibodies, CAT and SPAG detected CSA no longer detectable by PEG (1 anti-E, 1 anti-Jk^a by CAT; 1 anti-E, 2 anti-Jk^a by SPAG). Although more data are needed to draw firm conclusions, this study shows that all assays miss some CSA; in addition, SPAG offers the advantage of not detecting most CIA.

0046

AUTOMATED BLOOD TYPING (ABO,RH and PHENOTYPE) AND RED CELLS ANTIBODIES SCREENING WITH A NEW POLYVALENT AUTOMATED SYSTEM:THE "MITIS" SYSTEM

B.LAMY, C.TISSOT, C.HEYD. Régional Blood Transfusion Center, Besançon, France.

The MITIS system is composed of an automatic sample dispenser that can be used for the filling of microplate or filtration columns . The sampler is driven by a computer and the programm has been developped to let a total liberty of users parameters selection. The system can be used for isolated ABO Rh blood typing or phenotyping or red cell antibodies screening but these analysis can be combined.Blood group typing and phenotyping can be performed with both microplate and filtration columns systems (BioVue TM). Differents safety procedures eliminate all possibilities of sample exchange during all the processing. Samples,microplates and filtration columns are identified with a Codabar labelling.After centrifugation microplates are read with an automatic reader directly connected to the computer.More recently an automatic filtration columns reader has been developped so the different results can be automatically printed on the patients or donors blood group cards without manual intermediate step.The MITIS system is used in our laboratory for routine tests since January 1993. 36742 Blood groups and 7853 phenotypes (Rhesus,Kell) have been performed this year with the MITIS system.The analysis rate has been established at 64 ABO Rh typing per hour,96 Phenotypes per hour and 48 irregular antibodies screenings (with 3 red blood cells) per hour.The percentage of results rejection was found under 1% with tests performed in microplates.The automatic reading has been more recently introduced and the percentage of results rejection seems similars (results obtained on 948 irregular antibodies screenings).

0048

PROCESS MAPS FOR EFFECTIVE DOCUMENTATION

D.E. Nevalainen
Abbott Quality Institute®, Abbott Laboratories, North Chicago, Illinois, 60064, USA.

The development of high quality documents is the core process required for implementation of any Quality System. Flow charting (FC) or process mapping (PM) is basic to the development of functional documents. Process Analysis (PA) is a systematic procedure that documents and analyses, with precision, the work activities in a process or procedure. All work is a process, and any activity can be process mapped. FC is designed to bridge the gap between graphics and words. PM creates images of the logic behind the written descriptions of ideas and procedures. These images can be presented alone or in combination with text. PM or FC should serve as the basic template for preparation of all procedures by defining only the critical steps. User friendly software is available to make PM/FC easily accessable to everybody. Examples of computer generated process maps, and associated procedure documents will be presented using blood bank examples.

0049

INFORMATION SHARING IN OPERATIONAL QUALITY MANAGEMENT

E.B. Rossiter, B. Garrison *CITINGS* INFORMATION EXCHANGE, Richmond, VA, USA

A unique QA program now provides information about product and device problems in blood centers and transfusion services. All major blood collectors in the US provide information about their operational problems via the ***CITINGS* INFORMATION EXCHANGE™**. Monthly and quarterly reports are published, providing lot numbers of products and manufacturers' responses to customer problems. A review of reports since January, 1991 indicates that the most frequently reported problems have involved apheresis supplies and infectious disease test kits. Of the apheresis supply problems, only 10% concerned hardware; the remaining 90% involved disposable sets with loose or missing parts and leaking anticoagulant or blood containers. Infectious disease test complaints all occurred prior to 1993. Tests for anti-HBc were the subject of most reports, followed by anti-HIV-1 or 1/2 tests. There are relatively few reports of problems with anti-HCV tests, despite its being the newest test implemented by *CITINGS*™ members. This information, is also accessible via computer modem for text-based searching and retrieval, and can be used in QA programs by both vendors and customers.

0050

COMPUTERISED INFORMATION SYSTEM IN THE CROSS-MATCHING FOR THE PATIENTS WITH THE LOW TITRE RBC ANTIBODIES

M. Potočnik, P. Rožman, I. Bricl
Blood Transfusion Centre of Slovenia, Ljubljana, Slovenia

The haemolytic transfusion reaction (HTR) can be generally avoided by screening of the patient's blood for irregular RBC antibodies and consequent transfusion of ABO compatible blood. In certain cases, the routine pretransfusion testing can fail in detection of antibodies in very low titre. This can result in a delayed HTR. Presuming that such samples were once upon a time tested and found positive, the information transfer from the past blood transfusions or pregnancies is essential to prevent delayed HTR.

Normally such data are kept at various places and hospitals. The information system was therefore developed in our Blood transfusion centre to prevent similar accidents, caused by poor information transfer.

Before the implementation of the new computer assisted cross-matching system, in average 3 serious delayed HTRs were registered yearly (out of 60.000 units transfused to 25.000 patients). None has been registered after the implementation of the system.

The introduction of computerised information on allosensitized patients proved to be helpful. The current data bank of sensitised patients is growing and we also expect to include the data from other blood banks and hospitals in near future. Computer information system definitely plays a crucial role in ensuring safe transfusion even in the cases of "disappeared" RBC antibodies.

0051

Quality Assurance of Anti-D Quantitation

Fleetwood PJ, Knight RC, North London Blood Transfusion Centre, Colindale Avenue, London NW9 5BG, UK; McNeill D, Blood Transfusion Centre, Lancaster LA1 3UJ, UK.

In the UK, anti-D levels in both antenatal patients sera and in donor plasma collected for immunoglobulin production, are quantitated by an automated bromelin - methyl cellulose method against a national anti-D standard. In 1989 a quality assurance scheme was re-introduced; since then 19 exercises have been completed. There are 4 exercises annually, with 4 samples containing anti-D on each occasion. Three National meetings have been held to discuss problems in anti-D quantitation.

An improvement in the UK performance has been noted with less intralaboratory variation than previously.

The returned results are analysed and a score is calculated for each sample in the exercise, in terms of multiples of range between the median and the quartile in the same direction. A cumulative plot of the sum of these scores for each exercise, over a two year period, gives a graphical representation of each participants performance over time.

In the UK 15 regional transfusion Centres particiate, plus centres in Eire, Slovenia, Australia (3) Sweden and France.

0053

IN VIVO CLOTTING FACTOR (CF) RECOVERY AFTER INFUSION OF SOLVENT/DETERGENT TREATED FROZEN PLASMA (S/D-FFP). D Ciavarella, M Horowitz, D Wuest, K Grima, New York Blood Center, Valhalla, New York, USA

In-vivo CF recovery after S/D-FFP infusion was studied in 7 patients with fibrinogen (Fbg) depletion (< 1 g/L) after intensive plasma exchange. Percent recovery data (patients) are shown below, as are CF values from 3 lots of S/D FFP (% normal). Of interest are the low levels of antiplasmin (AP), protein C, and XI in the S/D FFP. This complicates interpretation of the very high mean and SD values for recovery of these factors in patients. Side effects were seen in 4 patients: hives (1), nausea/epigastric distress (3).

	RECOVERY			S/D FFP		
	mean	(SD)	median	lot1	lot2	lot3
Fbg (mg/dL)	107	20	106	189	232	225
II (%)	61	31	70	103	106	129
V (%)	123	34	137	73	93	109
VII (%)	106	55	112	86	83	110
IX (%)	135	78	102	80	95	102
X (%)	103	43	117	82	92	98
XI (%)	129	103	116	61	83	77
AT III (%)	107	34	113	98	113	93
Plmg (%)	116	40	102	84	99	94
C (%)	140	78	196	55	68	37
AP (%)	225	115	181	17	17	25

0054

INTRODUCTION OF VIRUS INACTIVATED PLASMA IN NORWAY

B.G. Solheim[1], J.L. Svennevig[2], P. Pederson[3], B. Schei[3]
Red Cross and National Hospital Blood Centre, Surgical Dept. A, Dept. of Anaesthesia, Rikshospitalet, Oslo Norway.

Despite strong exclusion criteria for blood donors as well as extensive testing of all collected blood units, there is still a risk of transmitting virus diseases associated with the use of fresh frozen plasma (FFP). Therefore FFP has been substituted in Norway by Octaplas which is a standardized coagulation active human plasma product, virus inactivated by solvent/detergent (S/D) method. Octaplas is applied in volumes of 200 ml.

Initial clinical trial: In 1992 we performed a clinical study to test the tolerability and efficacy of Octaplas. The material consisted of high risk elective open heart surgery patients; 46 prospective patients requiring Octaplas (20) or no plasma (26) and 20 consecutive patients receiving FFP. The choice of plasma preparation (Octaplas versus FFP) did not influence the post-operative course, and Octaplas corrected adequately both changes in coagulation factors and plasma colloid osmotic pressure without exhibiting bioincompatible properties such as complement activation. No signs of virus transmission were observed in patients receiving Octaplas.

Routine clinical use: As a consequence of our initial clinical trial, preliminary results of clinical trials in the USA and clinical experience in Germany, our Directorate of Health decided that FFP should be substituted by Octaplas, produced from Norwegian plasma. The change was effective from April 1993. Through 1993 more than 16,000 portions of Octaplas have been transfused in Norway with only one serious side effect due to citrate intoxication. One portion Octaplas of 200 ml represented an adequate substitute for 1 unit FFP in routine clinical use. In addition Octaplas maintained adequate levels of Antithrombine-3 (AT-3) in a patient on prolonged treatment with extra corporeal membrane oxygenator. This contrasts with our previous experience which shows a considerable need for specific AT-3 replacement in such patients.

0055

INVESTIGATIONS ON AUTOLOGOUS PLASMAPHERESIS AND INTRAOPERATIVE AUTOTRANSFUSION IN MAJOR ORTHOPAEDIC SURGERY

H.P. Wendel, W. Heller
Dept. of Thoracic- and Cardiovascular Surg., Univ. of Tuebingen, Germany

Fourteen patients who were autotransfused intraoperatively within the context of major orthopaedic surgery received, in addition to the autologous erythrocyte concentrate, fresh frozen plasma (FFP) that had been taken from them prior to surgery. The comparative group consisted of twelve patients who were also given autotransfusion during orthopaedic or accident surgery, and who additionally underwent homologous FFP substitution. The patients with autologous plasma transfusion could already be investigated during preparation for surgery in the plasmapheresis stage. Antithrombin III (AT III), alpha$_1$-antitrypsin, alpha$_2$-macroglobulin, kallikrein inhibition capacity and alpha$_2$-antiplasmin were investigated as parameters of the inhibitory system. In addition, prekallikrein (PK) and kallikrein-like activity (KK) as components of the kallikrein-kinin system, as well as plasminogen underwent observation with respect to the fibrinolytic process. The significant rise in KK after the second plasmapheresis is striking; it is stronger still after a third. Here it is clearly a case of contact phase activation. Further, a distinct drop in C1-inhibitor activity is to be observed. In the context of plasmapheresis a drop is above all to be found in plasminogen and in the inhibitors AT III, alpha$_1$-antitrypsin and alpha$_2$-macroglobulin. By the beginning of surgery the patient can recover as a rule.The plasma thus gained remains stable for the most part during storage at -40°C. Taking purely elective surgical interventions into consideration, intraoperatively comparable courses are generally to be found with no essential differences between the two groups. In the autologous plasma group the requirement of FFP could be covered completely intraoperatively with autologous plasma, two of the fourteen patients needing additional homologous erythrocyte concentrate. In the homologous plasma group all the patients had to be substituted intraoperatively with homologous FFP, eight of the twelve patients required additional homologous blood whereby the FFP unit value was identical.

0056

TRANSFUSION OF VIRUS-INACTIVATED PLASMA : ACCUMULATION AND CLEARANCE OF METHYLENE BLUE -PHOTOOXIDIZED FIBRINOGEN

J.U. Wieding, M. Unterhalt
University Hospital, D-37075 Göttingen, Germany.

Prior in-vitro studies demonstrated the disturbance e.g. of fibrin polymerization and clot retraction due to the photooxidative alteration of fibrinogen, a problem which is inevitable during methylene blue treatment of plasma (MB-FFP) for inactivation of lipid-enveloped viruses. Since most patients receiving plasma generally suffer from complex disturbances of hemostasis, we recently took advantage of monitoring a patient with inherited FXI -deficiency preoperatively receiving MB-FFP transfusions.
After transfusion of 29 units of 244±15 ml MB-FFP over 5 days, the factor XI levels increased from 1 to 46%. This increase of FXI agrees with its half-life as well as the average of 76% in MB-FFP as compared with normal plasma. Fibrin(ogen) and its immunologically detectable derivatives increased from 2.6 to 4.25 g/l after a total of 17.8 g fibrinogen had been transfused to the patient with initially appr. 8.9 g fibrinogen. The percentage of fibrinogen not normally clottable by thrombin (Clauss' test) was on average 20.5% in the transfused MB-FFP and reached ca. 12.4% in the patient. Interestingly, although the thrombin times were distinctly elongated in all MB-FFP units, they were not elongated in the patient. This finding possibly indicates an increased clearance of photooxidized fibrinogen. Notably, two thirds of circulating fibrinogen were transfused and roughly 13 g were cleared during 5 days. Fibrin(ogen) degradation products significantly increased 5-fold up to 350 mg/l indicating a reactive fibrin(ogen)olysis in the patient.
In conclusion, the clearance of methylene blue -photooxidized fibrinogen by fibrin(ogen)olysis or the reticuloendothelial system might be altered in comparison to that of 'native' fibrinogen from conventional fresh-frozen plasma. These and other problems of MB-FFP require further examinations.

0058

HEPARIN-ASSOCIATED THROMBOCYTOPENIA (HAT): ISOLATION OF THE ANTIBODY AND CHARACTERIZATION OF A MULTIMOLECULAR PF4-HEPARIN COMPLEX AS THE MAJOR ANTIGEN.

A. Greinacher[1], B. Pötzsch[2], J. Amiral[3], V. Dummel[1], A. Eichner[1], C. Mueller-Eckhardt[1]
1. Institut für Klinische Immunologie und Transfusionsmedizin, Justus-Liebig Universität, Giessen, 2. Abteilung für Hämostaseologie und Transfusionsmedizin, Kerckhoff-Klinik, Max-Planck-Institut, Bad Nauheim, FRG, 3. Serbio, Research-Laboratories, Gennevilliers, France.

Sera of 35 patients with HAT, strongly reactive in the serotonin release assay (SRA), were assessed in a platelet factor 4 (PF4)/heparin ELISA. Both tests correlated closely ($p = 8.44 \times 10^{-5}$), but one positive serum in the SRA was negative in the ELISA. We have isolated the HAT antibody by absorption and elution of HAT sera using human endothelial cells. Eluates gave similar results as the sera in the ELISA ($p = 3.04 \times 10^{-6}$), which also correlated very closely with the SRA ($p = 1.45 \times 10^{-7}$). This demonstrates that HAT antibodies bind to the same epitope on platelets and on endothelial cells. High heparin concentrations released PF4 in a dose dependent manner from microtiter plates if PF4/heparin, but not if PF4 alone, was covalently linked. Concomitant to the release of PF4, binding of HAT antibodies to PF4/heparin decreased, as indicated by median optical density (OD) OD 0.947 in the presence of buffer to OD 0.181 in the presence of 100 IU/ml heparin similar to the OD when PF4 alone was coated (median OD 0.203). Binding of 3 eluates was not inhibited by high heparin concentrations and they reacted also with PF4 alone. We conclude that multimolecular PF4/heparin complexes represent the major antigen in HAT, which are present on platelets and endothelial cells. This multimolecular complexes form immune complexes after HAT antibody binding which concommitantly alterate platelets and endothelial cells. This may explain the thromboembolic complications in HAT.

0059

DETECTION OF HAPTEN INDUCED IMMUNE THROMBOCYTOPENIAS BY THE BEADS IMMOBILIZED PLATELET ANTIGEN ASSAY (BIPA), CC. Loeliger, J. Hiller and P. Kuehnl, Dpt. of Transfusion Medicine and Transplantation Immunology, University of Hamburg, FR Germany.

Thrombocytopenia (TP) in the adult patient is caused by different mechanisms. The rapid differentiation of antibody induced TP's from bone marrow insufficiency and thrombosis associated TP is essential. We used a monospecific enzyme immuno assay with platelet antigens immobilized to immunomagnetic beads by monoclonal antibodies (MoAB) for the detection of immunoglobulin G (IgG) antibodies against HLA class I and platelet specific antigens CD41a, CD42a, CD42b and CD49b. In principle, 5 µl of magnetic beads, to which 0.5µg anti-HLA/CD-MoAB were coupled, were incubated with anticoagulated donor blood in the presence of 1.2% non-ionic detergents to capture their HLA/ platelet antigen molecules. The precoated beads were used to detect antibodies in the patient's serum by a second enzyme linked antibody to human IgG.
In 26 sera (20%) of 131 patients with TP, we found autoantibodies, which did not react with platelets from panel donors. Such antibodies seemed to be directed against antigenic haptens (penicilline, entercocci antigens in two cases) attached to CD41a, CD42a or CD49b rather than against the platelet antigens themselves. In 5% (7 sera) allospecific platelet antibodies (anti-HPA-1a, 5b) could be detected and 20% (26 patients) were negative. Autoantibodies, which reacted also with donor platelets, often showed multispecificity (57%).
The BIPA can detect and differentiate clinically relevant platelet antibodies even in thrombocytopenic patients, were the platelet count is below the necessary amount for standard immunofluorescence analysis, as it also detects unbound antigen-antibody complexes in the plasma of TP patients. It's short assay time renders it also useful for diagnosis prior treatment in even life threatening TP.

0060

FREQUENCY OF PLATELET ANTIBODIES AGAINST HPA-5b IN SPANISH PREGNANT WOMEN

A. Ribera[1], R. Parra[1], D. Gallardo[1], P. Pérez[1], J. Rodríguez[2], M. Pujol[3].
1 Banc de Sang de l'ICS. Barcelona; 2 Hospital Provincial. Pontevedra; 3 Hospital Germans Trias i Pujol. Badalona.

HPA-1a incompatibility is the most common and clinically relevant cause of neonatal alloimmune thrombocytopenia (NAIT) in caucasians. On the other hand, HPA-5b is involved in about 15-20% of NAITs, most of which presenting a mild severity.
In this study we screened 800 women at delivery for the presence of HPA-5b antibodies using the monoclonal antibody immobilization of platelet antigens (MAIPA) assay. In adition, 50 HPA-1a negative women (selected from 2017 women previously typed) were searched for the presence of HPA-1a antibody using the immunofluorescence test, but no one was detected. In contrast, 12 women of the former group presented HPA-5b antibodies of IgG class. Even that feto-maternal incompatibility was present in all cases, no NAIT was detected. Seven (58%) of the immunized women were primiparous.
In summary, HPA-5b immunization without NAIT in HPA-5b negative spanish women is not rare (2%) and is frequently observed in first pregnancies. These findings could be useful to stablish the best strategy for the prevention of new cases of NAIT.

0061

ANTI-Ko^a AS THE CAUSE OF NEONATAL ALLOIMMUNE THROMBOCYTOPENIA

H. Kroll[1], V. Kiefel[1], W. Muntean[2], C. Mueller-Eckhardt[1]
[1]Institute for Clinical Immunology and Transfusion Medicine, Justus Liebig University, Gießen, [2]Childrens Hospital, University Graz

Neonatal alloimmune thrombocytopenia (NAIT) is caused by maternal immunization against the fetal platelet alloantigens Zw^a or Br^a, but very rarely against others. Antibodies against the Ko^a antigen on glycoprotein (GP) Ib$_\alpha$ have so far been found in multiply transfused patients and are considered to be of IgM class. NAIT due to anti-Ko^a was described only twice. We report here on two additional cases.
Patient 1 was delivered spontanously as the 3rd child of healthy parents at 42 weeks of gestation (wg; 3950g, Apgar 9/10). Post partum platelet count of 53G/l decreased to 11G/l on day 4. Increasing signs of hemorrhage required transfusion of maternal platelets 3 times before the platelet count normalized at the age of 2 months. In case 2, the woman had her 2nd pregnancy. At 29 wg, hemolytic disease of the fetus due to anti-CD was treated by intra-umbilical transfusion. Subsequently fetal death occurred and a platelet count of 3G/l was found.
Initial serological crossmatch of maternal serum with paternal platelets in MAIPA assay (monoclonal antibodies against GP Ia/IIa, IIb/IIIa and Ib/IX) was negative since platelets were stored without protease inhibitors. When cryopreserved platelets were tested in immunofluorescence and platelet agglutination maternal serum showed strong anti-Ko^a of IgG, but not of IgM class. DNA typing of the parents demonstrated Ko^a incompatibility.
The presented data emphasize that anti-Ko^a of IgG class is more frequent than suspected and may cause severe cases of NAIT. For the serological diagnosis, platelet immunofluorescence, platelet agglutination and MAIPA assay are appropriate. However, proteolytic degradation of the antigen bearing glycocalicin fragment of GPIb$_\alpha$ should be inhibited.

0063

PROCESS VALIDATION FOR THE PREPARATION OF LEUKODEPLETED PACKED RED CELLS

T. Kearns[1]; M. Genatt[1], C. Bunch[1], J. Whitbread[1], K. Wilkins[2], E. Maynard[2], P. Ball[2], C. Lerenard[3], N. LeGoff[3], F. Pascale[1], N. Besso[1], and H. Brandwein[1]
Scientific & Laboratory Services Dept., Pall Corporation, Glen Cove, N. Y.[1]; Portsmouth, U. K.[2]; St. Germain en Laye, France[3]

The recent implementation of process validation for the preparation of leukodepleted packed red cells (prc) has included 1) use of the Pall BPF4 filter products, 2) training on the use of Nageotte hemocytometers (for quantitation of low leukocyte residuals) and 3) coordinating the collection of process validation data at 70 blood banks/blood centers in the U. S. and Europe.

Within these 70 blood banks, leukodepleted prc's of varying ages were prepared in either CPDA-1 or other anticoagulant/additive systems (AS-1, AS-3, SAG-M). All filtrations were performed according to standard BPF4 instructions for use which were integrated into each center's current S.O.P. for prc preparations. Post-filtration samples were drawn and counted for leukocyte residuals.

The data collected show that within this group of results (n=1124), there was a very high consistency of postfiltration leukocyte residuals for all blood centers, prc ages, and anticoagulants. Over all, the mean residual for these 1124 filtrations was 1.35 x 10^5 leukocytes/unit, with 100% of the filtrations having post-filtration residuals of less than 5 x 10^6 leukocytes, and more than 99% of the filtrations with residuals of less than 1 x 10^6 leukocytes.

These results demonstrate that the consistently low levels of leukocytes (in prc) needed for optimal patient benefits can be reliably and reproducibly achieved via the use of BPF4 filters and good manufacturing procedures, including adherence to well documented S.O.P.'s and process validation.

0064

AN IMPROVED METHOD FOR WHITE CELL COUNTING IN WHITE CELL DEPLETED RED BLOOD CELLS

D. Prati, P. Rebulla, C. Capelli, P. Bosoni, G. Sirchia. Centro Trasfusionale e di Immunologia dei Trapianti, Ospedale Maggiore, Milano, Italy.

Background: Current filters for white blood cell (WBC) removal from red blood cells (RBC) provide residuals close to the lower limit of accurate detection of most sensitive counting methods (0.1 WBC/µl). Aim: To set up a method with better sensitivity than those currently used for counting WBC in leukodepleted RBC. Materials and Methods: 42 RBC suspensions with known WBC concentration (0.005-5 WBC/µl) were prepared by adding known numbers of WBC to 1-2 days old RBC (Hct=60±5), each previously filtered through three Pall BPF4 filters. Ten ml of each suspension was added to 40 ml of 3% wt/v paraformaldehyde in H_2O, pH 7.4. After spinning at 800 *g* X 10 min, the supernatant was discarded and the pellet resuspended to 500 µl with Plaxan solution containing 0.5% Triton x 100. The suspension was loaded in a Nageotte chamber, and after 15 min one grid (50 µl) was examined with an optical microscope. The number of WBC/µl in native sample was calculated as follows:

$$\frac{\text{WBC in the sample} - \text{WBC in the diluent RBC}}{10{,}000} \times 10$$

Results: The correlation coefficient (r^2) between observed and expected concentrations of WBC was 0.92. The estimated count ranged from 0.006 to 0.017 in 5 samples expected to contain 0.01 WBC/µl. Comments: These preliminary results indicate that this method could be applied to the evaluation of high efficieny filters for WBC removal.

0065

MECHANISM OF MACROAGGREGATE FORMATION IN RED CELL CONCENTRATES STORED IN A NEW ADDITIVE SOLUTION

S. Chiba, T.A. Takahashi, N. Urushibara, M. Akino, S. Sekiguchi
Hokkaido Red Cross Blood Center, Sapporo, Japan.

Since 1993 the Japanese Red Cross has adopted a new additive solution for red cell concentrate (RC), MAP (mannitol-adenine-phosphate), which is a modified SAGM solution. However, frequent macroaggregate formation in MAP-additive RC (MAP-RC) has become a problem. We investigated the mechanism of macroaggregate formation in MAP-RC and sought method to reduce the frequency of such formation. During 3-week storage at 4°C, macroaggregates were formed in 30% of the buffy coat-poor RC (BP-RC) prepared by the conventional method without MAP, but in 100% of MAP-RC.

Electron microscopic observation of the macroaggregates showed that red cells were trapped in a network structure and enzyme treatments indicated that the network was made of DNA that leaked from granulocytes. The granulocytes stored in the MAP solution, however, formed macroaggregates only if plasma was added to the cell-suspension medium. Immunoblotting analysis indicated that fibrinogen and fibronectin were the constituents of the macroaggregate in addition to the DNA. Pre-storage filtration of MAP-RC with a leukocyte-removal filter (PALL BPF4) or preparation of BP-RC with the top & bottom system completely prevented the macroaggregate formation in the MAP-RC. These results indicated that reduction of leukocytes in MAP-RC to less than $1x10^8$/bag is necessary to prevent macroaggregate formation.

0066

EFFECT OF LEUKOCYTE-DEPLETED BLOOD ON CMV DISEASE AFTER HEART TRANSPLANT

A. Bracey, R. Radovancevic, B. Radovancevic, B. Zeluff, W. Vaughn, H. McAllister, O.H. Frazier
Texas Heart Institute, Houston, Texas, USA.

Purpose. CMV infections remain a major complication after heart transplant (HT). We conducted a pilot study to assess whether transfusing leukocyte-depleted blood into CMV-positive HT patients (pts) reduces CMV-related morbidity.
Methods. Nine CMV-positive pts received only leukocyte-depleted blood. Leukocytes were removed from red blood cells by BPF4 filtration after varying periods of storage. Platelets were filtered at the bedside with PL-100 filters. Sixteen historical CMV-positive HT pts served as controls. CMV disease was detected through biopsy or clinical patterns: febrile illness with 4-fold increase in CMV IgG, presence of CMV IgM, leukopenia (<4000/ml), thrombocytopenia (<100000 /ml), or a positive urine culture.
Results. The groups were comparable with respect to donor CMV serostatus, age, sex, induction of immunosuppression, and incidence of rejection. The median number of transfusions in the treated group was significantly lower than that of the control pts (11 vs. 14; p=0.045). No HT pts receiving leukocyte-depleted blood had CMV disease, compared with 4 control pts who did. In one control pt CMV disease occurred despite a CMV-negative donor. CMV disease did not occure with the CMV positive donor in 6/7 of the control pts or 8/9 study pts.
Conclusion. Our result suggests that the use of leukocyte-depleted blood in HT pts may decrease incidence of CMV disease. Further study of a larger patient population is warranted.

0068

DETECTION OF HIV-INFECTION AMONG HIGH RISK INDIVIDUALS BY PCR IS FREQUENT PRECEDING ANTIBODY CONVERSION BUT ABSENT IN PERSISTENTLY ANTIBODY NEGATIVE PERSONS

J.G. Huisman[1], G. Mientjes[2], S. Bruisten[1], F. de Wolf[3], P. van Delft[1], J. Goudsmit[3], R.A. Coutinho[2]
1. Central Laboratory of the Netherlands Red Cross Blood Transfusion Service, Amsterdam, 2. Municipal Health Service, Amsterdam, 3. Academic Medical Centre, Amsterdam, The Netherlands.

Human Immunodeficiency Virus (HIV-1) can be detected before antibody conversion in serum, plasma or peripheral mononuclear cells (PBMC) using nucleic acid amplification (PCR, NASBA™). For viral safety of blood and bloodproducts the length of the period between detection of HIV nucleic acid sequences and HIV antibody has been the subject of many studies. We have studied retrospectively, the prevelance of HIV-PCR reactions in PBMC and serum before seroconversion in 23 drugusers (IVDU) and 15 homosexual men. We also studied the prevelance of HIV-PCR reactions in subgroups of seronegative IVDU (n=40) and homosexual men (n=67), selected on the base of reported high risk behaviour.
In the IVDU seroconverters 5 out of 23 (22%) were HIV-PCR positive before seroconversion. Three of them were also HIV-p24-antigen positive. In the homosexual men seroconverter group 2 out of 15 (13%) were HIV-PCR and HIV-p24-antigen positive before seroconversion. In 40 antibody negative high risk IVDU and 67 antibody negative high risk homosexuals, none was HIV-PCR positive. In conclusion, silent HIV infection for a limited period is observed in IVDU and homosexual men and has to be taken into account in countries with high incidence of HIV-infection. Screening for p24 and HIV-nucleic acid sequences may detect silent infection and reduce risk.

0069

P-24 HIV ANTIGEN SCREENING IN DONATED BLOOD, EXPERIENCE FROM THAILAND

C. Nuchprayoon, S. Tanprasert, S. Thanomchat
National Blood Centre, Thai Red Cross Society, Bangkok, Thailand

Having at least 10 cases of transfusion associated HIV infection from fully screened blood been reported in the country, the National Blood Centre, Thai Red Cross Society, Bangkok, started on September 1,1991 to screen all units of donated blood using P-24 HIV antigen as well as anti-HIV assays. Abbot recombinant anti-HIV1 plus 2 sandwich EIA or Wellcozyme anti-HIV1 plus 2 sandwich ELISA was used for initial anti-HIV screening. Positives were confirmed by Western blot. Abbot HIV Ag-1 monoclonal or coulter HIV P-24 Antigen Assay was used for initial antigen screening. Positives were confirmed by neutralization tests. Blood was collected from healthy non-paid voluntary donors, male and females aged 17-60 years, excluding homosexuals, prostitutes, drug abusers etc. There were 534,022 donations during a period of 24 months (September 1,1991-August 31, 1993).The results are as follows:

	AntiHIV Status	P-24 Antigen Positive Initial (ELISA)	After Neutralization
Sept.1991-Aug.1992	Positive (1,107)	21(1.90%)	14(1.30%)
	Negative (263,985)	113(0.04%)	8(0.003%)
	Total (265,092)	134(0.05%)	22(0.008%)
Sept.1992-Aug.1993	Positive(1,058)	27(2.60%)	15(1.41%)
	Negative(267,872)	45(0.016%)	9(0.003%)
	Total(268,930)	72(0.026%)	24(0.008%)

The finding of 1 antigen positive in 30,000 antibody negative donated blood suggested that routine P-24 antigen screening in addition to anti HIV is mandatory to ensure safe blood supply in a country of high HIV prevalence like Thailand.

0070

PCR-POOLSCREENING, A NEW APPROACH TO PREVENT VIRUS-TRANSMISSION BY "WINDOW-DONATIONS". N. Ielie, T. Cuypers, H. Zaaijer, H. Reesink, H. Huisman. Central Lab. Bloodtransfusion Service, Amsterdam The Netherlands.

Objective: To study the feasibility of PCR-testing of pools of seronegative donations for HBV-DNA, HCV-RNA and HIV-RNA as an alternative to individual screening of donations for HIV-antigen, ALT and anti-HBc.

Introduction: In the Netherlands about 850,000 blooddonations are collected yearly . The mean yearly incidence of seroconverting repeat blooddonors in the Netherlands is 5.4 for HIV, 10.2 for HBV and yet unknown for HCV. Based on 6-months intervals between donations and mean-windowperiods of 6 weeks for HIV, 8 weeks for HBV and 14 weeks for HCV we can estimate the risk of infective window-donations: e.g. for HIV 1:500,000 donations.

Methods: We have compared p24 HIV-antigen and HIV-RNA endpointtitres in preseroconversion samples of a patient with primary HIV-1 infection as measured in Abbott p24 ELISA and cDNA-PCR

Results: HIV-1 RNA and p24 antigen endpointtitres in plasma

day	-7	-5	-4	-3	0(seroc)	9	15
HIV-1 RNA	400	3600	3100	2600	9200	110	80
p24 antigen	4	40	40	20	10	0	0

Conclusion: In most preseroconversion samples HIV-RNA titres were 100-fold higher than p24 antigen titres. Thus poolscreening 1:10 is one log more sensitive than p24 antigen screening of individual donations.Moreover the pools can be applied to HBV-DNA and HCV-RNA screening by PCR (we observed a very high HCV-RNA titre in a HCV window donation). This new approach is a more specific and economic option than the in some countries introduced ALT, anti-HBc or p24 antigen screening. Pool-screening for HBV-DNA may prevent posttransfusion hepatitis B by HBsAg mutants. PCR poolscreening prevents the current loss of plasma- products prepared from plasmapools contaminated by window donations.

These may have a 100-1000 fold higher viral load than normal seropositive donations. Ultimately PCR poolscreening may be applied to cell products.

0071

DISTRIBUTION OF HIV-1 IN BLOOD FROM INFECTED DONORS

R.R.Stromberg[1], T-H.Lee[2], J.Heitman[2], D.R.Henrad[3], M.P. Busch[2]

1Am Red Cross, Rockville,MD, 2Irwin Mem Blood Ctrs, San Francisco,CA, 3Abbott Diag, Abbott Pk,IL. USA

Quantitative DNA-PCR and RNA-PCR methods were used to study the compartmentalization of HIV-1 (HIV) in 450 mL whole blood (WB) units from 6 asymptomatic sero-positive donors. Provirus was confined to leukocytes (10-100 copies/10^6wbc); HIV-RNA was present in cell-free plasma (100-3000 copies/100μL). Both remained stable for 4 weeks at 4C. Leukodepleted (6$\log_{10}$) and serially washed (5X) red cell ghosts were negative for HIV DNA and RNA. However, leukodepleted (5$\log_{10}$) and washed platelets (5X) had high levels (100-100,000 copies/mL platelet rich plasma) of bound viral RNA. Further studies on smaller WB samples found purified platelets positive for HIV RNA (negative for DNA) on 50/50 seropositive subjects. The level of platelet associated HIV RNA exceeded the levels of cell-free RNA detected in the plasma using anti-gp41/gp120 coated immunocapture beads (IC). The platelet associated RNA signal was stable for at least one week at 20-24C and 30 days at 4C. Platelets from 3 seronegative donors adsorbed virus from 5 seropositive plasmas as well as IC beads. In panels of frozen plasma from sero-converting plasma donors (6) and gay men (3), the RNA signal from platelet associated HIV peaked in parallel with free HIV (IC beads), then stabilized at levels predictive of long term clinical course. It is concluded that platelet associated HIV is an important component of viremia which may be useful for prognosis and therapeutic monitoring.

0073

BLOOD DONATION - THE VIEWS OF UNIVERSITY STUDENTS

JE Cocks,[1] RJ Hawker,[2] GS Gabra[2].

[1]The Medical School, Birmingham University & [2]West Midlands Regional Blood Transfusion Centre, BIRMINGHAM. U.K.

6.7% of the 3.2 million eligible population of the West Midlands region (5.3 million) are regular blood donors. If more of this younger section of the community could be encouraged to donate, a potentially longer lasting donor panel would be established. A questionnaire was distributed to 333 randomly selected individuals from local universities. The majority (91%) were in the desired age range of 18-24 years (58% male/42% female) and were full-time mixed course students. 13% were existing donors, suggesting that students were possibly more informed and better motivated than the average population. 81% of these donors carried donor-organ cards compared with 38% of non-donors. Non-donors suggested that positive motivating factors for blood donation included: awareness of family need for blood (56%), peer (pressure) group visits (35%), reassurance of the absence of pain (40%), regular information by a personal approach on the times and dates of sessions (43%). Only 30% of the non-donors could give a good estimate of how long it took to give blood suggesting that they were not adequately informed on the process of blood donation. Major reasons for non-attendance were ignorance of session(47%), apathy(29%) and fear of needles(21%). Genuine reasons such as inability to attend or presumed medical grounds were less frequent and the medical reasons were often unfounded. 17% of students liked the idea of being given nominal-value free gifts. Attending with other donors (a friend) as well as altruism featured strongly as positive motivating factors by donors and 95% indicated that they would continue after leaving university. Their reasons for not donating regularly were cited as a lack of communication or advertising.

We conclude: recruitment strategies for universities should include: 1] a greater awareness of the need for, and uses made of blood; 2] conveniently scheduled, well advertised sessions; 3] dissemination of information to reduce the perceived anxiety and fears from the process of giving blood. These would be combined with the establishment of a specific donor retention system.

0074

DONOR OPINION ON TREATMENT AND COMMUNICATION: ARE WE GIVING OUR DONORS THE RIGHT TREATMENT ?

Achterhof L, Broers AME, Los APM, Smit Sibinga CTh.
R.C. Blood Bank Groningen-Drenthe, NL.

Attention to donor experiences and opinions forms a fundamental aspect of donor management. Information on the opinions of donors on reception and treatment can serve as a positive feedback and contribute to the improvement of donor policy.

METHOD: Postal questionnaire, sent to a random selection of donors, shortly after their visit to a donor-site. The sample (n=5,174), covers all (regional) donor-sites of the Blood Center. Format of questionnaire: structured questions with request for explanation on given answers and suggestions for improvement.

RESULTS: Response: 3,981/5,174 (78%). Most donors (>80%) judge the ambiance, reception, and treatment before, during, after donation as (very) pleasant. A few are not satisfied (<1%). Insufficient privacy at donor interview is mentioned by 12% of the (younger) donors in regional (mobile) donor-sites. Insufficient information is mentioned by 11% of younger donors. Respondents illustrated their answers with valuable written comments. All results are related to specific circumstances (location of donor-site, staffing).

CONCLUSION: The high response rate indicates great concern and good motivation. Results suggest overall a right approach and treatment. Information from written comments initiates and stimulates improvement of policy on privacy and information especially to the younger donors.

0075

DOCUMENT IMAGING FOR BLOOD BANKS. N.D.Kalmin, J.Orrell, V.Clegg and R.Maxey. South Texas Regional Blood Bank, San Antonio, TX. U.S.A.

Microfilming of documents, such as donor history cards, has been the standard method of maintaining "paperless" storage of records. There are many limitations to using microfilm such as: documents need to be in correct order prior to filming, copies are often unclear, maintenance of a library is time-consuming, retrieval can be slow, and the system is expensive.

Through the use of inexpensive computer software and readily available hardware, our center is able to automatically catalog and store images of donation history cards on optical disks. Each optical disk can hold 120,000 card images. Key personnel can recall and reproduce a copy of any donation history card in less than a minute.

In addition, information on gallon donors, blood drive efficiency, and inventory levels are examples of data that is currently provided to departments in formats that are loaded directly into microcomputer data bases. Various other reports and correspondence are being evaluated with a view towards storage on optical disks.

Video taped computer literacy and proficiency training courses have been developed by MIS personnel to train all blood bank departments on the potential use of this technology for record keeping in their areas. The goal is to reduce reliance on paper files throughout the organization.

0076

FORECASTING BLOOD DONORSHIP IN A EUROPEAN COUNTRY
C. Politis, J. Yfantopoulos
Hellenic Red Cross Blood Transfusion Centre, Athens, Greece.

Forecasting is a quantitative technique aiming at an estimate of a future value of a variable on the base of past and current information. In this study, to predict blood donorship we used a single equation regression model for different sources of blood collection during the period 1974-1990. We have also estimated the annual rate of growth of blood given by three categories of blood donors. The results of our study show that, during this time span domestic blood collection is doubled. This is primarily attributed to the increasing rates of blood donorship from the patient's environment and secondly to volunteers. The contribution of the armed forces remained as a third, relatively smaller, source of blood donorship. In order to assess the relationship between the three domestic sources of blood, we estimated partial correlation coefficients. The results reveal:i) A rather high degree of correlation between the blood from the armed forces and the blood from the patient's environment is estimated (r=0.56). A possible explanation may be a side complementary relationship between the two sources of blood donation. ii) The voluntary blood collection shows a less strong relation with the Army (r=0.44) and the relatives' blood (r=0.40). These findings support the hypothesis of a lacking comprehensive blood policy to encourage voluntary blood donation, while emphasis was imposed on patients' relatives to give blood.

0078

MEASUREMENT OF INTERLEUKIN-6 PRODUCTION BY MONOCYTES FOR IN VITRO SAFETY TESTING OF HEMOGLOBIN SOLUTIONS
W.K.Bleeker, E.M.de Groot, P.J.den Boer, J.C.Bakker. and L.A.Aarden
Central Laboratory of the Netherlands Red Cross Blood Transfusion Service, Amsterdam, The Netherlands

The main barrier to clinical application of hemoglobin solutions as blood substitutes are the potential side effects. Therefore, we are conducting an extensive safety study of our hemoglobin solution, including in vivo and in vitro testing. Because the Mononuclear Phagocyte System (MPS) plays a primary role in host defence and inflammation, we evaluated the activation of human monocytes as an in vitro toxicity assay.

Interleukin-6 (IL-6) production was measured after 24 hours incubation of test samples with heparinized whole blood. The assay was very sensitive for bacterial endotoxin (10 pg/ml). Hemoglobin solutions that had not been prepared under aseptic conditions also induced high IL-6 production. Pretreatment of hemoglobin samples with the detergent Triton X114 (a procedure that effectively removes endotoxin) completely eliminated the IL-6 inducing capacity of the hemoglobin solutions.

We conclude that the measurement of in vitro IL-6 production by monocytes provides a very sensitive assay for testing hemoglobin solutions on contamination with bacterial products. Furthermore, it is concluded that pure modified hemoglobin itself neither induces nor inhibits IL-6 production by human monocytes.

0079

VASOCONSTRICTION CAUSED BY CELL-FREE HEMOGLOBIN: THE RATE OF ONSET OF HYPERTENSION AND INCREASED RENAL VASCULAR RESISTANCE IN A PORCINE RESUSCITATION MODEL.
J. Hess, V. Macdonald, C. Gomez, V. Coppes. Walter Reed Army Institute of Research, Washington, DC, USA 20307-5100.

We have produced human hemoglobin (Hb) and chemically modified human Hbs, in sterile formulations and of high purity, to advance the development of hemoglobin-based oxygen carriers for the emergency resuscitation of hemorrhagic shock. The intravascular infusion of these Hbs caused systemic and pulmonary hypertension and a marked increase in systemic, pulmonary, and renal vascular resistance in a porcine model of resuscitation from hemorrhagic shock. In an effort to understand these vasopressor reactions better, the magnitude and rate of onset of hypertension and renal vascular resistance were compared during resuscitation with human Hb purified by anion exchange chromatography (HbA_0) versus resuscitation with isooncotic human albumin (HSA) and the nitric oxide (NO) synthase inhibiter l-nitroarginine methyl ester (l-NAME, 10 mg/kg). Hypertension and increased vascular resistance occured within one minute of the initiation of Hb infusion, at a time when the intravascular concentration of Hb was 0.05 millimolar and Hb at nanomolar concentrations was diffusing out of the vascular space. The blood pressure rose to levels equivalent to those seen with full volume resuscitation and full pharmacologic blockade of NO synthesis. Additional Hb did not raise pressure further. This suggests that vasoconstriction is a pharmacologic effect of Hb.

0080

THE EFFECTS OF HEMOGLOBIN SOLUTIONS ON RENAL FUNCTION AFTER AN EXCHANGE TRANSFUSION AND AFTER HEMORRHAGE COMBINED WITH A MILD PERIOD OF ISCHEMIA. P.T. Biessels, G. Rigter, J. Agterberg, W. Bleeker and J.C. Bakker, Central Laboratory of the Netherlands Red Cross Blood Transfusion Service, Amsterdam, the Netherlands.

The present study was performed to measure the effects of purified (SFHb) and modified hemoglobin (polyHb) solutions on the renal function after an exchange transfusion (ET) and after a hemorrhagic shock (HS) combined with a period of ischemia.
Clearance of inulin and para-aminohippuricacid (PAH) in anesthesized rats were used to measure the glomerulair filtration rate (GFR) and the renal plasma flow (RPF), respectively. Exchange of 1/3 of the blood volume with either SFHb or polyHb resulted in an increase in GFR and RPF, urine volume, mean arterial blood pressure (MAP). These values tended to control values within 40 min. After an ET with albumin (control) there was only a small increase in GFR and RPF. After hemorrhage of about 35 % of the blood volume, indicated by a decrease in MAP of at least 60 %, followed by an ischemic period of 30 min, resuscitation with SFHb caused a decrease in GFR and RPF. MAP and urine flow increased, but urine flow stopped at the end of the experiment, i.e. after 2 hr. After resuscitation with polyHb a small decrease RPF occurred, but tended to control value within 60 min. Albumin caused no decrease in GFR and RPF, but the restoration of the MAP was not complete, i.e. max. 80 % of the starting value. The efects on the tubular function were studied by measuring the amount of N-acetyl-ß-glucosamidase (NAG) excreted into the urine. After infusion of SFHb a clear increase in NAG excretion was found, both after an ET or hemorhage. However, infusion of polyHb caused only a small increase in NAG excretion after an ET and did not differ from the control, albumin.
Conclusion: purified and modified Hb solutions caused no impairment of renal function after an ET or HS. Purified, but not modified Hb solutions, impaired renal function after HS, possibly by obstruction of the kidneys by the αß dimers of the Hb molecule.

0081

CLINICAL TRIALS WITH HUMAN POLYMERIZED HEMOGLOBIN POLY SFH-P.
S.Gould, L. Sehgal, H. Sehgal,
E. Toyooka, G. Moss.
Michael Reese Hosp., Univ. of IL,
Chicago, Northfield Labs, Evanston, IL

Clinical trials with tetrameric hemoglobin solutions have documented vasoconstriction and renal dysfunction. We report the results of a therapeutic dose of tetramer-free Poly SFH-P.

30 volunteers received Poly SFH-P over a dose range of.125-.6g/kg. The Poly SFH-P had a [Hb] of 8g/dl and P_{50} of 30 torr. The 8 recipients of the highest dose level received 50±8.0g (Mean±S.D.), equivalent to a 1-unit red cell transfusion, with a maximum individual dose of 63g. The resultant plasma [Hb] was 1.2±.2g/dl. The O_2 extraction ratios for Poly SFH-P (27.5±3.9%) and red cells (26.1±5.6) showed equivalent efficacy. Data for all 30 recipients showed no vasoconstriction or renal dysfunction.

	Pre-Infusion	Post-Infusion
Heart Rate(bpm)	62±9	61±10
MAP(torr)	95±12	100±13
Inulin Clearance (ml/min/m^2)	52±13	51±12

CONCLUSION Poly SFH-P is safe and effective in man at a therapeutic dose. Clinical trials in trauma patients are now in progress.

0083

FEBRILE REACTIONS TO PLATELET TRANSFUSION : EFFECT OF PREPARATION METHOD AND IL-6 LEVEL OF THE PLATELET CONCENTRATES (PC).
L.Muylle[1], E. Wouters[2], M.E.Peetermans[2],
1.Blood Transfusion Center Antwerp, Red Cross, Edegem, Belgium,2.Hematology Department, University of Antwerp (UZA), Edegem, Belgium.

Cytokines exhibiting in vitro pyrogenic activity, such as IL-6 increase in PC during storage. High levels of IL-6 are associated with transfusion reactions. As the IL-6 level is related to the white cell (WC) content of PC during storage, early removal of WC is expected to prevent reactions. Therefore two methods for preparation of PC were compared : the platelet rich plasma method (PRP-PC) with a high WC content and the buffy coat method (BC-PC) with a low WC content. In order to prevent reactions due to transfusion of WC all PC were depleted of WC at the bedside. 324 platelet transfusions in 46 patients were studied.

	PRP-PC	BC-PC	
Transfusions n	204	120	
Transfusion reactions (%)	15 (7.4 %)	3 (2.5 %)	*
PC:WC (10^9/unit)	1.34 ± 0.80	0.13 ± 0.09	*
PC:IL-6 ng/l	45 ± 118	< 4	**

* $p < 0.05$; ** $p < 0.001$
Transfusion reactions were correlated with the PRP-PC method ($p<0.05$), the total WC content ($p<0.05$) and the IL-6 level ($p<0.0001$).
In conclusion, febrile transfusion reactions can be related to the IL-6 level in transfused PRP-PC. The low WC content of BC-PC is associated with undetectable IL-6 levels and a reduced transfusion reaction rate.

0084

HEMAGGLUTINATION ASSAYS FOR THE DIAGNOSIS AND PREVENTION OF IgA ANAPHYLACTIC TRANSFUSION REACTIONS
S.G. Sandler, R. Eckrich, D. Malamut, D. Mallory
American Red Cross Blood Services, National Reference Laboratories, Rockville, MD, USA

Using a passive hemagglutination assay (PHA), we detected class-specific anti-IgA in 76.3% of 80 IgA-deficient patients with a history of an anaphylactic transfusion reaction, and in 21.7% of 97 IgA-deficient blood donors or their IgA-deficient family members. Using a passive hemagglutination inhibition assay (PHIA), we confirmed IgA-deficiency (<0.05 mg/dL) in donors of 525 plasma containing blood components that were transfused without acute clinical reactions in 48 IgA-deficient recipients with anti-IgA and/or a history of an anaphylactic transfusion reaction. The frequency of IgA-deficiency with class-specific anti-IgA among 32,376 random blood donors was 0.08% (1/1200).

The strategy of using PHA to detect anti-IgA, and PHIA to measure IgA is a safe practice for the diagnosis and prevention of IgA anaphylactic reactions. However, the relatively high frequency of anti-IgA in healthy IgA-deficient persons, compared to the rarity of anaphylactic transfusion reactions, reflects the lack of specificity of anti-IgA by PHA for identifying persons who are truly at risk for significant IgA anaphylactic transfusion reactions. The consequence is an over-diagnosis of IgA anaphylactic transfusion reactions (when anti-IgA is only coincidental) and an over-estimation of the number of people presumed to have a lifetime requirement for IgA-deficient blood products.

0085

ADVERSE REACTIONS TO PLATELET TRANSFUSIONS ARE REDUCED BY USE OF PLATELET CONCENTRATES DERIVED FROM BUFFY COATS.

K.Oksanen[1], F.Ebeling[1], R.Kekomäki[1], E.Elonen[2], L.Sahlstedt[2], L.Volin[2], G.Myllylä[1].
1 Finnish Red Cross Blood Transfusion Service, Helsinki,
2 Third Department of Medicine, Helsinki University Central Hospital, Helsinki, Finland.

We closely observed 155 platelet transfusions to leukemia patients: 46 transfusions to 23 patients with standard (STD) random donor platelet concentrates (PCs), 23 (12 patients) with leukocyte-depleted (L-D) PCs, and 86 (24 patients) with leukocyte-depleted PCs derived from pools of buffy coat (BC). The L-D PCs and the BC PCs contained less than 10^6 leukocytes per unit of PC. The overall incidence of adverse reactions was 83% with STD PCs, 65% with L-D PCs, and 24% with BC PCs. Febrile transfusion reactions occurred in 50% with STD PCs (61% of patients), 22% with L-D PCs (25% of patients) and in 4.6% with BC PCs (21% of patients). Urticarial skin reactions were observed in 46%, 52%, and 19% (48%, 83%, and 29% of patients), and pulmonary reactions in 4%, 4%, and 0% (8%, 8%, and 0% of patients), respectively. The corrected platelet increments (CI) at 18 hours were higher after BC PCs (9.44) than L-D PCs (6.67) or STD PCs (6.75) (p=0.001). BC PCs that were filtered prior to storage resulted in better mean CIs than those filtered after three days´ storage (10.3 vs. 8.0, p=0.046). We conclude that BC PCs produce fewer and milder adverse reactions as well as better CIs than those obtained with the platelet-rich plasma method. Early filtration of BC PCs may result in better CIs.

0086

DEFINITIVE DIAGNOSIS OF POST TRANSFUSION GRAFT-VERSUS-HOST DISEASE USING HIGHLY POLYMORPHIC MICROSATELLITE MARKERS

S. Uchida, Y. Yahagi, L. Wang, K. Tokunaga, Y. Mitomi, K. Tadokoro and T. Juji

Japanese Red Cross Central Blood Center, Tokyo, Japan.

A new method of using highly polymorphic microsatellite repeat sequences for definitive diagnosis of post-transfusion graft-versus-host disease(PT-GVHD) has been established. Genomic DNA was extracted from blood, skin and nail and subjected to polymerase chain reaction(PCR) for five different markers. And then the amplified fragments were analyzed by polyacrylamide gel electrophoresis with the same condition for sequencing. The results demonstrated the replacement of patient DNA types with donor types on the occasion of PT-GVHD. 12 definitive cases were diagnosed by this system from 26 samples that we were requested to analyze since October 1992 till December 1993. Eleven patients out of twelve died through a typical clinical course of fever, erythema, liver dysfunction and pancytopenia. Another case recovered by administrating anti-CD3 antibody (OKT3) and Cyclosporine A. As a rapid, sensitive and easily applicable method, this system could be a useful tool for the clinical diagnosis of PT-GVHD.

0091

TRANSMISSION OF HTLV-II BY HTLV-I SCREENED BLOOD PRODUCTS. M. Rios[1], R. F. Khabbaz[2], J.E. Kaplan[2], D. Kessler[1], W. Hall[3], and C. Bianco[1]. 1New York Blood Center, New York, NY, Centers for Disease Control, Atlanta, GA, 3 Rockefeller University, New York, NY, U.S.A.

HTLV-I and HTLV-II were the first human retrovirus identified. Concerns about transmission of HTLV-I by transfusion lead to the licensing of blood donor screening tests by the U.S. FDA in December, 1988. At that time, screening for HTLV-II was considered an indirect benefit of the screening for HTLV-I because of the extensive cross-reactivity between antibodies to the two virus. Recent reports suggest that HTLV-I based assays may not detect some individuals who may be infected by HTLV-II. In addition, some authors have indicated that HTLV-II may be associated with disease. In order to assess the implications of these observations, we have reviewed cases of lookback for HTLV-II at our institution. We identified 6 cases of HTLV-II transmission by 5 donors. Four of the 5 donors and 4 of the recipients were tested by PCR amplification of HTLV-I and HTLV-II sequences. The HTLV-II subtype of 4 donor-recipient/pairs was determined by PCR amplification of the *env* region and was the same in each pair (3 were HTLV-IIa and 1 was HTLV-IIb). Three of the implicated donors had donated 1 to 5 times after HTLV-I screening was introduced, and had negative screening test results. The manufacturer modified the screening assay for HTLV-I in mid 1993, in an attempt to increase sensitivity for HTLV-II. An analysis of samples below the assay cut-off and of Western blot patterns of reactive samples suggest that the modifications led to decreased assay specificity without detectable change in assay sensitivity. In conclusion, HTLV-I tests have inadequate sensitivity for HTLV-II screening. The development of specific combined tests for HTLV-I and for HTLV-II may constitute a more effective approach to the prevention of HTLV transmission by transfusion.

0092

PCR ANALYSIS OF HTLV-INFECTION IN FRENCH BLOOD DONORS

C. Defer*, F. Descamps*, M. Maniez*, J.M. Lemaire, A.M. Couroucé and the Retrovirus Study Group of the French Society of Blood Transfusion. *CRTS Lille FRANCE.

To verify the criteria of HTLV seropositivity by Western-blot (WB), 185 blood donors repeatedly reactive by HTLV ELISA, selected according to the WB pattern were tested by polymerase chain reaction. The primer pairs used were SK110-111 (pol) and SK44-45 (tax) which amplify both viruses HTLV-I/II, SK54-55 (pol) and SK58-59 (pol) are HTLV-I and HTLV-II specific, respectively.

Western- blot pattern			N°	PCR results	
rgp21	p19	p24	tested	Negative	Positive
+	+	+	13	0	12 (I) 1 (II)
+	+	-	23	22	1 (I)
+	-	+	19	19	0
-	+	+	27	27	0
+	-	-	8	0	0
-	+	-	46	46	0
-	-	+	49	49	0

Conclusion : Due to a possible false positive rgp21 reactivity, a minimum of 3 bands on rgp21, p19 and p24 is necessary to conclude to HTLV-infection. When rgp21 reactivity is associated with a gag band alone (p19 or p24), it is necessary to discriminate between false and true positive. No HTLV-infection was observed in the absence of rgp21 reactivity.

0093

HTLV-I/II EPIDEMIOLOGY AMONG THE BLOOD DONORS IN CONTINENTAL FRANCE.

J.M.LEMAIRE[1], J.PILLONEL[2], A.M.COUROUCE[3], and the French Blood Banks.
1C.R.T.S. Montpellier, 2Réseau National de Santé Publique, Saint-Maurice, 3I.N.T.S. Paris (France).

OBJECTIVES : 1) To establish the prevalence of the HTLV-I/II antibodies among blood donations in continental France since systematic screening became mandatory on July 15th 1991.

2) To study the epidemiological characteristics of the infected Blood Donors.

RESULTS: 1) The prevalence decreased from 0.39 for 10 000 donations in 1991 (70/1 809 651) to 0.21 in 1992 (75/3 524 586).

2) Among the 145 HTLV positive Blood Donors, only 3 (2 %) were HTLV-II : 3 men, including 2 former intravenous drug addicts.

The remaining 142 were HTLV-I positive (the sex-ratio was 0.56) :

Birth place :

- endemic areas of high HTLV-I prevalence	61
- continental France	73
.sexual partner(s) born in endemic areas	39
.other risk factors	11
.unknown risk factors or no inquiry	23
- unknown or in other country	8
	142

CONCLUSION : The HTLV prevalence is low among the french Blood Donors. HTLV-I in continental France is linked to the diffusion of this virus in the endemic areas, and HTLV-II infection to drug addiction.

0094

RELATIVE SENSITIVITY OF 5 ANTI-HTLV-I ELISAs.

H. Vrielink[1], C.L. van der Poel[1], H.W. Reesink[1], W.P. Schaasberg[2], P.N. Lelie[2]. 1)Red Cross Blood Bank Amsterdam, 2)Central Lab Blood Transfusion Service Amsterdam, The Netherlands.

Objective: The relative sensitivity of 5 commercially available ELISAs for anti-HTLV-I was evaluated in 30 serially diluted anti-HTLV-I positive sera.

Methods/serum panel: Twofold serial dilutions of 30 anti-HTLV-I sera (10 asymptomatic blood donors, 10 patients with adult T-cell leukemia/lymphoma, 10 patients with HTLV-I associated myelopathy) were made with human AB serum and tested in ELISAs A, B, C, D and E. Statistical analysis of the relative sensitivity was performed by probit analysis (Finney DJ. Probit analysis. Cambridge: Cambridge University Press, 1971) and expressed as relative potency.

Results: Relative potency (95% C.I.) of the ELISAs of the various manifacturers in respect of each other.

	B	C	D	E
A	0.4 (0.3-0.6)	0.4 (0.3-0,6)	0.4 (0.3-0.7)	0.7 (0.5-1.0)
B		1.0 (0.7-1.5)	1.2 (0.8-1.7)	1.8 (1.2-2.6)
C			1.1 (0.8-1.6)	1.7 (1.2-2.5)
D				1.5 (1.0-2.3)

Conclusions: Probit analysis showed that ELISAs A and E were significantly less sensitive as compared to B, C and D.

0096

PERIODICALLY VARIING INTERFACE POSITION REDUCES WHITE BLOOD CELL (WBC) CONTAMINATION IN PLATELET PHERESIS WITH THE BLOOD CELL SEPARATOR AS 104

R. Moog[1], G. Schramek[2], T. Weißwange[3], N. Müller[1], H.-J. Neumann[3], V. Thierbach[2],
1 Inst. Transfusion Medicine, Univ. Essen, Germany,
2 Inst. Transf. Medicine, Univ. Leipzig, Germany,
3 Fresenius, St. Wendel, Germany

The aim of the study was the evaluation of optimal parameters of a new software with automatically varying interface position (VIP) to reduce the WBC-contamination in platelet concentrates (PC) obtained with the Fresenius blood cell separator AS 104.

The separation (whole blood volume 3600 - 3900 ml) was divided into n cycles with collection phase (interface position IFP=5:3) and transfer phase (IFP=8:0). Different numbers of cycles (n=3, 4, 5, 7, 10) and different transfer volumes (100, 150, 200, 250, 300ml) were investigated. Platelets were counted electronically. WBC in PC were counted manually in Neubauer or Nageotte-chamber.

Separation efficiency with standard software 4.62 is 1 to 4%-points higher than with the evaluated protocols. WBC-contamination in PC with VIP was lower than in standard PC (median in standard separation Leipzig 5.5x10^6 and Essen 2.7x10^6). Using protocols with 3, 4 or 5 cycles with 100 ml transfer volume in Leipzig WBC-median was decreased to 0.23, 1.1 and 1.3 x 10^6, resp. Separations with 3 cycles with 200 ml transfer volume in Essen produced a WBC-contamination below the detection limit of the Neubauer chamber (1.4 x 10^6) in more than 70% of the cases (mean 0.7x10^6).

WBC-contamination in PC obtained with VIP platelet pheresis is up to 80% lower than with the standard procedure. The reduction of separation efficiency can be compensated by slightly increasing the separation time or the blood flow rate.

0097

PLASMAPHERESIS AND INTERFERON REDUCE INTERFERON INHIBITOR FACTOR IN MULTIPLE SCLEROSIS PATIENTS RESPONDING TO THERAPY.

R. Medenica, S. Mukerjee, K. Alonso, G. Lazovic, T. Huschart, W. Corbitt, C. Solak, P. Long. Cancer Immuno-Biology Laboratory, Hilton Head Island, S.C., USA.

Sera from certain patients (pts) suffering from multiple sclerosis (MS) inhibit anti-viral, immuno-modulatory and proliferative activity of interferon (ifn) [as previously demonstrated by our group]. We named this factor interferon inhibitor factor (IIF). To determine what role IIF plays in the treatment of MS, we removed or reduced this factor from the pt's circulation during courses of plasmapheresis (PP). 24 pts with chronic progressive MS were treated by PP on Day 1 followed by ifn on Days 1, 2 & 3. These courses were repeated every 28 days x 4. IIF and ifn were measured in the serum before and after PP and in extracted plasma. With successive PP, IIF decreased in the sera to completely disappear in the responders. In all responders, circulating ifn level (CIL) increased. Ifn in the PP bag initially increased (average 2000 U/ml) and decreased after PP (average 500 U/ml). In the 3 pts that progressed with PP therapy, serum IIF remained high and no CIL was detected. In summary, decrease in IIF results in increase in CIL. At the same time, ifn levels in the PP bags increases constantly in the beginning in those pts who respond to PP therapy and then it decreases with successive treatment of PP. There is a direct relationship betwee the reduction of IIF, an increase in interferon serum level, and clinical response in PP-treated MS pts.

0098

THROMBOTIC MICROANGIOPATHY: ELEVEN YEARS EXPERIENCE

M.Réti, V.Harsányi, A.Mód, K.Kilián, J.Szabó, J.Kádár, S.Hollán
National Institute of Haematology, Blood Transfusion and Immunology, Budapest, Hungary

In the past eleven years 21 cases (20 patients) of thrombotic microangiopathy have been treated with plasma exchange (PEX) in our institute. Adjunctive drug therapy included dipyridamole, salicylate, corticosteroid and vincristine. The mean age was 29 years. 17/20 patients were female, 2 were pregnant. The mean initial laboratory data were: Plt: 14 G/l, Htc: 0,23, LDH: 1959 U/l. All patients had negative Coombs test. Fragmentocytes could be observed in the peripheral smears of all cases. 18/21 cases had neurologic symptoms. 8/21 cases had some degree of azotemia, but only 1 needed dialysis. 76 % (16/21) of patients responded following PEX. Response was prompt, the initial increment in Plt count above 50 G/l occurred after a mean of 3 PEXs, and a complete remission was obtained after a mean of 10 PEXs. Following cessation of PEX short-time relapse occurred in 2 patients (3 occasion), but all these episodes responded to re-treatment with PEX. Late-relapse (after 18 months) occurred only in 1 patient, but complete remission was achieved again. All responders but one are alive in full remission with a mean duration of follow-up of 65 (24-131) months. One patient in the responder group died of acute cardiac failure 2 days after her 4th PEX, at which time her Plt count was 140 G/l. There was no evidence of TTP at autopsy . One patient had 2 pregnancies, the 1st 19 months, the 2nd 57 months after her TTP. Both pregnancies ended in normal deliveries, no relapse occurred either during pregnancies or after. Albumin was used in 4 PEXs of 2 patients due to the very serious side effect of FFP. One of them died some hours after her 2nd PEX done with albumin. The other patient had a dramatic fall in Plt count, but complete remission was achieved after 5 PEXs using FFP again. 24 % (5/21) of cases who failed to respond died, 2 of them within 48 hours of the 1st PEX. Not even a partial haematological response was achieved in the non-responder group. The PEX/day ratio was 0.92 in the responder group, 0.95 in the non-responder group during the first 4 days, 0.76 in the responder group and 0.97 in the non-responder group during the whole period. When no Plt increment occurred after 4 PEXs, the prognosis was very poor.

0099

SEVERE HYPERVISCOSITY IN LOUIS-BAR SYNDROME: SYNCHRONIZED THERAPY WITH PLASMAPHERESIS AND STEROIDS.

C. Perotti[1] L. Torretta[1], L. Costamagna[1], L. Salvaneschi[1], V. Monafo[2]
1Servizio di Immunoematologia e Trasfusione, 2 Pediatric Dept. Univ. of Pavia, IRCCS Policlinico San Matteo, Pavia, Italy.

Louis-Bar syndrome (Ataxia-Teleangectasia - AT) is a heterogeneous autosomal recessive disorder characterized by cerebellar ataxia, oculocutaneous teleangectasies, cancer susceptibility and immunodeficiency both humoral and cellular. Humoral deficiency is marked by IgA and IgE deficit, with combined IgM increase in 80% of cases. Such condition predisposes to infections. Relevant clinical evidence due to hyperviscosity may occur in patients with elevated IgM plasmatic levels. We report a case of AT with a severe hyperviscosity syndrome treated with plasmapheresis, synchronized with drug therapy in order to maintain low IgM levels as long as possible. A 6 year-old girl affected by AT (diagnosis at 20 months) was admitted to our Centre because of hyper-IgM, undetectable IgG and IgA. Continuously increasing IgM level caused a severe hyperviscosity syndrome with gengival bleeding, disseminated petecchiae and somnolence. Plasma exchange (PE) was carried out with a Dideco BT 810 blood cell separator, generally employed in donor plasmapheresis because of its low extracorporeal volume (150 ml). Two single volume plasma exchanges were performed in a week, with 5% albumin in saline 0.9% solution as replacement fluid. After PE, therapy was conducted with i.v. immunoglobulins to prevent infections and with alternate day prednisone. Promptly clinical symptoms related to hyperviscosity withdrew and IgM level decreased from 10.5 to 3.8 g/dl and further to 2.6 g/dl over the next two months. Expected IgM rebound effect was not observed, despite a reduction of prednisone dose to 0.75 mg/kg every other day. The young patient is stable at 12 months, with no complications. PE had not been experimented in young patients with AT, in whom acute severe hyperviscosity may be difficultly dominated with steroid therapy alone. The adeguate synchronism of plasma exchange and steroid therapy proved a successful therapeutic approach in the management of this syndrome and in the control of its acute complications.

0101

LEUKOCYTE DEPLETION OF RANDOM SINGLE DONOR PLATELET TRANSFUSIONS DOES NOT PREVENT SECONDARY HLA-ALLOIMMUNIZATION AND REFRACTORINESS: A RANDOMIZED PROSPECTIVE STUDY

K. Sintnicolaas[1], M. van Marwijk Kooij[2], H.C. van Prooijen[2], B.A. van Dijk[3], W.L.J. van Putten[1], V.M.J. Novotny[4], A. Brand[4].
1Red Cross Blood Bank/Dr. Daniel den Hoed Cancer Center, Rotterdam, 2University Hospital Utrecht, 3University Hospital Nijmegen, 4University Hospital Leiden, The Netherlands

We studied the value of leukocyte depletion of platelet transfusions for the prevention of secondary HLA-alloimmunization in patients with a high risk of prior immunization induced by pregnancies. Seventy-five female patients with hematological malignancies, mostly acute leukemia, and a history of pregnancy were randomized to receive either standard random single donor platelet transfusions (mean leukocytes $430x10^6$ per transfusion) or random single donor platelet transfusions leukocyte depleted to less than $5x10^6$ leukocytes per platelet transfusion (mean $2x10^6$) by filtration. Of the 62 evaluable patients refractoriness to random donor platelets occurred in 41% (14 of 34) of the patients in the standard group and in 29% (8 of 28) of the patients in the filtered group (p=0.52); lymphocytotoxic antibodies developed in 43% (9 of 21) of individuals in the standard group and 44% (11 of 25) of cases in the filtered group. The time towards refractoriness and development of HLA-antibodies was similar for both groups. We conclude that leukocyte depletion of random single donor platelet products to $<5x10^6$ per transfusion does not reduce the incidence of clinical refractoriness due to boostering of anti-HLA antibodies.

0102

LEUKOCYTE DEPLETION OF BLOOD COMPONENTS IS COST-EFFECTIVE IN THE TREATMENT OF AML.

K.Oksanen[1] and E.Elonen[2].
1 Finnish Red Cross Blood Transfusion Service, Helsinki, 2 Third Department of Medicine, Helsinki University Central Hospital, Helsinki, Finland.

Leukocyte-depleted (L-D) platelets (PCs) and red cells (RBCs) (< 10^6 leukocytes per unit) were given to 65 and standard (STD) components to 50 patients with acute myeloid leukemia (AML). Two of 65 (3%) and 11 of 50 (22%) patients became refractory to random PCs. The extra costs for the hospital were FIM 70,- /unit of L-D PC, 280,- /unit of L-D RBC, and 374,-/unit of HLA-compatible PC. If the consumption of PCs and RBCs in STD and L-D groups had been equal, the extra costs of L-D vs. HLA-typed PCs would have been similar, and the extra cost of L-D RBCs (280,-/unit) would favour STD components. However, the need for PCs and RBCs was higher in STD group (51 vs. 32 units of PC and 8 vs. 6 units of RBC per treatment cycle), although the doses of cytostatic agents were equal. With the observed consumption, the cost of L-D components was 77% of the cost of STD components. The other benefits of leukodepletion (avoiding CMV infection, febrile reactions, and possible immuno-modulation) further favour the use of L-D components.

0103

PLATELET CONCENTRATRES PREPARED BY THE PLATELET-RICH PLASMA METHOD, FILTERED AND SUBSEQUENTLY STORED FOR 8 DAYS.

M.N.Boomgaard, C.H.Palfenier, I.E.Pankalla-Blandeau, H.A.Veldman, C.W.N.Gouwerok, D.de Korte, J.A.Loos.
Central Laboratory of The Netherlands Red Cross Blood Transfusion Service, Amsterdam, the Netherlands.

The effect of pre-storage filtration of platelet concentrates (PC) prepared by the platelet-rich plasma method on platelet function, morphology, metabolism and activation was studied immediately after filtration and during an 8 day storage period.

A pool of 20 PRP-PC was split into 4 equal volumes; 3 were filtered over a PL50HF (Pall), a PL-10A (Sepacell) or a Bio P10 (Biofil) filter, the fourth served as a control. After filtration the PC filtered by either the PL50HF or the Bio P10 filter contained about 7 x 10^4 leukocytes, while in the PC filtered by the PL-10A filter it was even less (0.8 x 10^4), in the control PC leukocyte contamination was 59 x 10^6. Platelet loss induced by the filters was about 13% for the PL50HF and the PL-10A filter and 19% for the Biofil filter, resulting in a mean post-filtration platelet content of 295 x 10^9. During storage pH, PO_2, PCO_2, and lactate and glucose concentration were equal in the filtered and the unfiltered units. Also no differences were observed between filtered and unfiltered PC in aggregation upon stimulation with collagen and/or ADP, adhesion capacity to collagen and fibrinogen in flowing blood, nucleotide content and nucleobase release of the platelets, the expression of activation dependent antigens or platelet morphologoy as observed light-microscopically and by the swirling effect.

PC prepared by the PRP-method can be filtered and subsequently stored for 8 days without detrimental effect on platelet viability, function, metabolism or activation.

0104

IN-PROCESS FILTRATION OF PLATELET CONCENTRATES FROM POOLED BUFFY COATS USING A NEW FILTER DEVICE

H. Klüter[1], M. Klinger[2], M. Bauhaus[1], H. Kirchner[1]
Institute of Immunology and Transfusion Medicine[1] and Institute of Anatomy[2], University of Lübeck, Medical School, Lübeck, Germany

Leukocytes in platelet concentrates (PC) have been shown to be associated with poor PC storability and increase the risk for HLA-alloimmunization after platelet substitution. We studied the impact of pre-storage white-cell depletion on PC storability and the practicability of this method in daily routine. PC were prepared from pooled buffy coats (BC). Eight ABO-identical BC were pooled in a 2-liter PVC-bag within 8 hours after whole-blood donation, mixed and divided into two identical fractions (n= 14). After soft-spin centrifugation the platelet-rich plasma was transferred either directly (fraction A) or (fraction B) through a standard leukocyte filter (PL-50 HF, Pall) into the storage bag (PL-732, Baxter) and stored under routine conditions. On days 1, 3, 5 and 8, samples were withdrawn for cell count determination, for biochemical analyses and for morphological study of the ultrastructure. The filtered group showed a significant ($p<0.01$) leukocyte reduction (51 vs 0.04 x 10^6) and a lower platelet content (268 vs 240 x 10^9). Both groups did not differ in various biochemical parameters and morphometric analyses showed good preservation of intracellular structures in both preparations. In a second series we investigated a new type of leukocyte filter (Autostop BC, Pall) that stops automatically when red cells enter the filter material. The study design was in accordance with the first series. White-cell reduction was >99.9% (72 vs <0.04 x 10^6) and platelet loss was within the range of the first series (10%). Laboratory testing revealed good platelet preservation during the whole storage period. We conclude that pre-storage leukocyte depletion can be easily performed but has no impact on platelet storability when methods for preparation of PC with low leukocyte contents are used. However, the benefit of modern pre-storage filtration devices like the Autostop BC should be studied further, since the role of soluble HLA-antigens and other leukocyte mediators are not completely known.

0106

EFFECT OF PLATELETS ON LEUKODEPLETION OF RED CELLS BY FILTRATION

[1]R.R.Stromberg, [1,2]R. Gonzales
1American Red Cross, Rockville, MD, 2Walter Reed Army Medical Center, Washington, DC. USA

We studied the effect of platelet concentration (PC) on filtration of single red cell (RC) units. "Platelet Enriched" (PE) and "Platelet Poor" (PP) Adsol® RC units were prepared from pooled whole blood (WB) by adding platelet concentrate from the PP to the paired PE unit. For PC differences (Δ) between PE and PP of ~1 $\log_{10}$, there were no significant differences in post-filtration wbc levels.

Filter Type	Δ Plt/unit, $\log_{10}$	WBC/unit, PE/PP
Pall RC50 (n=4)	1.2	1.9/1.4 ($x10^7$)
Pall BPF4 (n=6)	0.8	1.1/1.6 ($x10^5$)
Asahi R500 (n=5)	0.9	1.7/2.9 ($x10^6$)

In a second study (n=3), multiple PE and PP (Δ~1 $\log_{10}$) RC, prepared from pooled WB, were passed through a single filter (BPF4). Wbc levels were measured in each 100 mL of filtrate. Differences were observed after 400 mL had passed through the filter; higher residual wbc levels in the PP RC.

	400 mL	600 mL	800 mL
PE (wbc/mL)	$1x10^2$	$6x10^2$	$2x10^3$
PP (wbc/mL)	$1x10^2$	$3x10^3$	$6x10^3$

We conclude that, for the filters studied, removal of platelets from WB will not affect the residual wbc level for single units. This work however, supports and extends the studies of Steneker, et.al. (*Transfusion* 33:42 1993), who found that platelet-filter interactions are involved in wbc removal, as indicated when large RC volumes are filtered.

0107

DOES PLASMA INFLUENCE THE EFFICIENCY OF LEUKOCYTE FILTRATION?

E. Ledent[1,2], G. Berlin[1].
1 Dept. of Transfusion Medicine and Clin. Immunology, and 2 Dept. of Cell Biology, University Hospital, Linköping, Sweden.

Our effort to make "pure" blood products results in erythrocyte concentrates (RBC) with a low number of platelets as well as a small amount of plasma. We have studied if the amount of plasma of RBC influences the efficiency of leukocyte depletion by filtration.

Two units of fresh whole blood were pooled, mixed and split into two equal units, a control unit and a test unit. RBC was obtained by centrifugation (2500 *g*, 11.5 min). The control RBC was suspended in 100 ml of SAGMAN solution, according to our standard protocol, whereas 5 or 10 ml of SAGMAN was substituted with an equal amount of autologous plasma in the test unit. After an over-night storage at +4°C, filtration through a RC50 filter (PALL) at a slow flow rate (2 h) was performed. The pre-filtration number of platelets was counted in a Bürker chamber and the number of leukocytes after filtration in a Nageotte chamber. The amount of plasma was determined by weighing.

Results (mean±SEM):	5 ml (n=8)		10 ml (n=10)	
	Test	Control	Test	Control
Amount of plasma (ml)	12.3±1.1	6.7±1.1	15.2±0.9	5.1±0.8
Platelets $x10^9$/unit	1.6±0.4	1.7±0.6	1.7±0.4	1.9±0.3
Leukocytes $x10^6$/unit	6.9±2.4	36.5±6.7	1.9±0.5	30.0±9.1

Our results show that the amount of plasma in the RBC plays an important role for the outcome of leukocyte depletion by filtration. By adding 5 or 10 ml of plasma to the standard SAGMAN product we found a significant decrease in the number of leukocytes after filtration (p=0.002 and p=0.013, respectively; paired t-test). No difference was found in the number of platelets of the test and control units.

0108

LEUCOCYTES REMOVAL FROM RED CELL CONCENTRATES (RCC): PERFORMANCE OF BPF4 FILTER (Pall)

G Baldini, S Roncaglia, G Milanti, P Marchegiano
Blood Transfusion Service.Policlinico of MODENA-ITALY

RCC in SAGM solution were prepared from CPD whole blood by centrifugation at high speed 3500gx10 min (Standard RCC, n=9) or at low speed (1100gx6 min) (Platelet Depleted RCC, n=9). All 18 RCC units were filtered accordingly to BPF4 manufacturer's instructions. White blood cell (WBC) counts on post filtration samples were performed in Nageotte chamber. RESULTS (mean values reported)

	STANDARD RCCs (n=9)	Platelet Deplet. RCCs (n=9)
Prefiltration		
WBC x10e8	24.63	12.28
PLT x10e9	61.50	11.07
Postfiltration		
WBC x10e6	0.051	0.210
PLT x10e6	2100	1160
WBC Reduction Capacity	99.99	99.87

CONCLUSION:Performance of BPF4 filter was satisfying in both groups of RCCs. A correlation between platelet load prior to filtration and WBC reduction capacity was observed (r=0.706,p=0.01). Platelet adhesion to filter material may account for the observed increase in BPF4 filtration efficiency when comparing Standard RCCs with Platelet Depleted RCCs ($p < 0.05$).

0109

EVALUATION OF AN INTEGRAL FILTER FOR LEUCOCYTE-DEPLETION AND SUBSEQUENT STORAGE OF SAG-M RED BLOOD CELLS

S.E.Rogers[1], D.Edmondson[1], M.J.Goodrick[1], D.Pamphilon[1], V.Franck[2], A.Reppucci[2]
[1]Regional Transfusion Centre, Bristol, UK and [2]Baxter R&D, Nivelles, Belgium.

Prestorage leucocyte depletion of blood components may reduce the incidence of adverse reactions and improve product quality. We have studied a bottom and top system with an integral third generation leucocyte filter. Whole blood was collected from 30 healthy donors; 20 into the Optipac^{LS}-Integral Filter System and 10 control units (C) into Optipacs. Ten test units (A) were buffy coat (BC) depleted and then filtered after 72 hours, 4°C storage and ten (B) were BC depleted and filtered at room temperature within 8 hours of collection. All units were stored at 4°C for 42 days and sampled weekly. Average leucocyte counts were 0.33 x 10^6 (A), 2.6 x 10^6 (B) and 460 x 10^6 (C). We found no significant differences in lactate, pH and glucose between the three groups. Similarly there were no differences in Na^+, K^+, 2,3-DPG, ATP and % haemolysis. Autologous *in vivo* 24 hour recovery studies were done in 8 healthy volunteers whose red cells were processed as in B and reinfused after 35 days storage. Good recovery (mean >80%) was found using single and double isotope-label methods. The Optipac^{LS} achieves effective leucodepletion without detriment to *in vitro* or *in vivo* storage parameters.

0111

BACTERIAL SCREENING OF PLATELET CONCENTRATES. IS IT FEASIBLE AND DESIRABLE?

C.F. Högman[1], J. Gong[1], M. Engstrand[1], M. Lundholm[2], I. Gustafsson[2], O. Åkerblom[1]
Departments of 1Clinical Immunology and Transfusion Medicine and 2Clinical Microbiology, University Hospital, Uppsala, Sweden

In 3 years we have detected 4 infected platelet concentrates (PCs), giving clinical complications, in approximately 10,000 therapeutic doses of transfused PC. The contaminating bacteria have been *B. cereus, B. subtilis, E. aerogenes, P. mirabilis* and pneumococci. The storage time before transfusion has been 4, 3, 1, and 3 days. The origin most likely appeared from the environment in 3 cases and from the donor in 1 case.

In an experimental study platelet concentrates (PCs) prepared from pools of 4 buffy coats using 30% plasma in a platelet additive solution were inoculated, 11 with 50-98 colony forming units (CFU) per ml, 11 with 0.3-9 CFU/ml and 11 uninoculated as controls. The BacT/Alert system for automated blood culture was used: pediatric bottles, aerobic culture only, and compared with a manual blood culture method and quantitative culture. Positive test was obtained at 132 sampling occasions from large-inoculum PCs and in all small-inoculum PCs with viable bacteria; uninoculated PCs were negative. The time for detection was 6-16 h in the BacT/Alert tests, longer in the other tests.

Bacterial contamination is a risk in PC transfusions.The BacT/Alert technique seems to be a rapid, reliable and labour-saving method for routine PC testing.

0112

PHOTOCHEMICAL INACTIVATION OF BACTERIA IN PLATELET CONCENTRATES

H. Londe,[1] R. Alfonso,[2] M. Janda,[2], L. Corash[1], and L. Lin,[1] [1]Steritech Inc., Concord CA; [2]Calif. Depart. of Health Services, Berkeley CA, U.S.A.

Previously we have demonstrated the efficacy of an 8-methoxypsoralen (8-MOP) mediated photochemical decontamination (PCD) technique to inactivate high levels of a broad spectrum of bacteria in platelet concentrates (PC) with adequate preservation of *in vitro* platelet function (**Blood** 82: 205a, 1993). The objective of this study was to further evaluate this technique using a model that mimics routine blood banking procedures. *S. epidermidis*, a common gram-positive contaminant, and two highly virulent gram-negative strains, *K. pneumoniae* and *P. aeruginosa* were used. $10^{2.5}$- $10^{3.1}$ cfu/ml of these bacteria were added to freshly prepared CPDA1 platelet rich plasma (PRP). PC were prepared from contaminated PRP using standard procedures and resuspended in a balanced salt isosmolar (pH 7.2) synthetic medium S2.22 containing 23 µg/ml 8-MOP and 15% plasma. Proliferation of these bacteria was determined following 2, 5, and 18 hr of storage at 22°C. The highest levels of *S. epidermidis*, *K. pneumoniae*, and *P. aeruginosa* reached after 5 hr of storage were $10^{3.0}$, $10^{4.8}$, and $10^{2.9}$ cfu/ml, respectively; and after 18 hr of storage: $10^{5.3}$, $10^{8.7}$, and $10^{4.3}$ cfu/ml, respectively. Treatment of these contaminated stored PC with 3 Joules/cm^2 of UVA, a condition shown to adequately maintain *in vitro* platelet function, inactivated all bacteria with the exception of *K. pneumoniae* for which $10^{7.4}$-$10^{7.7}$ cfu/ml were inactivated. These results suggest that 8-MOP mediated PCD treatment, when carried out within 18 hr following preparation of PC in a blood bank, is an effective means to prevent bacterial proliferation in PC during 22°C storage.

0113

REDUCTION OF BACTERIAL CONTAMINANTS - EFFICACY OF A COLLECTION SYSTEM WITH AN IN-LINE LEUKOCYTE REMOVAL FILTER

A. Ali[1], L. Bardossy[2], P. Lyn[2], H. Richardson[2], M. Blajchman[1,2]
[1]The Canadian Red Cross Society & [2]Department of Pathology, McMaster University, Hamilton, Ontario. Canada.

Evidence that the early removal of leukocytes (LKC) from donated blood is of benefit to transfusion recipients has increased interest in collection systems with in-line LKC filters. However, this pre-storage removal of LKC might negate the removal of bacterial contaminants. Thus the following studies were conducted. Known loads of a coagulase negative *staphylococcus* (ATCC 29971) were inoculated into fresh red cells collected into Leukotrap® Red Cell Storage Systems (Miles Inc.). After varying intervals, half of each unit was transferred to the additive pack via the in-line LKC filter (bag F) and half was transferred, without filtration, directly to a pack that had been added using a sterile docking device (bag NF). Samples for bacterial culture in the Bactec 9240 blood culturing system (Beckton Dickinson) were taken pre and post inoculation and after transfer to the NF and F bags. The bags, then stored at 4 °C, were sampled daily for 5 days, then weekly up to 42 days. Incubation prior to filtration was done at both 22 °C and 4 °C. At a bacterial load of 10^2 CFU/mL of red cells, all post-transfer samples from the NF bags were positive regardless of incubation period or temperature. In contrast, there was a marked reduction in the number of organisms grown from the F bags following 4 to 6 hours incubation at 22 °C and after 8 hours incubation all F units (n=11) were still negative after 42 days storage. At 4 °C there was some, but much less, inhibition in bacterial growth in the F bags. These data indicate that there is a time and temperature dependent process involved in the removal of organisms and that, with optimal use, in-line LKC filter blood collection systems can enhance the removal of contaminating bacteria.

0114

A POSSIBLE ROLE OF LEUKOCYTE FILTERS TO PREVENT TRANSFUSION-TRANSMITTED *Trypanosoma cruzi*

Wendel, S.[1,2]; Takaoka, D.T.[2]; Jancso, M.M.[2].; Mariano, M.[1]; Fragata Filho, A.A.[3]; Pereira-Chioccola, V.L.[3] and Lourenço, A.M.[3]
1- Hospital Sírio-Libanês - Blood Bank, São Paulo, Brazil
2- Centro de Imunologia e Imunogenética, São Paulo, Brazil
3- Lab. Xenodiagnóstico, Instituto Dante Pazzanese, São Paulo, Brazil

Leukocyte filters are currently used to provide leukocyte-poor blood products, to prevent HLA-alloimmunization or non-hemolytic febrile reactions. In addition, a possibility to decrease the incidence of CMV and HTLV-I/II transmission by cellular components has also been described. We carried out a preliminary study in order to establish a possible role of leukocyte filters in preventing transfusion-mediated *T. cruzi* infection.

MATERIAL AND METHODS: Trypomastigote forms (Y strain) were spiked into whole blood units (n= 3), achieving a final concentration of ± 50 parasites/ml, and filtered with IMURGARD IG500 filters (Terumo, Japan). Aliquots of each sample (pre- and post-filtration) were inoculated intraperitoneally into female A/Sn mice (± 10 parasites/mouse), in a total of 18 animals (9 pre- and 9 post-filtration). In addition, 2 mice were inoculated with non-contaminated whole blood.

RESULTS: All the animals that received pre-filtered blood became infected, with the onset of parasitemia occurring at day 9,33 ± 0,71, and maximum parasitemic levels at day 12,67 ± 0,50. 3/9 animals died up to day 26 post-inoculation (p.i.). Of the group that received filtered blood, 6/9 animals became infected (p= 0,20), with onset and peak of parasitemia occurring at day 11,67 ± 1,97 (p= 0,011*) and 15,50 ± 2,07 (p= 0,004*), respectively; 2/6 infected animals died up to day 26 p.i. 3/9 of the mice that received filtered blood did not become infected up to day 26 p.i.. As expected, no infection was observed in the 2 mice inoculated with non-contaminated whole blood.

CONCLUSION: These very preliminary results show that in animals challenged with a high number of parasites (as compared to chronic chagasic patients, who have approx. 0,1 to 1 parasites/ml), a certain level of protection could be achieved by blood filtration; i.e., in the group of mice inoculated with filtered blood, a delay in the onset as well as in the peak of parasitemia was observed among the mice that became infected (6/9); in addition, 3/9 of the mice did not become infected, suggesting that a lower number of parasites could be present in the post-filtration samples, opening a new horizon in the field of prevention of *T. cruzi* transmission by blood transfusion.

(*) Mann-Whitney test

0116

INTRAOPERATIVE AUTOTRANSFUSION IN UROLOGIC CANCER SURGERY BY USING MEMBRANE FILTERS

C.Güdemann; M.Wiesel; G.Staehler
Dep. for Urology, University Heidelberg; Germany

The benefit of autologous blood is the reduction of complications associated with homologous blood products. The intraoperative mechanical autotransfusion (IAT) is a technique widely employed and established in many operative disciplins. In urology, IAT did not become a routine technique yet. One reason for this may be the opinion that IAT is generally thought to be contraindicated in presence of malignancy. In experiment it was shown, that it was possible to separate cells of urological tumor cell line from salvaged blood by use of a membrane filter.[1,2] In 1992, 22 patients underwent major urologic cancer surgery at our hospital with the use of IAT. The intraoperative blood loss ranged from 200 ml to 3700 ml (mean blood loss 985 ml). Mean cell saver blood was 720 ml. The salvaged blood was not transfused but filtered using a membrane filter. Cell saver blood samples were taken before and after passing through the membrane filter and were examined for tumor cell by immunoenzymatic assay for cytoceratin 18 or prostate specific antigen. In 14 of 22 cases tumor cells were found in the unfiltered samples, but no tumor cells were found in the samples after filtration.

1 Osawa T; Nippon-Hinyokika-Gakkai-Zasshi 1992; 83(8); 1276-83
2 Miller GV: Br J Surg 1991; 78; 713-715

0117

QUALITY CONTROL OF DIFFERENT METHODS OF AUTOLOGOUS BLOOD SALVAGE IN CARDIAC SURGERY

B.H. Walpoth[1], B.N. Walpoth-Aslan[1], R. Rogulenko[1], P. Spaeth[2], U. Althaus[1]

Dept. of Thoracic and Cardiovascular Surgery[1], SRK Central Laboratories[2], University of Berne, 3010 Bern, Switzerland

Several methods of autologous blood salvage during cardiac surgery have been described.We assessed the quantitative and qualitative aspects of non-processed and processed blood at the end of cardiopulmonary bypass (CPB) namely by: Centrifugation, haemofiltration and sedimentation. The remaining CPB blood was either returned directly to the patient or processed by the 3 methods described above. Volumes, Haematocrit, Thrombocytes, Protein concentrations as well as activated clotting time (ACT) and Heparin content were measured:

	CPB Blood	Centri-fugation	Haemofil-tration	Sedimenta-tion
Volume (ml)	1383	419 *	604 *	546 *
Haematocrit (%)	21	58 *	52 *	48 *
Protein Total (g/l)	44	41	115 *	31
Thrombocytes (10^9/l)	130	165	202	52 *
ACT (sec)	678	634	713	951
Heparin (u/ml)	3,8	1,5 *	4,9	3,0
Heparin / Volume	2800	600 *	2800	1600 *

(mean values; * = p < 0,05 to unprocessed CPB blood)

Haemoconcentration, water and waste removal are significant in all three processing modalitites when compared to the blood at the end of CPB. The total amount of heparin, plasma haemoglobin and complement (C3a) retransfused to the patient calculated by volume is significantly lower in centrifuged or sedimented blood.

Processing of CBP blood is advisable in all cases when compared to the non-processed product before retransfusion to the patient. Not only due to the increase in haemotocrit and plasmaproteins but also because of removal of heparin and waste products.

0118

SURGICAL TRANSFUSION ASSISTANCE, HOMOLOGOUS AND AUTOLOGOUS : A SERVICE FROM THE BLOOD TRANSFUSION CENTRE

H. Guntzberger, A-M Ammeux, L. Noel
Centre de Transfusion des Yvelines, Centre Hospitalier de Versailles.France

To optimize surgical transfusion therapy a "transfusion assistance team" from the Blood Transfusion Centre (BTC), beside training and advising on homologous transfusion, is closely involved in routine with surgical teams (STs) through autologous transfusion (AT). The various AT technics are available to define the transfusion solution best adapted to each patients. Concurrently to pre-deposit , a service is provided in 15 hospitals or clinics to prepare washed and filtered red cell concentrates (RBC) from intra and post operative sanguineous losses. In all cases, according to agreements, the BTC supplies instruments, disposables, and monitors and runs a quality assurance program with the STs. For STs with low activity or limited experience the manipulation is carried out by the BTC team on appointements.

In 1993, 908 patients benefited of this service and received a mean 2.6 RBC equivalent units from peri-operative blood salvage. Centralised data on usage of autologous or homologous RBC for each patient can be analysed according to type of surgery, and ST.

This comprehensive involvement of the BTC in surgical transfusion, created a working relationship with STs that benefits the practice of homologous transfusion as well as optimises the use of AT technics. Future developments will aim at an improved quality assurance and clinical evaluations.

0119

INTRAOPERATIVE AUTOTRANSFUSION DURING VASCULAR SURGERY.

L.Claeys, Cl.Bartels, S. Horsch.
Dept. of Surgery, Acad. Hospital Cologne-Porz, P.O. 90 06 80, G-51116 Cologne, Germany.

We use a small, disposable set for intraoperative autotransfusion(IAT), it requires no additional equipment and enables fast retransfusion.
This system was used in 986 patients, 120 underwent venous thrombectomy, 866 aortoiliac surgery, n=275: aneurysma resection; n=591: aortic occlusive disease. We autotransfused 1180 lit. of blood and transfused 860 units of homologous blood. Only 28 pat. undergoing venous thrombectomy required an average of 2,6 units banked blood, 358 pat. undergoing aortic surgery required an average of 2,2 units banked blood. To control the quality of the blood, we studied the following parameters: Hb, Hct, platelet count, bilirubin, fibrinogen:

	preop.	IAT-set	1°D.postop	2°D.	3°D.
Hb	13,2	9,8	11,4	11,8	11,5
Hct	39,8	30,2	34,3	33,2	33,7
Plat.C.	243	98	196	221	260
Bil.	0,48	0,44	1,02	0,75	0,50
Fibr.	405	260	307	335	417

The coagulation-function tests stayed within normal or therapeutical range. There was no evidence of increased bleeding, consumption coagulopathy or renal failure. Using this set for IAT we did not have problems in handling it. Maximal Hct. decrease and platelet declination occured 24 to 36 hours postoperatively. With IAT-techniques a majority of patients can undergo surgery without homologous transfusion.

0121

INCIDENCE OF TRANSFUSION-TRANSMITTED INFECTION

T.A. Callaghan, M.T. Brennan, J.A.J. Barbara, M. Bailey, G. Century, D.R. Howell, M.C. Contreras.
North London Blood Transfusion Centre, UK.

Aims To determine the incidence of transfusion-transmitted viral disease in recipients of blood and blood components and to assess the effectiveness of current measures to minimise disease-transmission.
Methods Serum samples are collected from patients 9 months following transfusion and tested for any evidence of infection by hepatitis B and C, human immunodeficiency virus and human T-cell leukaemia virus. Where a sample tests positive, a pre-transfusion sample is also tested to differentiate pre-existing infection from seroconversion. Patients with confirmed seroconversion are recalled, counselled and questioned about other risk factors. Archived samples from the involved donations are also re-tested. If a sample is reactive, the donor is recalled and retested; if no sample is reactive, all donors are retested.
Results Follow-up of 1,077 patients, corresponding to 4,259 units of transfused blood, has been completed. No case of transfusion-transmitted disease has been identified. This is in keeping with the estimated low level of risk in the UK (1).
Conclusion The incidence of transfusion-transmitted disease in London is very low. To achieve statistically valid data, follow-up of further recipients, to correspond to a total of at least 20,000 transfused units, is planned.

1. Barbara J.A.J. Current Medical Literature: Virology 1993:2(3)67-73.

0122

NATIONAL GUIDELINES FOR DEFERRAL OF DONORS AND BLOOD PRODUCTS WITH A POSITIVE SCREENING TEST.

C.L. van der Poel[1], H.W. Reesink[1], P.N. Lelie[2], C. Dudok de Wit[3]. 1) Red Cross Blood Bank Amsterdam, 2) Central Lab RC Blood Transfusion Service, 3) Blood Transfusion Council of the NRC, Amsterdam, The Netherlands.

Objective: To develop national uniform guidelines for donors and blood products with an initially (IRST) or repeatedly reactive screening test (RRST).

Methods: A working group of representatives from blood banks, confirmatory labs and the government designed guidelines for deferral of donors and the handling of blood products with an IRST or RRST.

Results: National guidelines were accepted in March 1993: 1) All blood products with an IRST should immediately be blocked and not be used for transfusion until tests are repeated. 2) Blood products with an RRST should be discarded and future donations of donors with an RRST must be blocked automatically. 3) If confirmatory assays (Immunoblot, antigen test, PCR) show the RRST to be non-specific, the implicated donor is unblocked and future donations can be used for transfusion. 4) RRST-donors with a positive or repeatedly indeterminate confirmatory test, or donors with RRST on more occasions are notified and definitely deferred. In 1993, among 88,562 blood donations, 4/72, 4/114, 8/125, and 2/206 were found confirmed positive/RRST for HBV, HIV, HCV and HTLV respectively. Effects of the national guidelines on donors with unconfirmed RRST will be given.

Conclusion: National guidelines for donors and blood products with RRST are important to guarantee optimal safety of the blood supply.

0123

Evaluation of an enzyme immunoassay for Syphilis antibodies as a method for screening blood and plasma donations.

D H Lewis; P Berry;
Centocor Diagnostics Inc (UK Division), Mercia House, Broadford Business Park, Shalford, Guildford, Surrey, UK.

A commercially available enzyme immunoassay for Treponema pallidum IgG class antibodies (CAPTIA Syphilis-G, Centocor Inc, Diagnostics Division) was evaluated in three major United States blood/plasma centers.

A total of 9,325 partly selected donors were tested by the CAPTIA assay in comparison with the RPR test, and 6,106 of these were also tested by an automated haemagglutination procedure. Donors giving a repeatably reactive result in any test were confirmed using an FTA-Abs test. Donors were tested by CAPTIA mainly as plasma specimens, but a subset of 4,272 donors was also tested as the paired serum specimens.

The CAPTIA assay detected 99.48% of confirmed reactive donors (n=196) compared with 66.84% detected by the RPR test. The haemagglutination procedure detected 89.52% of confirmed reactive donors, (n=105). The specificities of all three tests were similar, giving reactive predictive values of: CAPTIA, 87.39% (plasma) to 100% (Serum); RPR, 83.97%-85.27%; Haemagglutination, 95.52%-96.80%. The CAPTIA and RPR assays showed consistency between initial and repeat tests. The haemagglutination procedure gave a high initial false reactivity rate. The CAPTIA assay was highly reproducible and performed well with high volume specimen-handling instrumentation.

0124

B19 PARVOVIRUS INFECTION IN BLOOD DONORS

H. Shiraki, M. Tsujimura, K. Matsushita, H. Sato, K. Okochi and Y. Maeda
Fukuoka Red Cross Blood Center, Fukuoka, Japan

Human B19 parvovirus (B19) discovered in the sera of blood donors in 1975 has been shown to be as the causative agent of erythema infectiosum and associated with rheumatoid arthritis-like disease.
In normal persons, the features of B19 infection are that the infection is usually acute, the period of viremia is short, and the appearance of virus specific antibodies follwed by brisk marrow recovery. Accordingly, current infections with B19 can be diagnosed by virus detection in blood samples. Therefore, we tested for the presence of B19 antigens and IgG/IgM antibodies in blood samples (approximately 440,000) donated at the Fukuoka Blood Center from June in 1991 to December in 1993, by using counter-immunoelectrophoresis or ouchterlony method. The confirmation of test results was performed with a DNA bybridization for B19 antigens and captured-ELISA for B19 specific antibodies. In this seroepidemiological study, 1)we detected the B19 antigens in sera from 15 blood donors in this period, 2)the detection of B19 antigens in blood samples was concentrated in the period between February in 1992 and January in 1993 (5 in Feb.-Apr., 4 in May-Jul., 3 in Aug.-Oct. and 3 in Nov.-Jan.), 3)this period (Feb. in 1992-Jan. in 1993) was coincident with the prevalence period of erythema infectiosum in the area at the Fukuoka Blood Center. These observations suggest that the donor screening of B19 antigens in the prevalence period of erythema infectiosum is effective for prevention of B19 infection by blood products.

0126

CHIMERISM AFTER BLOOD TRANSFUSION, PCR APPLIED AS DETECTION TECHNIQUE

J.G.A. Houbiers, C. Nieuwenhuys, A. Brand
Dept. of Immunohaematology & Blood Bank, University Hospital Leiden, the Netherlands

Blood transfusion (BT) modulates the immune system. The mechanism of their immunosuppressive effects has not been elucidated, although transfusion of leukocytes seem crucial. In animal models tolerance for the alloantigens of the transfused blood is associated with persisting donor cells: chimerism. To investigate whether donor leukocyte chimerism is established after BT we have chosen the polymerase chain reaction (PCR). Discrimination between donor and recipient is only feasible in case of DNA amplification of polymorphic genes. The second exon of the ß-chain of HLA-DR is very polymorphic, whereas genes on the Y-chromosome are unique to males. In dilution experiments of male (DR4/DR7) in female blood we could detect 1 male (and DR7 and DR4) cell in 500.000 female (or non DR7/4) cells. Southern blotting and dot blotting confirmed the specificity of the amplified DNA.

Preliminary results in 5 female patients show disappearance of transfused male leukocytes from peripheral blood below detection levels in 4 to 6 days. Samples, 7 to 12 days and three months after BT, contained no detectable Y-chromosome DNA. Samples, taken every 2 hr showed quick disappearance of donor cells from peripheral blood: after 3 hr less than 1:10,000.

0127

LOW MONONUCLEAR CELL CONTENT IN STORED, BUFFY COAT-DEPLETED SAGM-SUSPENDED RED CELLS

F. Knutson, C.F. Högman
Department of Clinical Immunology and Transfusion Medicine, University Hospital, Uppsala, Sweden

Leucocyte depletion of red cells to <5 x 10^6 leucocytes per transfusion reduces considerably the risk of HLA immunization. However, in some reports the incidence of immunization has been low even with less effective leucodepletion than filtration. A possible reason could be that the number of the most immunogenic, mononuclear cells is strongly reduced already by the removal of buffy coat and that storage may cause further reduction. Using flow cytometry (Ortho Cytoron) and monoclonal antibodies we have studied the content of CD3, CD14, CD19, and CD45 positive cells in buffy coat-depleted, SAGM suspended red cells (Opti System, Baxter). Buffy coat-removal resulted in the following reduction of cell contents: CD3: 93%, CD19: 88%, CD14: 99.3%. Most of the remaining cells were CD45 positive. After ≥7 days no cells showing any of these markers could be detected (<1 x 10^6/l). The whole content of a unit of 10-day stored red cells was concentrated approximately 100-fold using a Ficoll-hypaque technique, but still with negative result. Thus, all white cells remaining in stored red cell units were granulocytes.

We conclude that <10^6 intact mononuclear cells remain in ≥7-day stored SAGM red cells, when initially leucoreduced with the Opti System method of buffy coat-removal.

0128

ULTRAVIOLET-B (UVB) LIGHT ALTERS T-CELL EXPRESSION OF ICAM-1 AND CD 28. Mosunjac M, Lackey DA, Hillyer CD. Department of Pathology, Emory University, Atlanta, GA, USA.

UVB light can alter the in vitro immune responsiveness of T-cells and has been used to decrease both HLA-alloimmunization and graft versus host disease (GVHD). We studied the effect of UVB light on cellular adhesion molecule expression by T-cell enriched peripheral blood stem cell (PBSC) products using 10 mJ/cm^2, a dose that allows CFU-GM growth. PBSC were obtained from 5 normal donors; antigen presenting cells (APC) were isolated by plastic adherence, and T-cells (CD3+) by magnetic bead separation (purity>98.5%). Following irradiation (2x10^6 cells/mL; 10 mJ/cm^2; 302 nm; 0.3 mW/cm^2), T-cells were cultured in RPMI, 0.2% PHA and 10% FCS (37°C) with APC (5 T-cells : 1 APC; irradiated and unirradiated) for 48h and proliferation determined by ^{3}H-thymidine uptake. UVB irradiated T-cells had a near 95% reduction in thymidine uptake while UVB irradiated APC supported the proliferation of unirradiated T-cells as shown below (* p<0.05):

	T+APC	T+APC^{UVB}	T^{UVB}+APC
% control	100%	79±13.87*	5.84±2.2*

ICAM-1, LFA-1, 2, and CD28 were analyzed by FACS at 0, 24, 48 and 72h post irradiation of enriched T-cells (ICAM-1 required coincubation with 0.2% PHA). There was no change in LFA-1 or 2 in either irradiated or unirradiated cells. There was significant downregulation of ICAM after 72h, and of CD28 expression after 48h (mean channel fluorescence ± sd; *p<0.05):

	0 mJ/cm^2	10 mJ/cm^2
ICAM-1	429±76	308±73*
CD28	513±91	383±20*

Downregulation of ICAM-1 and CD28 may be an important mechanism by which UVB alters T-cell activation and abrogates the T-cell response to PHA, and could be used to immunomodulate contaminating T-cells in allogeneic PBSC to abrogate GVHD.

0129

CYTOKINE PROFILES OF STORED CPDA-1 WHOLE BLOOD

A. Zielonki, R. Grunenberg, M. Becker, J. Krüger
Institute of Transfusion Medicine, University of Cologne, D-50924 Cologne, Germany

Many sequential changes of blood constituents have been documented during storage. For instance the number of leucocytes was found to decrease steadily from (5±1)x10^3 to (3±1)x10^3 cells/µl (M±SD) over a period of 28 days. All of the leucocytic cells degenerate with storage time releasing an increasing amount of antigenic material and immunomodulatory factors. These may cause transfusion reactions. Therefore over a storage period of 35 days cytokine concentration of whole blood units were examined. Plasma samples were collected at weekly intervals and the levels of IL-1β, TNF-α, TNF-β, GM-CSF and IL-6 were determined by ELISA techniques (HB, R&D Systems). IL-1β, TNF-α and TNF-β increased from 1.3, 1.2 respectively 2.7 pg/ml to peak levels after 5 weeks of 5.2, 3.0 and 25.0 pg/ml plasma. Il-6 and GM-CSF were below the sensitivity of the tests at day of collection and peaked after 1 week of storage with 1.1 respectively 3.0 pg/ml. After 5 weeks the levels had decreased beyond detection.

These data indicate that at any time of storage ILs are released and that they may reach biologically significant plasma concentrations. Therefore cytokine mediated transfusion reactions may also be abolished by prestorage leucoreduction.

0130

ANALYSIS OF MUTATIONS IN THE BLOOD-GROUP H GENE IN DONORS WITH H-DEFICIENT PHENOTYPES

P.H. Johnson[1], M.K. Mak[2], S. Leong[2], R. Broadberry[3], G. Duraisamy[4], A. Gooch[5], M. Lin-Chu[3], Y. Makar[5], Y. Okubo[6], E. Smart[7], E. Koepsall[8], M. Ewers[9].

[1]M.R.C. Blood Group Unit, London, UK; [2]R.C.B.T.S., Hong Kong; [3]Mackay Memorial Hospital, Taipei, R.O.C; [4]Pusat Perkhidmatan Darah, Kuala Lumpur, Malaysia; [5]N.B.T.S., Lancaster, UK; [6]Osaka R.C.B.T.S, Japan; [7]Natal B.T.S., Durban, SA; [8]Blutspendedienst Hessen, Frankfurt, Germany; [9]Inst. Transfusionsmedizin, Aachen, Germany.

The single coding exon of the H gene (Larson *et al.* PNAS 1990;87:6674) was analysed for mutations by denaturing gradient gel electrophoresis, single stranded conformational analysis and direct sequencing of four overlapping PCR products. Only a single synonymous base change (Thr^{274}) was detected in over of 200 donors of normal ABH phenotypes. In contrast, 9 different coding mutations were detected in approximately 60 H-deficient secretors and non-secretors and their immediate families. Mutations were found throughout the exon, the majority concentrated in the 3'domains. They comprise base substitutions (eg Trp^{267}→Cys, Asp^{278}→Asn) and one and two base deletions (TTT→T, codon 294; CTG→CT, codon 330). The only group in which no coding mutations were detected are the classical Bombays of Indian origin.

The products of these alleles most likely represent a series of independent mutational events that give rise to the range of H-deficient phenotypes observed by serologists. The results provide further evidence in favour of the two homologous genes hypothesis for H and Se (Oriol *et al.* Am J Hum Genet 1981;33:421).

0131

THE FREQUENCY OF A NEW 0 ALLELE, NAMED 0^B DEFINED BY ABO GENOTYPING IN A DANISH POPULATION

N. Grunnet[1], R. Steffensen[1], E. Bennett[2], and H. Clausen[2]
1Regional Center for Blood Transfusion and Clinical Immunology, Aalborg Hospital, DK-9100 Aalborg, Denmark, 2School of Dentistry, University of Copenhagen, DK-2200 Copenhagen N, Denmark.

Traditional blood group AB0 serology is based on immunoreactivity with the carbohydrate determinants A, B, and H antigens. Recent advances at the DNA level of the AB0 genes have provided a molecular genetic model for the AB0 polymorphism. This genetic model has to-date only been tested on a limited basis. The present study was initiated to evaluate the universality of the proposed genetic model on a larger group of serologically defined AB0 phenotypes. 300 healthy Danish blood donors were analysed (A: 50, B: 50, AB: 50, 0: 150) by PCR amplification followed by diagnostic restriction enzyme cutting. In all cases of A, B, and AB at least one allele of correctly predicted status was found. However, in 0 phenotype individuals, 11 out of 150 carried one allele discordant to the proposed genetic model. This novel 0 allele (7.3% allele frequency) was further characterized by diagnostic restriction enzyme analysis in two positions divergent between A and B alleles (all 11) and by DNA sequencing of the two major exons (6 cases). This novel 0 allele is termed 0^B as it typed as B in nucleotide position 526, and as A in positions 703, 796, and 803, in contrast to the most predominant 0 allele termed 0^A, which types as A in all 4 positions. The structural defect in the 0^B allele appears to be an additional substitution at nucleotide position 802.

The results clearly demonstrate that with the addition of the two distinctly different 0 alleles, 0^A, 0^B, the previously proposed molecular genetic basis of the AB0 polymorphism is quite valid. More important the determined characteristics of these two 0 alleles have practical implications in AB0 genotyping, because it establishes within the limits of the number of samples tested that AB0 genotypes can be assessed directly by non-allele specific PCR amplification and restriction enzyme analysis.

0132

THE IMPORTANCE OF THE CHIDO/RODGERS BLOOD GROUP IN XENOTRANSPLANTATION FROM NONHUMAN PRIMATES J.M. Moulds[1], D.L. Merritt[2]. [1]Univ Texas Medical School, Gulf Coast Regional Blood Center, Houston, TX, USA

Due to the shortage of human organs, xenotranspl anatation is again being investigated as a viable option, eg. transplantation of a baboon liver to a human. Because the liver is critical for the production of the fourth component of complement (C4), we investigated whether the C4-related blood group antigens (Ch/Rg) were similar between primates and humans. Our studies included: plasma C4 allotyping by agarose gel electrophoresis immunofixation, immunoblotting utilizing monoclonal Ch1 and Rg1, plasma inhibition of human polyclonal anti-Ch or -Rg, C4 quantitation by radial immunodiffusion (RID) and Southern blot analysis of the C4 genes using Nla IV and a C4d specific probe. A total of 11 baboons, 5 chimpanzees, 5 cynomolgus, 1 rhesus and 2 African green monkeys were investigated. All animals had C4 levels comparable to man but only the chimps exhibited distinct C4 bands on allotyping. The chimp C4 was shown by immunoblotting to carry the Ch1 epitope but not Rg1. However, the chimp plasma completely inhibited both anti-Ch and -Rg from a human source. Although all the primates had plasma C4, none other than the chimps inhibited the human anti-Ch or -Rg suggesting that most differ antigenically from man. Since the Ch and Rg antigens lay in the thioester bond site of C4, these antigenic differences may relate to functional differences and thus influence the efficacy of liver xenotransplantation.

0133

MOLECULAR CLONING AND TERTIARY STRUCTURE OF THE LW BLOOD GROUP GLYCOPROTEIN

P. Bailly[1], P. Hermand[1], I. Callebaut[2], H.H. Sonneborn[3], J-P. Mornon[2], J-P. Cartron[1]
1INTS and INSERM U76, 6 rue Al. Cabanel, Paris, France, 2CNRS URA09, UP6/UP7, 4 Pl. Jussieu Paris, France, 3Biotest AG Reseach Dep, Offenbach, F.R.G.

The LW blood group antigens reside on a 42-kDa erythrocyte membrane glycoprotein which was purified by immunoaffinity and partially sequenced. From these limited structural informations, a specific PCR-amplified DNA fragment was generated and used to screen a λgt11 human bone marrow cDNA library. Two forms of cDNA were isolated, the first encoded a single spanning transmembrane protein of 270 amino-acids including a 29 amino acids peptide signal and 4 potential N-glycosylation sites, the second encoding a shortened protein form of 236 residues devoid of transmembrane and cytoplasm domains. That the protein encoded by these clones were LW gene products was deduced by raising a rabbit antibody against the 15 N-terminus amino acids of the predicted protein which reacted on immunoblots with authentic LW glycoprotein and in indirect agglutination test with all human erythrocytes except those from LW(a-b-). Most interestingly, the LW protein was found to exhibit strong sequence similarities (overall identities are within the range of 30%) with the intercellular adhesion molecules ICAM-1, -2 and -3 which are the counter-receptors for the lymphocyte function-related antigens LFA-1. The extracellular domain of LW consists, like that of ICAM-2, of two immunoglobulin-like domains and the critical residues involved in the binding of LFA-1 to ICAMs were partially conserved in LW.

0134

FUNCTIONAL ROLES FOR GLYCOPHORIN A AND BAND 3 AS TRANSMEMBRANE SIGNALING MOLECULES. J. A. Chasis[1], S. McGee[1], D. Anstee[2], and N. Mohandas[1]; [1]Lawrence Berkeley Laboratory, Berkeley, CA USA, [2]International Blood Group Reference Laboratory, Bristol, England.

Although MN antigen bearing glycophorin A (GPA) and AB antigen-bearing band 3 have been well characterized structurally, the functional roles of these major erythrocyte proteins are not fully elucidated. The capacity of transmembrane receptors to associate with the cytoskeleton in response to ligand binding appears to be a key mechanism in signal transduction. We have previously shown that binding monovalent Fab of MoAb to the exoplasmic domain of GPA rigidifies the membrane and that GPA cytoplasmic domain plays a crucial role in this mechanical signal transduction. To study the effect of ligand binding to band 3 we measured ligand induced alterations in membrane material properties by ektacytometry. Binding of MoAb BRAC 18 to the exoplasmic domain of band 3 produced a dose-dependent increase in membrane rigidity. However, a bivalent interaction was required since BRAC 18 monovalent Fab did not rigidify the membrane but addition of rabbit anti-rat IgG to these cells induced a marked increase in membrane rigidity. Biochemical analysis showed that BRAC 18 binding resulted in oligomerization of band 3. We conclude that different mechanisms operate in mechanical signal transduction through GPA and band 3. GPA-ligand acts through alterations in the cytoplasmic domain of the GPA monomer while band 3 ligand induces signal transduction through oligomerization and clustering of band 3. These data imply that the blood group antigen bearing protein of the red cell membrane can also play an important role in regulating signal transduction and mechanical properties of the membrane.

0135

NOVEL GLYCOPHORIN B IN AN INDIVIDUAL WITH THE S-s-U- PHENOTYPE
M.E. Reid[1], C-H. Huang[1], O.O. Blumenfeld[2], 1New York Blood Center, 2Albert Einstein College of Medicine, New York, NY.

Red blood cells (RBCs) from a S-s-U- blood donor were agglutinated by a monoclonal anti-He (29E9, kindly provided by Gamma Biologicals, Houston). Since S, s, U and He are all carried on glycophorin B, a blood sample was obtained for analysis of DNA and RNA. These studies identified an allelic variant of the GYPB gene. An insertion of GYPA into the GYPB gene gave rise to the sequence defining the He epitope while concomitantly abolishing GPB-associated N antigenicity. This novel gene carries two splice site mutations: G->G transversion at the 3' end of exon V and a G->T transversion at the +5 position of intron 5. This resulted in ligation of exon 4 to exon 6 and gave rise to a new elongated hydrophobic sequence for membrane anchoring. Interestingly, although the novel gene has the linear sequence of nucleotides predicted to encode S and U antigens these determinants were not demonstrable on the RBCs.

0137

COMPARATIVE ANALYSIS OF DIFFERENT METHODS OF BONE MARROW (BM) CRYOPRESERVATION

L.Fregatova, S.Chavva, G.Platonova, B.Afanasiev

Clinical Centre of Advanced Medical Technologies, Petrov's Institute of Oncology, St.-Petersburg, Russia

Cryopreservation of BM is an essential step of the autologous BM transplantation.
Methods: We performed a comparative analysis of four different methods of cryopreserva-tion of BM: **(1)** Non-controlled freezing with 10% DMSO. The samples were frozer at -80°C. **(2)** Controlled freezing, using 10% DMSO. The freezing rate was -1°C/min>-14°C,-3°C>-80°C **(3)** Non-controlled freezing, using 6% HES, 5% DMSO and 4% human albumin as cryopro-tectants. The samples were frozen at -80°C. **(4)** A modification of technique (3), using 4% autologous plasma in the cryoprotective medium. After freezing, all samples were stored in liquid nitrogen.
The viability of BM cells after thawing was evaluated by a)counting vital trypan blue excluding cells and b)assaying the number of colony forming cells (CFU-GM, CFU-G, BFU-E).
Results: 1)The rate of vital cells was between 85%-92% with all four techniques. 2)There were no significant differences between techniques (2),(3) and (4) in the recovery of CFC, whereas uncontrolled freezing with 10% DMSO yielded unacceptable low of CFC.
Concluding from these results, we decided to use the technique (4) for routine freezing, as if it combines a low concentration of DMSO with cost effectiveness.

0138

CLONAL EXCESS DETERMINATION BY FLOW CYTOMETRY: AN INDICATOR FOR B CELL PURGING

A. Giulivi[1], P. Birch[1], V. Fuller[1], L.B. Huebsch[2]
[1]Canadian Red Cross Society, Ottawa, Ontario, Canada
[2]Hematology, University of Ottawa, Ontario, Canada

Clonal excess determination using flow cytometry is a rapid technique which can be used as an indicator for B cell purging and detecting minimal disease in the peripheral blood stem cell (PBSC) collections. In the Ottawa Regional Autologous Bone Marrow Trans-plant Program approximately 80% of our candidates are monoclonal B cell lymphomas. Flow cytometry provides a quantitative estimate of the B cell clonality using kappa/lambda (K/L) analysis and D value determination indicating the proportion of abnormal cells and disease status at the time of collection. The D value measures the channel differences in kappa and lambda light chain profiles and expresses this as a per-centage of the total number of cells. The K/L ratio and D values were determined on normal peripheral blood and PBSCs collected from 17 lymphoma patients. Each patient had recieved chemotherapy and daily G-CSF infusions for 9 days, with PBSC collections on days 8, 9, and 10. Normal peripheral blood kappa and lambda curves were superimposable with a D value of 3.7±1.8 and K/L ratio of 0.98±0.14. Of the 17 patients 13 demonstrated normal K/L ratios of 1.2±0.7 and D values of 2.4±1.8. Three of the patients exhibited abnormal D values averaging 19.1±13.7, but only one had an abnormal K/L ratio, indicating the ratio is a poor marker of clonal excess. Currently the patients with abnormal K/L ratios and D values are rejected from the transplant program, and their cells dis-carded. This exclusion could be avoided with a rapid determination of the D value then abnormal units could undergo purging of the contaminating malignant cells.

0139

COMPARISON OF SHORT TERM STORAGE PROCEDURES FOR UMBILICAL CORD BLOOD STEM CELLS (CBSC). A. Winkelstein[2], W.B. Rybka[1], P.J. Hamilton[3], R. Roscoe[2], E. Curry Johnson[3], R.A. Dracker[3], E.D. Ball[1]. 1Div. Hematol/BMT, University of Pittsburgh, 2Central Blood Bank, Pittsburgh, PA, and 3Biocyte Corp., Stamford CT, USA.

CBSC are a rich source of cells capable of reconstituting bone marrows after myeloblation. In the present study, different storage conditions were evaluated on the short term survival of CBSC. Cell survival at 22°C was assessed in ACD (15 ml/100 ml) and heparin (27 U/ml) anticoagulated specimens and in ACD specimens at 4°C and 22°C. Total mononuclear cell numbers (MNC), cell viability, CD34 cell numbers and colony formation were measured at 3, 24, 48, and 72 hours. The mean volume and total numbers of MNC collected at the time of delivery were 108 ml and 7.0 x 10^8 respectively. MNC remained comparatively stable throughout the 3 day incubation period in both anticoagulants. Total cell viability was better preserved in heparin. CD34+ cell numbers and total colonies did not significantly vary throughout the incubation. Likewise, indices from specimens held at 4°C did not significantly differ from those held at 22°C. These studies indicate that CBSC can be stored for 72 hours without appreciable stem cell loss indicating the feasibility of establishing "CBSC banks".

0140

COLLECTION AND CRYOPRESERVATION OF CORD BLOOD: A PILOT STUDY. A Shannon[1], C Bharucha[1], B Devine[2] and P Weir[2]. Northern Ireland Blood Transfusion Service[1] and Mater Infirmorium Hospital[2], Belfast, N.Ireland

Cord blood (CB) has been used successfully as a source of haemopoietic stem cells for transplantation in several patients. There is increasing interest in establishing banks of cryopreserved CB for allogenic use and has led to the formation of the European Cord Blood Bank Project. This study reports the practical aspects of collection by a team of midwives in a teaching hospital, transportation to the Regional Transfusion Centre (RTC) and cryopreservation. Midwives were trained in CB collection, a total of 70 procedures were analysed. Cryopreservation was performed using a standard controlled rate freezing programme currently used for stem cell storage. The cell counts were repeated after thawing at 40°C.

Mean volume collected was 73 ml (range 30-155), mean total nucleated cells 8.2 x 10^8 (1.8-33.0) and mean total mononuclear cells 4.1 x 10^8 (1.6-8.6).

Despite enthusiasm for the concept of establishing CB banks, no criteria have been agreed regarding appropriate material for transplantation or indeed patient eligibility for unrelated CB transplant. In the UK, RTC's have established standard operating procedures for National Bone Marrow Donor Registry and this study shows that it is feasible for an RTC to establish a CB bank. However, the resource implications are considerable and some form of centralisation is appropriate.

0142

AN EVALUATION OF RECOMBINANT HUMAN ERYTHROPOIETIN (rEPO) IN PREDEPOSIT AUTOLOGOUS BLOOD DONATION: A MULTI-INSTITUTIONAL DOUBLE BLIND STUDY.

S.Tachibana, K.Takahashi[1], S.Asano[2], S.Minami[3], Y.Shibata[4], N.Wakimoto[5], Y.Ikeda[6], H.Tsutsui[7]
1) Toranomon Hosp., 2) Hokkaido Univ., 3) Chiba Univ., 4) Tokyo Univ., 5) Teikyo Univ., 6) Keio Univ., 7) Kyusyu Univ., Tokyo, Japan.

Of 94 orthopaedic donor-patients in 22 different institutions in Japan, 78 were evaluated as a double blind study to determine the efficacy of once a week subcutaneous(SC) rEPO(KRN5702) administration for blood collection of total 1,200ml within three weeks.

The 78 patients were randomly allocated to two groups; K(40) receiving 24,000 IU of rEPO, and P(38) receiving only a placebo once a week for four weeks pre-operatively. Blood collection of 400 ml/week for three weeks began one week after a preparatory rEPO or placebo administration.

Homologous blood transfusion(HBT) was required in only 2.7% of the K group, while it was needed in 25.9% of the P group ($p<0.01$). At one week after the third phlebotomy, Hb level was not significantly decreased in the K group compared to the start of the study (12.3±0.6 to 12.0±1.3 g/dl), while it was decreased in the P group (12.5±0.6 to 10.4±0.8 g/dl). In the K group, 77.5% could donate 1,200 ml of blood within three weeks without Hb dropping below 11 g/dl, while only 10.5% of the P group could do so ($p=0.0001$).

Our results clearly indicated that a once a week SC administration of rEPO at a dose of 24,000 IU could improve post-phlebotomy anemia, and minimize HBT in elective orthopaedic surgery.

0143

RELATING AUTOLOGOUS DONATION TO TIMING AND CONTENT OF PATIENT TRANSFUSION EDUCATION.

MA Spivey, CJ Lancaster, CM Macchia, DA VandeMerwe, EK Jeter. Medical University of SC, Charleston, SC, USA.

In order to increase preoperative autologous donation, we conducted a randomized questionnaire survey of 200 post-op patients to assess timing and content of patient transfusion education. External education involved referring physicians and the news media. Only 22% reported receiving transfusion information at the doctor's office compared to 61% on the TV news. Internal education consisted of the informed consent process and a newly developed "Patient's Guide to Blood Transfusions" brochure. While 69% reported their surgeon discussed blood pre-op, only 30% indicated that alternatives were discussed. However, 78% of patients were aware of the alternatives. Only 14% recalled seeing the brochure which was available in the clinics. No more than 34% had $\geq$ 3 weeks advance notice of surgery to accommodate multiple autologous collections. Of these 34%, 38% had received information from their physician on alternatives. Of the 200 patients 5% donated blood autologously and 70% of these had discussed alternatives more than 3 weeks before surgery. We believe that verbal transfusion education in our locality is frequently too late and incomplete to allow for adequate pre-op autologous donation, and educational brochures are largely ignored without reinforcement. Our plans include distribution of brochures to referring physicians' offices with the recommendation that the brochure contents are briefly discussed with each pre-op patient.

0144

PREDONATION OF AUTOLOGOUS BLOOD, PLASMA AND PLATELETS IN OPEN-HEART SURGERY

J. Charvát[1], B. Nývltová[1], M. Rozehnalová[1], O. Nývlt[1], B. Charvátová[2]
1Institute for Clinical and Experimental Medicine, Prague, 2Faculty Transfusion Department, Prague, Czech Republic.

To reduce the need for homologous blood transfusion, 34 patients predonated 2 T.U. of blood and, using apheresis, an average 940 ml of FFP within 3-4 weeks before elective open-heart surgery. Twenty-one of these patients predonated platelets ($3.5 \pm 0.6 \times 10^{11}$) and 420 ml of FFP using Haemonetics PCS plus. There were no differences between the groups of 13 and 21 patients in age (53 and 55 years), sex and time of extracorporeal circulation (86 ± 20 and 73 ± 18 min, respectively). We observed no ischemic events, no circulation disorders or arrhythmia.

The blood loss in group A (13 patients without autologous platelets) was 982 ± 589 ml during the first 24 hours and 1129 ± 787 ml altogether. The patients received 1.9 ± 1.5 T.U. of homologous RBCs and 5.0 ± 2.9 T.U. of homologous FFP. Three patients (23%) required no homologous RBCs (criterion for transfusion was Hb < 10 g/dl).

The blood loss in group B (21 patients with autologous platelets) was 581 ± 201 ml during the first 24 hours and 635 ± 220 ml altogether. The patients received 0.9 ± 1.3. T.U. of homologous RBCs and 2.2 ± 2.1 T.U. of homologous FFP. Eleven patients (52%) needed no homologous RBCs. The two groups statistically differed in all the above parameters.

0145

AN AUTOLOGOUS BLOOD TRANSFUSION STRATEGY IN NEUROSURGERY : PREOPERATIVE ERYTHROCYTAPHERESIS

J.L. Beaumont[1], F. Kalfon [2], J.J. Fournel[1], P. Viars[2]
1- Transfusion Center, 2- Dept. of Anesthesiology , Hôpital Pitié-Salpêtrière, 75651 Paris Cédex 13 - France

The risk of transfusion-related viral infections promotes techniques intended to reduce such a risk. Preoperative erythrocytapheresis is an autologous blood collection technique which minimizes the inconvenients of repeated predeposit autologous donations. We considered to enrollement 33 patients who underwent neurosurgery with an estimation of blood loss of more than 800 cc. Erythrocytapheresis has been performed in the blood bank one day before surgery using a discontinue flow cell separator (PCS+ Haemonetics®). Patients who presented with anemia, unstable cardiovascular condition, bacterial infections and unsuitable peripherial venous state were excluded. The mean (± SD) collected red cells volume was 526 (±176) ml. The mean total blood loss was 1040 (± 52) ml. Homologous blood transfusion was avoided in 29 patients (87.9 %), 4 patients who underwent surgery for meningioma have received homologous red cells units in addition to their autologous blood. Preoperative erythrocytapheresis is a simple and well tolerated procedure. It can be proposed to withstand transfusion needs in case of programed neurosurgery when the delay before surgery is short and the anticipated blood loss is moderate. It reduces the risk of receiving homologous blood. Erythrocytapheresis participates in a global autologous blood transfusion strategy.

0149

NANOFILTRATION OF SD-TREATED FACTOR IX AND FACTOR XI CONCENTRATES : VIRAL VALIDATION AND PROPERTIES

M. Burnouf-Radosevich, P. Appourchaux, J.J. Huart, T. Burnouf

Centre Régional de Transfusion Sanguine, Lille, France

We have evaluated two new nanofiltration membranes, BMM Planova 15N and 35 N, with respective mean pore size of 15 and 35 nm, to eliminate viruses in CRTS-Lille highly purified, SD-treated factor IX and factor XI concentrates. Virus spiking experiments indicated that single dead-end nanofiltration on both membranes removed high challenging doses of enveloped viruses [human immunodeficiency virus (> 7.3 log), bovine viral diarrhoea virus (> 5.7 log), porcine pseudorabies virus (> 6.4 log)] as well as non-enveloped viruses, [reovirus type 3 (> 6.1 log), simian virus 40 (> 7.0 log), and bovine parvovirus (> 5.8 log)] in both concentrates. In addition, the 15 nm-membrane could remove poliovirus Sabin 1 (> 6.7 log), a small non-enveloped virus. In vitro tests and animal studies of the nanofiltered concentrates did not reveal any significant differences as compared to the non-nanofiltered material. Nanofiltration, which allows generic removal of viruses on the basis of their size, is a potential breakthrough for the improvement of the viral safety of plasma derivatives and, at least for these factor IX and factor XI concentrates, did not have an impact on the recovery and characteristics of the end-products.

0150

CLINICAL STUDIES WITH S/D PLASMA IN PATIENTS WITH TTP. J.Pehta, P.Sellers, M.S.Horowitz, New York Blood Center, NY, U.S., and The S/D Plasma Study Group.

We have evaluated the use of solvent detergent-treated (S/D) plasma in patients with both acute and chronic thrombotic thrombocytopenic purpura (TTP). Four patients with chronic TTP received monthly infusions of 1-3 units of S/D plasma or fresh frozen plasma (FFP) over a six month period. One additional patient with chronic TTP required weekly plasma exchange rather than infusion. The response to S/D plasma was compared to that of FFP by evaluating the rise in platelet count and length of remission after treatment. There were 28 infusions of S/D plasma. In two patients, who each received 3 infusions of S/D plasma, therapy was alternated with FFP. The remaining three patients received only S/D plasma (10 infusions and 12 exchanges), and these data were compared to each patient's prior response to FFP. Our results showed no clinical difference between infusion with FFP or S/D plasma:

mean	S/D plasma	FFP
platelet count (increase)	95,000	140,000
length of remission (days)	23	21.5

There were no adverse effects of infusion with S/D plasma or decrease in effectiveness over time. Thirteen acute TTP patients have also been treated with S/D plasma. Preliminary data show equal effectiveness of S/D plasma in reversing the clinical and hematologic abnormalities in these cases. Thus, S/D plasma appears as effective as FFP in the treatment of patients with TTP.

0151

DOUBLE VIRUS INACTIVATION OF FACTOR VIII CONCENTRATE (Octavi SDPlus) BY A COMBINED SD TREATMENT AND MODIFIED PASTEURIZATION

L. Biesert[1], S. Lemon[2], H. Suhartono[1], L. Wang[1], H.D. Brede[1], H. Rübsamen-Waigmann[1]

1Georg-Speyer-Haus, Frankfurt/Main, Germany,
2The University of North Carolina at Chapel Hill, USA

The inactivation of both transfusion-relevant viruses and a large number of model viruses by a heat step introduced into the manufacture of Octavi, a very high purity FVIII concentrate, has been studied following established EU-guidelines. In-process samples of Octavi obtained after the first virus inactivation step with solvent/detergent were stabilised, heated to 63°C in solution and then spiked with virus-containing cell culture supernatant. Samples taken at different times in order to obtain inactivation kinetics were titred on susceptible cells.

Virus	Genome	Envelope	RF*	Time
HIV-1	RNA	yes	≥9.0	<240 min
HSV-1	DNA	yes	≥5.7	<240 min
PRV	DNA	yes	≥5.3	<120 min
HAV	RNA	no	≥5.6	≤480 min
Polio-1	RNA	no	≥7.5	≤480 min

* RF: reduction factor

The inactivation kinetics demonstrated the presence of virus subpopulations of different heat sensitivity. The combination of SD treatment and a heating step performed under more stringent conditions than conventional pasteurization (63°C, 10 h) leads to a factor VIII preparation (Octavi SDPlus) with a higher safety standard than monoinactivated products.

0152

ENHANCEMENT IN THE USE OF UVC FOR TREATMENT OF BLOOD DERIVATIVES BY QUENCHERS, Sing Chin, Bolanle Williams, Paul Gottlieb, John Hamman, Bernard Horowitz, New York Blood Center, New York, NY, USA

The use of solvent/detergent mixtures and various forms of heat treatment to inactivate viruses has become widespread in the preparation of blood derivatives. Because viruses which lack lipid envelopes and/or are heat resistant {e.g., hepatitis A virus (HAV) or parvovirus} may be present, the use of two methods of virus inactivation/removal that operate by different mechanisms has been advocated. We now report on UVC irradiation for virus inactivation and the enhancement of its compatibility with proteins by quenchers. Treatment of an AHF concentrate or whole plasma with 0.1 J/cm^2 UVC resulted in the inactivation of 10^6 infectious doses (ID) of the bacteriophage M13; however, factor VIII recovery was 30% and 60%, respectively. Factor VIII recovery could be increased to ≥80% by inclusion of 200 μM of the flavonoid quercetin and 750 μM ascorbate, without affecting M13 kill. Similar results were obtained when 1.6 mM rutin was used alone. Flavonoids were selected because of their known reactivity with various radicals and active oxygen species. Treatment also results in the inactivation of $\geq 10^{7.7}$ ID of encephalomyocarditis virus, $\geq 10^{6.5}$ ID of vesicular stomatitis virus, $\geq 10^{3.0}$ ID of adenoassociated virus, and $\geq 10^{4.4}$ ID of HAV. In treatment of plasma, the recovery of other coagulation factors (I, V, VII, IX, and XI) typically was between 80 and 90%. We conclude that addition of UVC treatment to existing processes in the manufacture of blood derivatives would provide an added margin of safety, especially for non-enveloped or heat-stable viruses.

0153

HIV-1 RNA detection by NASBA; a new tool for detection of HIV-1 infection.

H.T. Cuypers[1], W. Kok[2], H.W. Reesink[1,3], H. Foolen[2], J.H. ten Veen[3], P.N. Lelie[1], and H.J. Zaaijer[1].
1. Central Laboratory of the Blood Transfusion Service, Amsterdam; 2. Organon-Teknika, Boxtel, the Netherlands; 3. Prinsengracht Hospital, Amsterdam.

Introduction. NASBA is a primer-dependent technology, that can be used for the continuous amplification of RNA in a single mixture at one temperature.
Aim. We studied presence of HIV-1 RNA in plasma from individuals in various stages of HIV-1 infection and in plasma from uninfected volunteer donors, using the experimental NASBA assay from Organon-Teknika.
Methods. The following panels were analyzed: A. 70 samples from 58 different HIV-1 infected individuals as confirmed by Western-blot assay and PCR-positivity for HIV-DNA in mononuclear cells. B. 29 samples from different volunteer blood donors, tested negative for anti-HIV-1/2 by third generation anti-HIV ELISA. We tested all samples in panel A and B in the experimental assay following the instructions of the manufacturer. Each sample was tested in duplicate in 2 different runs. Samples with inconsistent duplicate test results were repeated in duplicate.
Results. All 70 HIV-1 infected samples (100 %) in panel A tested positive for HIV-1 RNA in the NASBA, irrespective of the stage of HIV-1 infection; presence of HIV-1 p24 antigen and number of lymphocytes and leucocytes. In panel B initially 5 uninfected donor samples tested indeterminate (weak positive and negative). These 5 samples were negative in repeat testing.
Conclusion. The experimental NASBA assay detected HIV-1 RNA in the plasma of all HIV-1 positive individuals. This indicates that detection of HIV-1 RNA in plasma, using the sensitive NASBA concept, has the potential to be used as confirmatory-assay, irrespectively of stage of HIV infection.

0154

DETECTION OF HIV p24 ANTIGEN AND PLASMA RNA CAN IDENTIFY TRUE HIV-1 INFECTION AMONG EIA-REACTIVE/SEROINDETERMINATE SPECIMENS.

Denis R. Henrard, Jack Phillips, Bruce H. Phelps, Susan L. Stramer*, S. Swanda, and Ronald O. Gilcher*. Abbott Laboratories, N. Chicago, IL, * OBI, Oklahoma City, OK.

Methods: Two types of specimens reactive by HIV-1/HIV-2 rDNA EIA but indeterminate by Western blot (WB) were analyzed. One group consisted of 41 "true" EIA reactive samples obtained from 27 seroconverting individuals, and the other of 341 "false" EIA reactive blood donations. Samples were tested by p24 antigen (p24) EIA followed by neutralization, and for HIV-1 RNA by immunocapture-cDNA/PCR. Reactivity to p24 and gp41 or gp120/160 on FDA licensed Western blot was classified as positive.
Results: Among seroconverters, EIA+/WB- preceeded EIA+/WB indeterminate patterns, which lasted on average for 5.4 days and 8.5 days, respectively. All 13 EIA+/WB- samples were positive by p24 EIA. Fifteen of 28 (53%) EIA+/WB indeterminate samples were positive by p24 EIA. Eight of the 13 antigen negative samples and 6 of the 15 antigen positive samples were tested for plasma RNA; all (100%) were positive. Among blood donors, in contrast, of 233 EIA+/WB- and 108 EIA+/WB indeterminate samples, none were positive by p24 EIA.
Conclusion: p24 antigen can be useful to identify HIV infection among EIA reactive/WB negative specimens.

0155

CLINICAL HIV MONITORING USING QUANTITATIVE NUCLEIC ACID ANALYSES

S.M. Bruisten[1], M. Koppelman[1], M.C. Hermus[1], N. Cool[1], B. van Gemen[2], J. Frissen[3] and J.G. Huisman[1]
1. Central Laboratory of the Netherlands Red Cross Blood Transfusion Service, Amsterdam 2. Organon Teknika, Boxtel 3. Onze Lieve Vrouwe Gasthuis, Dept.Internal Medicine, Amsterdam, The Netherlands.

We developed competative polymerase chain reaction (cPCR) to measure the HIV-1 proviral load in peripheral blood mononuclear cells and the HIV-1 viral load in plasma. The reliability of the assay was compared to Q-NASBA™ (quanatitative Nucleic Acid Sequence Based Amplification, Organon Teknika) an isothermal amplification process for HIV-1 RNA in plasma and to the branched DNA test (bDNA-Chiron). In this test RNA is not amplified, but the detection probe is extensively branched which results in increased sensitivity. All three quantitation procedures were applied on plasma samples of a patient who experienced a primary HIV-1 infection. Blood samples were tested daily from one week before to one week after seroconversion. All three tests detected high levels of HIV-RNA from day -7 to +9. Peak levels were found at days -3 and -4. The absolute levels differed threefold: $3x10^7$, $1x10^7$ and $3x10^8$ RNA copies/ml plasma for respectively NASBA™, cPCR and bDNA. HIV-p24 antigen was detected from days -7 to day 0. Comparison of the three tests on longitudinal plasma samples (every 8 weeks) of asymptomatic HIV-1 infected individuals indicated the superior sensitivity of cPCR and NASBA™. Many subjects had RNA levels below cut off with bDNA ($<10^4$ RNA copies/ml). The absolute NASBA™ RNA levels were 0.5-1.0 log higher than cPCR ($2x10^3$ to $2x10^5$ RNA copies/ml). The viral burden results will be evaluated in perspective to the available clinical and immunological data to assess its usefulness as a direct parameter for primary infection and for disease progression.

0156

RISK OF HIV TRANSMISSION BY TRANSFUSION OF BLOOD COLLECTED FROM VERY RECENTLY INFECTED DONORS.

A.M. COUROUCE[1], J. PILLONEL[2] and the Retrovirus Study group of the French Soc. of Blood Transfusion.
1 INTS Paris, 2 R. N. Santé Publique Paris FRANCE.

The risk of post-transfusion HIV infection associated with the window period was estimated as follows from the data of the blood centers involved in the Retrovirus Study Group : One fourth of the anti-HIV negative donations collected in the past 12 months from regular donors found HIV positive was considered infectious according to previous reports. For first-time donors, this risk was estimated at 1 for 500 000 donations from a prevalence comparison with regular donors (HIV positivity, seroconversion pattern by Western-blot, other viral markers).
The estimated risks of HIV transmission, for a prevalence of 0.009 to 0.006% were the following :

	Regular	Total (CI 95%)
1991	1/500 000	1/500 000 ($1/1.5x10^6$-1/250000)
1992	1/600 000	1/580 000 ($1/2x10^6$ - 1/300000)
1993 1st sem.	1/900 000	1/800 000 ($1/8x10^6$-1/300000)

0157

PHOTOINACTIVATION OF HIV-1 with METHYLENE BLUE: DESTRUCTIVE EFFECTS ON REVERSE TRANSCRIPTASE AND VIRAL RNA

B.Bachmann, J. Knüver-Hopf, H. Mohr
DRK Blutspendedienst Niedersachsen, FRG

During the production of virus-inactivated fresh frozen plasma, the plasma is exposed to visible light in the presence of 1μM Methylene blue (MB). This procedure inactivates HIV-1 at up to $10^{6.32}$ $TCID_{50}$/ml in 10 minutes. To understand the mechanism of the inactivation we investigated the reverse transcriptase (RT) and the viral RNA.
While studying recombinant RT (Boehringer) alone we found that RT is totally inactivated after 30 min of photoinactivation with 1 μM MB. In the presence of template-primer (poly A/oligo dT) inactivation is nearly complete after 10 min (5% residual activity). This result leads to the conclusion that photoinactivation affects RT and RNA.
The best inactivation of the RT was found in virus resuspended in plasma or medium. In NaCl, the residual activity was 40% after 30 min of illumination. Although the virus retained its specific gravity after inactivation, western blotting showed a change in protein pattern. Also, a decrease in the amount of viral RNA was found with PCR. In summary, the photoinactivation of HIV seems to be an interplay of protein and RNA destruction.

0158

AUTOMATED HISTORY OF TEST RESULTS FOR SILENT RE-ENTRY OF HIV-ELISA FALSE-POSITIVE BLOOD DONORS.

C.L. Van der Poel, N. Schram, J.W. Landman, P.J. Ter Linden, and H.W. Reesink. Red Cross Blood Bank Amsterdam, The Netherlands.

Objective: To install on-line automated test history records (ATHR) for re-entry of donors with previously false-positive anti-HIV ELISA screening test results.

Background/methods: Before re-entry was officially approved, anti-HIV ELISA positive but Western Blot(WB) indeterminate or negative donors were assigned a product blocking code (PBC) in the Blood Bank donor database to discard future donations without notification (1985-1992). In 1993 a computer program was installed to generate on-line overviews of all previous screening and confirmatory test results dating back to 1986. The generated ATHR (n=6,943 records from 501 blood donors) were downloaded to a personal computer data base. By sorting the donors into categories based on the ATHR, silent re-entry was performed ie: removal of the PBC without notification.

Results: 156 / 501 (31%) donors, with previously ELISA positive, but WB negative results were silently re-entered in 2 working days.

Conclusions: ATHR are helpful in silent re-entry of donors with previously false-positive screening test results.

0160

USE OF THE SIMPLEX STRATEGY TO OPTIMIZE PREPARATION OF PLATELET CONCENTRATES FROM POOLED BUFFY-COATS

P. Rebulla, N. Greppi, G. Introcaso, G. Sirchia. Centro Trasfusionale e di Immunologia dei Trapianti, Ospedale Maggiore, Milano, Italy.

We used the simplex strategy (a technique that programs serial experiments according to the results of preceeding ones-Transfusion,1976;16:370) to identify centrifugation conditions associated with highest platelet yield and lowest white cell count and Hct in platelet concentrates prepared from buffy-coats (BC-PC). Pools of 4 buffy-coats were diluted with 400 mL of Plasmalyte-A (Baxter) into a 600 mL transfer bag and centrifuged at 22±2°C in a Sorvall RC-3C centrifuge equipped with an HG-4L rotor. Finally, the supernatant BC-PC was collected. The centrifuge displays the integer of time x speed (ω^2dt x 10^6). Platelets were counted with an automated counter, WBC with a Nageotte chamber. Hct was evaluated by Hb spectrophotometric determination. Platelet yield from the BC pool (PLT%), total WBC/unit and Hct were (median results; n=5 per ω^2dt value):

ω^2dt	*g*	rpm	min:sec	PLT(%)	WBC(10^6)	Hct(%)
1.1	67	480	7:48	*no cell sedimentation*		
1.8	135	680	6:18	*no cell sedimentation*		
2.2	225	880	4:48	*no cell sedimentation*		
2.4	119	640	9:24	*no cell sedimentation*		
3.5	206	840	8:00	65	216	0.250
4.3	315	1040	6:30	73	261	0.040
4.5	448	1240	4:54	72	382	0.040
4.5	233	800	11:00	68	271	0.100
6.0	291	1000	9:30	72	137	0.010
7.2	420	1200	8:00	73	190	0.020
7.6	745	1600	5:00	70	223	0.030
7.8	571	1400	6:30	69	59	0.020
9.5	392	1160	11:06	66	192	0.030
11.0	539	1360	9:36	58	24	0.010
12.0	709	1560	8:06	56	14	0.010

We conclude that ω^2dt values of 6-7.8 x 10^6 optimize platelet yield and minimize WBC count and Hct.

0161

OPTIMALIZATION OF COMPONENT PREPARATION

D.de Korte, C.H.Palfenier, I.E.Pankalla-Blandeau, H.A.Veldman,J.A.Loos
Central Laboratory Netherlands Red Cross Blood Transfusion Service, Amsterdam, the Netherlands.

Using a Compomat (NPBI,the Netherlands) we studied variation of centrifugation speed on composition of red cell concentrates (RCC), buffy coats (BC) and plasma, prepared from 530 ml whole blood (WB). Two programs were used;1.addition of plasma to BC via rinsing of BC compartment for preparation of platelet concentrates (PC); 2.just removal of BC. Centrifugation was performed during 8 min at various speed (Hettich Roto Silenta R/P, start phase 70 sec, brake 3, radius 28cm). The volume of the components varied only slightly, but at higher speed (>3000 rpm) RCC contained more platelets (Plt) and leukocytes (WBC), especially without rinsing. The recovery of haemoglobin in RCC was 90% after rinsing and >96% without rinsing. Below 2700 rpm the cellular contamination of the plasma became unacceptable. At the optimal speeds (2700-3000 rpm) 90 % of the Plt were in the BC and up to 90% (with rinsing) or 75% (without rinsing) of WBC, whereas RCC prepared with rinsing has WBC as low as 338 ± 83.7 x 10^6 and Plt <1 x 10^9. BC prepared without rinsing can be used for preparation of PC in synthetic medium.

	RCC				plasma	BC		
rpm	volume	Hb	WBC	Plt	volume	volume	WBC	Plt
2400	56	91	13	<1	42	22	87	70
2700	55	91	11	<1	41	21	88	88
3000	52	89	25	2	45	22	75	91
3300	51	89	26	10	46	21	74	86
3600	54	91	37	10	44	20	63	88

Results with rinsing, mean as percentage from WB; N=6 with a variation coefficient of maximal 20 %.

0162

STUDIES ON PLATELET AGGREGATES IN BUFFY COATS USED FOR PREPARING BUFFY COAT PLATELETS

N. Greppi, P. Rebulla, G. Introcaso, G. Sirchia. Centro Trasfusionale e di Immunologia dei Trapianti, Ospedale Maggiore Policlinico, Milano, Italy.

We routinely prepare platelet concentrates (PC) from pools of 6-7 buffy coats (BC) separated from blood units centrifuged at 5400 *g* x 6 min within 2-3 hrs of donation. BC are stored overnight under gentle agitation at 22±2°C, pooled in 400 mL of Plasmalyte-A (Baxter) and centrifuged at 570 *g* x 6.5 min. Finally, the supernatant BC-PC is collected. In spite of several practical and biochemical advantages of BC-PC *vs* PC from platelet-rich-plasma, we noticed that platelet yield was lower in the former (55-60% *vs* 70-75%). To investigate the causes of decreased yield in BC-PC we prepared smears from BC before and after 24 and 48 hrs of gentle agitation at 22°C and determined the number and size of platelet aggregates. Results were (median no. of aggregates per 20 microscopic fields at 100x; n=7):

BC age (hours)	*Number of platelets/aggregate* <5	5-10	10-20	>20	*PLT count* ($x10^3/\mu L$)
0	8	8	3	4	1099
24	21	1	0	0	1300
48	18	1	0	0	1382

This experiment showed that large platelet aggregates present in BC are partially dissolved during overnight rotation. In a second series of experiments (n=5) we resuspended BC samples in EDTA immediately after preparation, 24 and 48 hours after gentle rotation. This resulted in platelet counts in EDTA that were 147±15% of those performed in the absence of EDTA. These preliminary results indicate that approximately one third of BC platelets are trapped in aggregates, suggesting that platelet aggregation plays a significant role in limiting platelet yield in BC-PC.

0163

AN INCREASE IN BLOOD COMPONENT PREPARATION BY 15,000 A YEAR WITHOUT STAFF EXPANSION BY INTRODUCTION OF OPTIPAC™/OPTIPRESS™

M.H.J. Molijn, D.J. van Rhenen, P. v Toledo, J. Vermeij, Red Cross Blood Bank Rotterdam, Rotterdam, The Netherlands.

As our Blood Bank started in 1990 with the "Bottom and Top"-packs (BAT-packs), one of goals was the avoidance of staff expansion.
Whole blood units in BAT-packs were collected at 5 regular donor centers (Monday to Friday). All units were processed in two working stations in red cells, buffy-coats and plasma. Processing in each working station was performed by two technicians using 3 centrifuges and 6 OPTIPRESSES™. A fifth technician served as coordinator.
The units whole blood were processed in 2 categories: 1. blood collected from 8 am to 2 pm (25%), processed at the end of the same day at one working station. 2. blood collected from 2 pm to 8 pm (75%), stored at 20 °C, and processed the next morning.
In 1990 and 1991 75,000 units whole blood were drawn and processed with 5 technicians during 5 days per week and 4 hours per day. The two working stations processed on an average 75 units whole blood per hour.
In 1992 and 1993, 90,000 units whole blood were drawn and processed similar to 1990 and 1991. The processing of the units was performed with the same number of technicians within the same time as the first two years after introduction of the BAT-packs. The working stations processed on an average 90 units whole blood per hour.
The increase of 20% of whole blood units collected in OPTIPAC™ BAT-packs and processed in OPTIPRESSES™ did not give any staff expansion during the first 4 years after the implementation of BAT-packs. Apart from a greater efficiency, an increase in standardization and quality of blood products was obtained.

0165

CRYOPRESERVATION OF HUMAN RED BLOOD CELLS (RBC) USING HYDROXYETHYL STARCH (HES) AND LIQUID NITROGEN: AUTOLOGOUS RETRANSFUSION IN HEALTHY VOLUNTEERS

A. Sputtek , G. Singbartl , W. Schleinzer , P. Kuehnl

Dept. of Transfusion Medicine / Transplant. Immunology, University Hospital, Hamburg Dept. of Anaesthesiology, ENDO-Klinik, Hamburg, FRG

The cryopreservation of RBC in the presence of HES may be effective for stockpiling for use in civil or military disasters. But it can also be beneficial in other situations such as for rare blood groups and problems due to multiple antibodies. Frozen/thawed autologous RBC are of particular interest as a supplement to liquid storage for elective operations to extend the preoperative collection period.
In this study using 7 healthy volunteers, 500 ml of whole blood was replaced by a suspension of cryopreserved autologous RBC (hematocrit 43% ± 2% (v/v), HES concentration 11.5% (w/w), NaCl concentration 45 mmol/l). Viability of the RBC after thawing in terms of saline stability reached 92% ± 1%.
In all 7 cases the frozen/thawed autologous RBC were tolerated very well. The level of free plasma hemoglobin increased initially by a factor of 2, and then decreased within 20 h, accompanied by a restoration of haptoglobin. More than 85% of the HES was eliminated from the plasma within the first day.

0166

CONDITIONS FOR OPTIMAL CRYOPRESERVATION OF PERIPHERAL STEM CELLS.

Ineke C.M. Slaper-Cortenbach, Maria J.G.J. Wijngaarden-du Bois, Ada de Vries-van Rossen, Aster Vos, Anahid Zadurian and Anneke Blom.
Central Laboratory of the Netherlands Red Cross Blood Transfusion Service, Amsterdam, the Netherlands.

In our laboratory, separation and cryopreservation of hematopoietic stem cells for transplantation purposes is routinely being performed. Aim of this study was to investigate the optimal conditions for cryopreservation of peripheral blood stem cells (PBSC) and compare these data with the conditions for bone marrow derived stem cells. Although mobilization protocols are being composed in a way that the expected optimum of circulating stem cells is during the week, careful monitoring of the number of CD 34^+ cells may indicate optimal time of harvesting in a weekend. This urged us to investigate the possibilities to store leukocytapheresis products. Experiments showed that PBSC transplants can be stored for 1-2 days at 4°C before cryopreservation without an adverse effect on the recovery of living cells or CFU-GM numbers. Storage of PBSC is independent of the cell concentration. Prolonged storage of PBSC however, does influence the recovery of CFU-GM after cryopreservation. In contrast with bone marrow stem cells, controlled rate cryopreservation of PBSC results in a considerable reduction of CFU-GM after thawing, but is not further diminished when the cells were stored at 4 °C for 1 day prior to cryopreservation. Selection of $CD34^+$ progenitor cells prior to freezing might improve the post thaw recoveries.

0167

MODIFICATION OF A CRYOPRESERVATIVE FOR AUTOLOGOUS STEM CELL PRESERVATION

A. Giulivi[1]; J. Demone[1]; Bette Rutherford[1]; L. B. Huebsch[2]
[1] Ottawa Centre, Canadian Red Cross Society, Ottawa, Ontario, Canada [2] Hematology, University of Ottawa, Ontario, Canada

DMSO is the cryoprotectant most commonly used for autologous stem cell preservation. The potential adverse reactions of DMSO are well documented. To reduce potential reactions, it would be of benefit to reduce the amount of DMSO during storage. As one option, it was decided to investigate whether the current 20% DMSO solution could be replaced with a 10% DMSO/6% HES/4% Albumin solution. However, due to the non-availability of HES in Canada, the replacement of HES with Pentaspan (a licensed volume expander obtained from Dupont Pharmaceuticals), was investigated. Samples were obtained from 5 autologous bone marrow harvests (ABM), 3 stimulated autologous peripheral blood stem cell harvests (APBSC), and 2 non-stimulated peripheral blood stem cell donations (PBSC). Samples were frozen in the modified 12% Pentaspan/10% DMSO/8% Albumin solution. To assess viability, the following parameters were measured: WBC concentrations, percentage viability, and CFU assays. Data were compared to pre-freeze values. For ABM samples, WBC counts were 79-100% of pre-frozen, control values. Viability ranged from 88-100%. For APBSC samples, WBC counts were 83-100% of pre-values. Viability ranged from 84-90%. For PBSC samples, the WBC counts were 100% post freezing and the viability values were 93-95% of control. As expected, the CFU assays for all samples showed a decrease following storage, however, there was significant residual G, M, G/M, BFU-E, GEMM activity. To-date, seven autologous transplant patients have been reinfused (with little clinical toxicity) with cells frozen in the 12% Pentaspan/10% DMSO/8% Albumin cryopreservative solution and all have successfully engrafted as expected. Thus, this cryopreservative solution appears to be a viable alternative to the 20% DMSO solution.

0168

COMPARISON OF A 4% HYDROXYETHYL STARCH (HES) METHOD WITH THE 5% DIMETHYL SULFOXIDE (DMSO) TECHNIQUE FOR THE CRYOPRESERVATION OF PLATELET CONCENTRATES (PC)

A. Sputtek[1], B. Barthel[2], P. Kuehnl[1]

[1]Dept. of Transfusion Medicine / Transplant. Immunology, University Hospital, Hamburg, [2]Helmholtz-Institute for Biomedical Engineering , Aachen, FRG

As HES in contrast to DMSO is a well tolerated and biodegradable cryoprotectant, HES protected frozen / thawed PC need not be washed prior to transfusion. The purpose of this study was an *in vitro* comparison of an optimized HES technique (Sputtek et al., Cryo-Letters 8, 216-229, 1987) to a standard DMSO technique.
PC were obtained from 20 whole blood donations (10 donors). Cryopreservation did not markedly affect the platelet count (i. e. 88% ± 38% for HES, 102% ± 39% for DMSO). The mean platelet volume increased by 14% ± 22% and 7% ± 33%, respectively. The coagulation time measured by resonance thrombography (RTG) dropped by about 30%. However, ATP recovery, aggregation induced by ristocetin, and the inverse ratio of Hartert's P_R values derived from RTG for DMSO (55% ± 22%, 87% ± 27%, 45% ± 27%) were superior to the corresponding values found for HES (26% ± 14%, 41% ± 18%, 13% ± 8%).
In conclusion, although the HES protocol is effective, the DMSO protocol resulted in smaller changes after thawing.

0170

PRENATAL DETERMINATION OF FETAL RHc STATUS BY DNA AMPLIFICATION

C. Le Van Kim[1], I. Mouro[1], Y. Brossard[2], J.P. Cartron[1], and Y. Colin[1].
[1]INSERM U76, INTS, 6, rue Alexandre Cabanel, 75015 Paris; [2]CHP, 53 boulevard Diderot 75012 Paris

After anti-RhD, anti-Rhc is the most important red cell alloantibody which can cause hemolytic disease of the new born (HDN). Following the demonstration that the RH locus is composed of two genes (D and CE) encoding the D and C/c and E/e Rh polypeptides in RhD-positive donors, but only one (CE) in the RhD-negative genomes, PCR experiments have been developped to determine early in pregnancy the fetal RhD type in DNA from amniotic cells, chorionic samples (Bennett et al, 1993, N.Engl.J.Med.5, 329:607-610).
Taking into account the polymorphisms between the c and C alleles in exon 2 (Mouro et al, 1993, Nature Genet. 5:62-65), we have now developped two PCR based methods in order to detect the presence of the Rhc allele in fetal amniotic cells from homozygote CC women. The first assay involved restriction fragment lenght polymorphism (RFLP) based on the presence of an XhoI site in C transcripts. The second used c allele specific oligonucleotides (ASO).
Such determination together with the prenatal determination of fetal RhD type will help in the management of pregnancies at risk of RhD and Rhc hemolytic diseases.

0171

EVALUATION OF SCREENING KIT FOR FETAL BLEEDS USING AN IgM MONOCLONAL ANTI-D

B.A. Brick[1], J. McCabe[2], P. Pedreira[3], H. Polesky[4], I. Shulman[5]
1 Baxter Diagnostics AG, Düdingen, Switzerland, 2 Brigham and Women's Hospital, Boston, MA, 3 Jackson Memorial Hospital, Miami, FL, 4 Memorial Blood Centers of Minnesota, Minneapolis, MN, 5 LA County/USC Medical Center, Los Angeles, CA, USA

The evaluation of a new screening kit for the detection of D positive fetal bleeds in D negative mothers using an IgM monoclonal Anti-D (NELP 4) is described. The kit, based on the rosetting technique of Sebring and Polesky, was evaluated using 30 prepared samples to simulate a range of feto-maternal hemorrhages (FMH), and 134 random samples from D negative women who delivered D positive infants. One drop of a 3% saline suspension of the test red cells was mixed with one drop of Anti-D and incubated 1-10 minutes at room temperature. The cells were washed 3 times with saline and one drop of R_2R_2 Indicator Cells and one drop of the Enhancement Reagent were added. The cell mixture was mixed and spun for 15 seconds at 1000 rcf. The cell button was resuspended and read microscopically for the presence of rosettes. The presence of 5 rosettes within 5 fields represented a positive result. Positive samples from the random phase of testing were quantitatively tested by the Kleihauer-Betke procedure to determine the amount of the FMH. Of the prepared samples all 8 technologists were able to detect as positive a 15 and a 30 ml bleed. Ninety-two percent of 48 readings were positive with a prepared 5 ml bleed, 29% with a 2 ml bleed and no positives were detected with the simulated 0 ml bleed. Seven of 134 random samples tested had positive screen results. Results of the Kleihauer-Betke test with 6 of these samples showed bleeds between 5 and 40 ml. The seventh sample was reported as a 25 ml bleed by the test site but the screen was negative and the fetal bleed was reported as 1 ml by the reference site. This kit was reported as fast and easy to use by all sites. All technologists were capable of detecting an FMH of at least 15 ml using this kit. This screening kit would provide a quick and reliable method to determine if additional doses of Rh immune globulin would be required.

0172

QUANTITATION OF FETOMATERNAL HEMORRHAGE BY A FLUORESCENT MICROSPHERE METHOD

B.A. van Dijk, A.J.M. de Man, V.A.J.M. Kunst.
Blood Transfusion Service, University Hospital, Nijmegen, The Netherlands.

For quantification of fetomaternal hemorrhage (FMH) of D-positive red blood cells (RBC) in D-negative women the Kleihauer-Betke test is the commonly used technique. However, this method is difficult to quantitate and has a rather poor reproducibility. We developed a reliable and reproducible method for the quantitation of subpopulations RBC using fluorescent microspheres (Vox Sang 1988:55, 37-41). D-positive RBC sensitized in vitro with anti-D, were labelled with fluorescent anti-IgG coated microspheres and analyzed by fluorescence microscopy. The sensitivity level of the assay is one positive cell per 10.000 negative RBC (0.01%), which equals 0.2 ml of fetal RBC. To study FMH during pregnancy and delivery 1310 samples of 291 D-negative women who delivered D-positive infants were determined using this method. Also 356 samples of 78 D-negative women who delivered D-negative infants were determined as negative controls. In 12 (4%) of the pregnancies D-positive fetal RBC were found; 2 in the third trimester and 10 after delivery. The size of FMH ranged from 0.22-12.14 ml (mean 2 ml) fetal RBC. The incidence of FMH reported is much lower than the frequencies of 20-70% found with the Kleihauer-Betke technique. This discrepancy is explained by an overestimation of the FMH by the Kleihauer-Betke procedure.

0173

Human anti-idiotype antibodies from phage display libraries

H.M.Griffin*, B.D.Gorick# and W.H.Ouwehand*$
*Division of Transfusion Medicine and #MRC, University of Cambridge, UK, $NIBSC, Potters Bar, UK.

It has been recently reported that antibody fragments against human self antigens, including immunoglobulin idiotypes of a human antibody, can be derived from a human phage display library (Griffiths *et al. EMBO* J, 1993,12, 725-34). The library was composed of the rearranged V genes of peripheral blood lymphocytes from non-immunised donors (Marks *et al. J. Mol. Biol.*, 1991 222, 581-97). We selected this same library on the human IgG Rhesus D antibody Reg-A (Melamed *et al. J. Immunol. Meth*, 1987, 104, 245-51) in order to isolate single-chain Fv (scFv) fragments with anti-idiotypic activity. After three rounds of selection four scFvs were obtained which were reactive with Reg-A IgG in ELISA. Further studies with a panel of human monoclonal antibodies against Rh(D) indicated that all four clones produced scFvs directed against the variable domains of Reg-A. Subsequently, the four scFvs were tested for their ability to inhibit the binding of ^{125}I-Reg-A antibody to human red blood cells bearing the RhD antigen (cDE/cDE). The extent of inhibition of ^{125}I-Reg-A binding to the RhD antigen by the scFvs was determined by titration. One of the four scFvs (C3) showed 100% inhibition of binding suggesting it was anti-idiotypic, whereas the scFvs produced by the three other clones were unable to inhibit binding. The nucleotide sequence of the V_H and V_L genes of these four scFvs is being determined to further analyse the molecular basis of the idiotype-anti-idiotype interaction.

0176

STEM CELL TRANSPLANTATION AS A NEW TOOL FOR THE INDUCTION OF TRANSPLANTATION TOLERANCE IN ORGAN TRANSPLANTATION.

A. de Vries-van der Zwan, A.C. Besseling-Boersma and L.P. de Waal.
Central laboratory of the Netherlands Red Cross Blood Transfusion Service, Amsterdam, The Netherlands.

Induction of specific transplantation tolerance across major histocompatibility complex (MHC) barriers without long-term immunosuppressive treatment is a major goal in transplantation immunology.
The aim of the present study was to induce engraftment of full H-2 disparate donor bone marrow cells resulting in the development of transplantation tolerance. In a semi-allogeneic bone marrow transplantation model recipient mice were treated with anti-CD3 and received on the same day a low dose whole body irradiation (3 Gy). As a result, stable long-term chimerism was obtained.
Skin transplantation in chimeric animals performed two and six months after the conditioning regime showed indefinite survival of first and second grafts respectively. In addition, specific CTL non-responsiveness developed. Induction of transplantation tolerance can also be achieved in a fully allogeneic bone marrow transplantation model following sublethal irradiation (6 Gy).
We conclude that stem cell transplantation offers a new approach for the induction of transplantation tolerance in organ transplantation.

0177

HEPARIN-ASSOCIATED THROMBOCYTOPENIA (HAT): DIFFERENT EFFECTS OF VARIOUS INTRAVENOUS IgG PREPARATIONS ON ANTIBODY MEDIATED PLATELET ACTIVATION. A POSSIBLE NEW INDICATION FOR HIGH DOSE I.V. IgG.

A. Greinacher[1], U. Liebenhoff[2], V. Kiefel[1], P. Presek[2], and C. Mueller-Eckhardt[1]
1 Institut für Klinische Immunologie and Transfusionsmedizin, 2 Rudolf-Buchheim-Institut für Pharmakologie, Justus Liebig Universität, Giessen, FRG.

HAT is caused by an antibody which, in the presence of sulfated oligosaccharides, activates platelets via the Fc-receptor. We investigated platelet activation by HAT antibodies using normal platelets and platelets from a patient with Glanzmann's thrombasthenia (GT) lacking gp IIb/IIIa. Heparin and sera from patients with HAT stimulated GT platelets in the same manner as determined by ^{14}C-serotonin release and by changes in phosphorylation of p20 and p47. Platelet activation could be inhibited by Fc- but not by $F(ab')_2$-fragments of human IgG. The effect of four commercially available i.v. IgG preparations on the platelet activating effect of six HAT sera was investigated by ^{14}C-serotonin release. The inhibitory effect was strongly dependent upon the manufacturing process. At a concentration of 20 mg/ml only IgG that had been subjected to low pH and traces of pepsin sufficiently inhibited platelet activation (index:0.62). IgG treated with polyethylenglycol (i:0.35) or sulfitolysis (i:0.32) was less effective, whereas beta propiolactone-treated IgG almost completely lost the ability to inhibit platelet activation by the HAT antibody (i:0.23).
We conclude that inhibition of gp IIb/IIIa - fibrinogen interaction is insufficient for preventing platelet activation in HAT. This is, however, possible by high dose i.v. IgG, whereby inhibition of FcRII on platelets strongly depends upon the process by which the i.v. IgG preparation was manufactured.

0178

LONG-TERM TREATMENT OF MULTIPLE SCLEROSIS WITH IgG IMMUNOTHERAPY

E. Schuller*, P. Lambin, G. Deloche *, A. Gervais***

* Laboratory of Neuro-Immunology (INSERM) - Hôpital la Salpétrière - 47 Bd de l'Hôpital - 75013

** Laboratory of Immuno-Chemistry - INTS - 6 rue A. Cabanel - 75015.

Thirty-five definite multiple sclerosis (M.S) patients were treated in an open trial (1975-1993) with a standard dose preparation (5 grams of total IgG per week) by intra muscular or intravenous injection. This treatment was used in 35 patients : 35 for 3 years, 34 for 6 years, 33 for 8 years, 29 for 12 years, 25 for 14 years and 20 for 16 years. Using Kurtzke's disability scale (K score) and progression index ratios related to the duration of M.S., (K/A) and to the age of the patient (K/G) the results are :1) a significant deterioration only 16 years after entry.2) regarding current therapeutic results : improvement for 8 patients, deterioration for 18, and stability for 9. 3) a significant decrease of K/A and a great stability of K/G.

Neither age at M.S onset, age at entry, duration of M.S, nor the disability score at entry were factors modifying significantly the efficacy of the treatment. The comparison of these results with the previous predictive studies suggests a significant reduction of M.S progression, with an increase of the time to loss of functional independence. No side-effects were observed, and this immunotherapy, which is convenient for home treatment, may be proposed as an adjuvant long-term treatment.

0179

HLA-DR MATCHED DONORS AMONST MULTIPLE CONCOMITTANT TRANSFUSIONS PREVENT ALLO-IMMUNIZATION

JGA Houbiers[1,2], LMG van de Watering[1,2], CJH van de Velde[2], FHJ Claas[1], A Brand[1].

[1]Immunohaematology & Blood Bank, [2]Surgery, University Hospital, 2300 RC Leiden, the Netherlands

Blood transfusions can induce alloantibodies as well as have immunosuppressive effects. Lagaaij et al. showed that among recievers of one unit of packed cells those who matched one HLA-DR allele with the donor were significantly less frequently allo-immunized compared to completely HLA-DR mismatched blood recievers. It is not clear what will happen when multiple transfusion are given within a short period.

Therefore, we screening 50 colorectal cancer patients for IgG and IgM alloantibodies after transfusion of on average 3.7 units of packed cells. Those who had received solely completely HLA-DR mismatched blood (N=15) were more often alloantibody positive compared to patients who had received at least one units that was matched for at least one HLA-DR allel (N=35). This difference reached statistical significance for IgG alloantibodies. Although more often allo-immunized these mismatched patients recieved significantly less units of blood and encountered significantly less allogeneic HLA-A and HLA-B antigens.

1

0180

INFECTIOUS COMPLICATIONS AND IMMUNE FUNCTIONS IN PATIENTS AFTER GASTRO-INTESTINAL CANCER SURGERY AND BLOOD TRANSFUSION

L.Quintiliani[1], P.Iudicone[1], M.DiGirolamo[2], A.Buzzonetti[1], M.Guglielmetti[1], A.Pescini[1], P.Traietti[2], D.Monno[2].

1 National Blood Transfusion Center, Italian Red Cross - ROME

2 S.Giovanni Calibita Hospital - Isola Tiberina - ROME - ITALY

Blood transfusion (BT) has been shown to be associated with a high risk of bacterial infections in patients operated for colo-rectal cancer; the BT has been indicated as responsible for the enhanced susceptibility to infections because of its effect on the immune system functions. In this study the natural killer (NK) activity and the lymphokine synthesis by peripheral blood mononuclear cells (PBMC) of 78 patients affected by gastro-intestinal cancer (21 gastric, 26 colon, 31 rectal cancer) were evaluated before the tumor resection and 12-14 days after surgery. The patients were divided into sub-groups according to the post-operative infection occurrence or the requirement of BT. Before surgery, the immune responses of the patients who afterwards developed post-operative infections were comparable with those of the patients who did not.Similar results were found comparing transfused and untransfused patients. Following tumor resection, 23 out of 78 patients developed infections (5 gastric, 6 colon, 12 rectal cancer), 22 out of them were transfused. Infected patients showed a significant lower NK cytotoxicity as compared either to all patients without infections (P=0.005) or to the no infected transfused patients (P=0.008). On the contrary, no significant differences in the immune responses were found between transfused and untransfused patients. These results confirm the existence of a higher risk of infections in patients operated for gastro-intestinal cancer and perioperatively transfused, but they do not support the hypothesis that a negative immunomodulation of BT is responsible for that. The significant decrease of NK function, which is essential to combact bacterial infections, may be the result of factors different from BT, such as location and stage of the tumor, surgical trauma, anhestesia, blood loss.

0181

PERIOPERATIVE BLOOD TRANSFUSION IS NOT ASSOCIATED WITH A FALL IN NATURAL KILLER CELL (NK) OR LYMPHOKINE ACTIVATED KILLER CELL (LAK) ACTIVITY.

F.T.Cordingley, I.Caminschi, G.Sheridan, M.F.Leahy.
Haematology Dept., Fremantle Hospital, Fremantle Western Australia.

Blood transfusion is known to be immunosuppressive and perioperative transfusion has been associated with increased postoperative infections and with increased tumour recurrence. The mechanism of this immunosuppression is unknown.This study investigated the effects of allogeneic packed red cell transfusion on NK and LAK cell function and numbers in 57 patients undergoing elective hip and knee replacement surgery, 42% of whom received packed red cell transfusion.

We found a statistically significant severe reduction in NK and LAK cell cytotoxicity 3-8 days after surgery; mean NK activity falling from 33% to 18% ($p<0.001$) and LAK activity falling from 41% to 28% ($p<0.001$). This change was not related to age, non-steroidal antiflammatory drug therapy, operative blood loss, duration of surgery or to transfusion status, with no statistically significant difference between transfused and non-transfused patients in NK and LAK cell activity or numbers by multivariate analysis. When studied three months post-operatively, NK and LAK activity had recovered and were not significantly different from preoperative values.

Comparison between heavily transfused (4 or more units) and lightly transfused patients (3 units or less) showed a significant increase in postoperative LAK activity in the heavily transfused group (58% compared to 32%, $p=0.007$). This post transfusion increase in LAK activity has not been previously reported.

These results do not support the hypothesis that the immunosuppressive effect of blood transfusion is exerted through an effect on NK or LAK activity

0183

INACTIVATION OF INFECTIOUS HIV IN LARGE VOLUME SAMPLES OF HUMAN PLATELET CONCENTRATE.

D.N. Cook[1], L. Lin[1], R. Alfonso[1], C.-S. Sun[2], C.V. Hanson[3], C. Asuncion[2], and J. Chapman[2]. [1]Steritech Incorporated, Concord CA USA; [2]Baxter-Fenwal, Round Lake IL USA; [3]California Department of Health Services, Berkeley CA USA

To validate HIV inactivation in blood products, a method to detect a small number of infectious particles in large volumes (i.e. ≥ 50 ml) is required. In a prototype experiment, MT-2 cells were used to capture infectious virions from 4 ml of deliberately contaminated platelet concentrate (PC) with the subsequent detection of viral antigen expression after extended culture. HIV-1 in PC was inactivated with the novel psoralen S-70 (100 μM) and UVA (5J/cm²). After treatment, a PC containing HIV (1.2×10^6 TCID per ml) was incubated with MT-2 cells (1.2×10^6 cells per 4 ml sample) for 2 h at room temperature with gentle mixing. Cells were collected by centrifugation, washed to remove unbound virus, and resuspended in culture medium. Infectious virus was detected by measuring the increase in p24 antigen during culture. The results can be summarized as follows: **1)** S-70 treatment completely inactivated >1.2×10^6 HIV per ml in 4 ml as measured by extended 6-week culture of cells. **2)** As few as 40 HIV in 4 ml of PC were detectable one week after capture. **3)** HIV, including S-70 inactivated virus, adsorbed to MT-2 cells immediately after capture and gave rise to a substantial p24 signal. **4)** Live virus was distinguished from killed virus by the increase in p24 expression with time.

0184

INACTIVATION OF HUMAN IMMUNODEFICIENCY VIRUS TYPE 1 (HIV-1) IN HUMAN PLATELET CONCENTRATES (PC) USING A NEW PSORALEN DERIVATIVE (CP-38) AND ULTRAVIOLET-A LIGHT (UVA)

S.Sowemimo-Coker, N.Yerram, S.C.Park, T.Goodrich, S.Crandall, P.Forster, M.S.Platz* and R. Goodrich. Cryopharm Corporation, Pasadena, CA 91107, USA.
* Department of Chemistry, The Ohio State University, Columbus, OH 43210-1173, USA.

Inactivation of HIV-1 in PC was conducted under normal ambient oxygen tension using a new photosensitizer CP-38 and UVA at 22±2°C. Dose response and kinetics studies were conducted in order to determine the optimal conditions for complete inactivation of HIV-1 in human PC with preservation of normal platelet function. 5-7 logs of HIV-1 virus was added to standard units of human PC. The contaminated PC were incubated at ambient light for 10±2 minutes with different concentrations of CP-38 (50-300μg/mL). Following incubation, the PC were exposed to UVA at different fluences (4.32-51.84 J/cm²). Inactivation of HIV-1 virus was evaluated by an infectivity assay (syncitia formation using MT-4 cell line) and by p24 antigen capture assay. In parallel several in vitro platelet properties were monitored at the different photoinactivation conditions. Salient results showed complete inactivation of HIV-1 virus(5-7logs)at100-400μg/mL of CP-38 and UVA fluences of (25.92-51.84J/cm²). Under these conditions there was (1) no evidence of replication competent HIV-1 virus in the PC,and (2)no major alterations in the measured platelet in vitro properties. Screening studies showed that CP-38 was not cytotoxic to the MT-4 indicator cells. These studies demonstrate that high titers of cell-free HIV-1 in PC can be effectively inactivated under normal oxygen tension in plasma without the need for a synthetic plasma free platelet storage media.

0185

PHOTOCHEMICAL INACTIVATION OF HTLV-I -INFECTED CELLS BY MEROCYANINE 540 AND VISIBLE LIGHT

T.A. Takahashi, K. Kwon, M. Yano, H. Abe, S. Sekiguchi
Hokkaido Red Cross Blood Center, Sapporo, Japan.

We have investigated inactivation of HTLV-I-infected MT-2 cells, with merocyanine 540 (MC540) and visible light. A syncytia formation assay and rabbit infection assay were used for evaluation of HTLV-I infectivity in vitro and in vivo, respectively. MT-2 cells were suspended in RPMI1640 medium containing 5% fetal calf serum, and phototreated with MC540 (0-50 μg/mL) at a dose of 30 J/cm² from a tungsten halogen bulb. HTLV-I infectivity of cells was completely eliminated with more than 30 μg/mL of MC540. MT-2 cells phototreated with 50 μg/mL of MC540 were intravenously injected into rabbits (group A; four rabbits), each injection containing 1×10^7 cells. As a control, four rabbits (group B) were inoculated with the same number of untreated MT-2 cells. When antibody was measured by gelatin particle agglutination assay (PA), HTLV-I antibody appeared at the titers of 1:32-1:256 and 1:16-1:128 in groups A and B, respectively, 1 week after the injection. The PA titer in group B increased to 1:256-1:1024 at 2 weeks and remained stable for 4 weeks. In contrast, the titer in group A decreased to 1:16-1:128 at 2 weeks and to 1:8-1:16 at 7 weeks. PCR analysis showed that the HTLV-I genome was integrated into lymphocytes in group B, but not in group A. In conclusion, MC540 phototreatment reduced cell-associated HTLV-I infectivity of MT-2 cells, but the antigenicity of the cell still remained.

0186

VIRUS INACTIVATION BY METHYLENE BLUE/LIGHT IN THROMBOCYTE CONCENTRATES

A. Klein-Struckmeier and H. Mohr, German Red Cross, Blood Transfusion Service, Lower Saxony

Thrombocyte concentrates treated by methylene blue/light virus inactivation procedure established for fresh frozen plasma show some functional deteriorations. Decreased hypotonic shock reaction and a drop in aggregation response to collagen can be measured directly after treatment. The influence on pH-value and biochemical parameters such as glucose consumption, lactate production and potassium leakage is negligible even after 5 days of storage.

The step of this virus inactivation procedure affecting these functions most severely seems to be the 1 hour exposure to red light of a narrow emission bandwidth. Reducing light exposure time for better platelet protection has no negative effects on virus inactivation if platelets are stored in a plasma-poor (20 %) medium with only low quenching effect.

Two light sources with narrow emission bandwidth were compared with regard to virus inactivation efficiency and platelet function stability.The Baxter LED (peak at 660 nm) showed better results than a natrium element (peak at 590 nm) which provides very high energies leading to a quick decay of photochemical active methylene blue and to platelet lesion.

For further protection of platelets from damage during methylene blue/light virus inactivation different typ I and II quenchers were tested.

0189

SUPERIORITY OF ADJUSTED DOSE CONTINUOUS FACTOR VIII INFUSION (CIF) OVER BOLUS INJECTIONS OR FIXED DOSE CIF

U. Martinowitz, S. Schulman and D. Varon
The National Hemophilia Center, Sheba Medical Center, Tel-Hashomer, Israel.

We have investigated the pharmacokinetics, effectiveness, tolerance, safety and economy of adjusted dose CIF with a variety of factor concentrates: a) high purity f.VIII (Octavi®, Octapharma) in 31 cases, b) ultra-pure f.VIII (Monoclate P®, Armour) in 14 cases and c) f.VIII-von Willebrand factor concentrate (Haemate P®, Behringwerke) in 6 cases. The settings were: a) elective surgery (n-28), b) emergency surgery (n=7) and c) hemorrhage (n=16). The concentrates were reconstituted according to manufacturers' recommendations (undiluted) and infused via ambulatory mini-pump (Infumed™ 300 or 350, MedFusion Inc.). Prior to elective surgery a pharmacokinetic study was performed to assess the individual clearance in order to calculate the maintenance dose. In all surgical patients as well as in hemorrhage f.VIII:C levels for hemophilia A, VIII:RiCoF and vWF:Ag for vW patients were tested daily in order to adjust the infusion rate according to the clearance and desired level. Pharmacokinetic models predict a 30% decrease of f.VIII dose using CIF due to the elimination of the unnecessary high peak levels. This is true for fixed dose CIF but underestimate the saving in adjusted dose CIF. Adjustment of the dose according to the decreasing clearance (down to 50% for VIII:Ac in Octavi and Monoclate P, and 75% for VIII:RiCoF in Haemate P) increases the saving significantly. The average factor requirements for major surgery was 22000 units as compared to 75000 in the literature (average in 10 publications). Possible mechanisms for the decrease of the clearance will be discussed. Adjusted dose CIF is convenient for the patient and the medical staff, efficacious, safe and cost-effective, can be used as home treatment and save days of hospitalisation. The only side effect was frequent thrombophlebitis at the infusion site, which can be prevented by addition of heparin (2 unit/ml for Octavi, 4 units/ml for Haemate P and 5 units/ml for Monoclate P).

0190

HEMOPHILIA AND HIV : CHANGING RELATIONSHIPS BETWEEN PRODUCERS, PHYSICIANS AND HEMOPHILIACS

C. Smit, Netherlands Hemophilia Society, Badhoevedorp, The Netherlands.

The World Federation of Hemophilia congress in Stockholm in 1983 was the first congress which discussed the aids-problem in hemophilia. No one could imagine at that very moment the impact aids would have on the hemophilia community. Ten years later, more than five thousand hemophiliacs developed aids or died because of its complications. Also a considerable number of their sexual partners and children became HIV-infected. Aids had a devastating effect on the lives of numerous families and caused tremendous feelings of guilt by the family members who infused the missing clotting factors. Also some physicians had these feelings and retired from their work.
Aids changed the international hemophilia community from the cosy 'comprehensive care team' to the well-known grim pictures of the imprisonment of the leading hematologist Jean-Pierre Allain in France and - less well-known - the protesting hemophiliacs and their families in the U.S.
Not only in France, Germany and the United States, but also in The Netherlands the increasing tension in the hemophilia community can be felt when it concerns the lack of recognition of their problems from the side of the government.

In this paper the increasing tensions within the international hemophilia community will be further explored.

0193

FLOW-CYTOMETRIC QUALITY CONTROL FOR STEM CELL SEPARATION

J. Zingsem[1], S. Serke[3], V. Weisbach[1], R. Zimmermann[1], T. Zeiler[2], R. Eckstein[1]

1 Abt. für Transfusionsmedizin, Friedrich-Alexander Universität Erlangen, 2 Abt. f. Transfusionsmedizin und Gerinnungsphysiologie, Philipps-Universität Marburg, 3 Abt. Innere Medizin und Poliklinik m.S. Hämatologie und Onkologie, Universitätsklinikum Rudolf Virchow, Freie Universität Berlin, FRG

One of the most important prerequisites for successful separation of pripheral blood derived haematopoietic stem cells (PBSC) is the precise determination of the optimized separation days. As we previously demonstrated that neither PLT counts nor WBC counts are of predictive value for the amount of colony forming cells (CFC), we started a daily monitoring of CD 34-positive cells using a FACS-Scan® (Becton Dickinson) or a Cytoron® (Ortho) to determine the beginning of the separation series. In addition to routine cell counts and CFU testing we assessed the number of CD 34^+ in the PBSC concentrates to ascertain the number of separations needed for each patient. Due to the strong correlation of CD 34^+ cells to CFC it is possible to predict the number of CFC collected within two hours after finishing the PBSC separation and to calculate the efficiency of the separation for quality control.

0194

LARGE VOLUME LEUKAPHERESIS (LVL) FOR PERIPHERAL BLOOD STEM CELL COLLECTION.

M Torrabadella, L Massuet, A Cabanillas, E Argelagués and C Martín-Vega.
Banc de Sang de l'ICS. Barcelona. Spain.

Numerous leukapheresis (LK) procedures must usually be performed to collect enough cells to ensure engraftment. The aim of this study was to analyze the effect of LVL in order to reduce the number of LK procedures. Over a period of 11 months, we performed 34 LVL for 16 peripheral blood stem cell (PBSC) collections after mobilization with chemotherapy and G-CSF, in 14 patients. Mean age was 21 years (range 5-46), and there were 7 men and 7 women. Eight patients had haematologic malignancies and 6 had solid tumors. Vascular access was by double lumen subclavian or jugular vein catheters. LK were performed in a continuous-flow blood cell separator (COBE). The blood ACD-A ratio was 24:1 with 5000 and 3000 u of heparin added to the first and second 500 mL ACD, respectively. The blood flow rate averaged 103 mL/min in adults (range 60-124), 48 mL/min in children (range 25-55) and an average of 26 L of blood in adults (range 14-36), 14 L in children (range 10-19) was processed per procedure. The procedure time averaged 275 min (range 165-480). We observed no side effects with LVL while processing the patients blood volume to 7-fold. The minimum target dose of $3x10^8$ MNC/kg, $2x10^6$ CD34/kg and $5x10^4$ CFU-GM/kg was reached after 2 LVL (range 1-4). **Conclusions**: the addition of heparin to the ACD-A allows high blood volume to be processed without citrate toxicity symptoms. One or 2 LVL are effective for the collection of sufficient of PBSC. The increase of blood flow rate means that a greater volume of blood can be processed in the same length of time.

0195

USE OF THE HAEMONETICS MCS TO COLLECT PERIPHERAL BLOOD STEM CELLS FROM NORMAL SUBJECTS.

E. Burgstaler[1], A. Pineda[1], D. Ciavarella[2], R. Weinstein[3], H. Smit Sibinga[4]. 1Mayo Clinic, Rochester, MN, 2Hudson Valley Blood Services, Valhalla, NY, 3St. Elizabeth's Medical Center of Boston, Boston, MA, 4Haemonetics Corp., Braintree, MA, USA.

The highly mobile Haemonetics MCS has been used successfully to collect platelets (plt) and plasma. In this multicenter study, we report on the use of the MCS modified to collect peripheral blood stem cells (PBSC) from normal subjects. Evaluations included mononuclear cell (MNC), colony forming units-granulocyte macrophage (CFU-GM) and $CD34^+$ contents, and product purity. Twenty normal subjects underwent 3-hour leukapheresis via peripheral veins, using dual access with gravity flow reinfusion bag (RB). The procedures used the 225 ml bowl, a non-surge collection of buffy coat 40 ml into the red cell layer and plasma returned to the RB as it left the bowl. One to two times per procedure, the buffy coat product was routed through the bowl to collect a concentrated MNC product. Mean values included 6648±1019 ml of blood processed in 182±12 minutes (36.7 ml/min) at anticoagulant ratios of 10-12:1. Mean preprocedure counts were: 5.9±1.4 x $10^3/\mu L$ WBC, 2.2±0.5 x $10^3/\mu L$ MNC, 40.1±3.7% hematocrit, and 243±58 x $10^3/\mu L$ plt. The mean product was 156±61 ml and contained 73±14%, 8.0±2.5 x 10^9 MNC, 3.2±2.5 x 10^5 CFU-GM (n=19), and 0.3±0.3% $CD34^+$ cells (n=12). Mean MNC and CFU-GM collection efficiencies were 67±14% and 58±24% respectively. Mean RBC and plt contamination was 17.4±9.6 ml and 5.1±1.8 x 10^{11} respectively. The MCS is capable of efficiently collecting PBSC from normal, unstimulated subjects.

0196

ANALYSIS OF PERIPHERAL BLOOD PROGENITOR CELL COLLECTION BY THE FRESENIUS BLOOD CELL SEPARATOR AS 104 IN A CONTROLLED LABORATORY SET UP AND DEVELOPMENT OF A PROCEDURE FOR ENRICHMENT OF PERIPHERAL STEM CELLS BY COUNTERFLOW ELUTRIATION.

J. Kwekkeboom, D.E.P. Buurman, J.A. Loos, and I.C.M. Slaper-Cortenbach.
Central Laboratory of the Netherlands Red Cross Blood Transfusion Service, Amsterdam, The Netherlands.

The collection efficiency of peripheral blood stem cells by the Fresenius Blood Cell Separator AS 104 was analyzed in a laboratory setting using pooled units of donor blood, which were supplemented with mobilized stem cells obtained from patients. Upon separation, more than 99% of erythrocytes (n=8) and 87% to 93% of platelets (n=9) were recovered in the "return" fraction, which is normally continuously reinfused into the patient. The machine harvested 24% (range 18% - 28%; n=6) of the leucocytes passing by, and 34% - 50% of mononuclear cells, indicating that a preferential harvesting of low density cells occurred. Collection efficiency of myeloid precursors (CFU-GM) was equal to that of mononuclear cells. Enrichment of progenitor cells from leukapheresis material by counterflow centrifugal elutriation was investigated using an equipment with disposable chambers. The majority of CD34+ cells and CFU-GM was found to co-elutriate with monocytes. Elutriation fractions containing more than 90% of CD34+ cells and CFU-GM were depleted of 50% to 70% of lymphocytes and 20% to 30% of granulocytes. Further depletion of contaminating cells from the progenitor cell fraction by rosetting of cells with beads is being investigated.

0198

TRANSMISSION OF HEPATITIS C VIRUS BY ANTI-HCV NEGATIVE BLOOD TRANSFUSION.

C.L. van der Poel[1], H. Vrielink[1], H.W. Reesink[1], H.L. Zaaijer[2], H.T.M. Cuypers[2], P.N. Lelie[2], 1) Red Cross Blood Bank Amsterdam, 2) Central Lab RC Blood Transfusion Service Amsterdam, The Netherlands.

Background: Open window transmissions of HCV have not yet been described.

Case report: A case of acute post-transfusion hepatitis C was reported to the Blood Bank. A recipient received 3 red cell transfusions. Six weeks after transfusion the patient developed acute icteric hepatitis C (ALT > 1000 IU/L). Implicated blood donations were traced by automated blood bank registration system. In the Blood Bank a serum sample from every blood donation is kept frozen since 1984; stored sera from implicated donations (all negative by ELISA-2) were re-tested by cDNA-PCR and ELISA plus RIBA-3. One implicated donation was strongly PCR positive in duplicate but anti-HCV negative by 3d gen assays. The donor was recalled and was found (13 weeks after the implicated donation) to have become anti-HCV positive (ELISA and RIBA-3), a thawed sample of an earlier donation of the donor was anti-HCV and PCR negative. No risk factors for HCV infection were found, except a 24 hour admission to an emergency ward after a car accident, 4 weeks before the implicated donation. The donor received no blood products at that time, only an IV drip. 8 months after the infectious transfusion, the donor is still PCR and RIBA positive, whereas the recipient became PCR negative but remained RIBA positive.

Conclusions: This is the first reported case of an open window transmission of HCV by blood products.

0199

TRANSMISSION OF HEPATITIS C BY BLOOD FROM ANTI-HCV POSITIVE DONORS (LOOK-BACK STUDY)

U.Foberg[1], B.Ekermo[2], U.Mathiesen[3], A.Widell[4], A.Frydén[1].
Departments of 1Infectious Diseases, 2Blood Centre and 3Internal Medicine, University Hospital, Linköping, 4Laboratory of Clinical Virology, Malmö General Hospital, Sweden

Objective: The recipients of blood products from 14 anti-HCV screening positive donors were retrospectively traced and tested to assess the contagiousness of the donors. Methods: Donors and recipients were tested for anti-HCV with 2nd generation ELISA and recombinant immunoblot assay (RIBA-2). HCV-RNA was tested for with polymerase chain reaction (PCR). HCV-genotyping was performed with PCR using type specific primers. Results: 10 RIBA-2 and PCR HCV-RNA positive donors had donated blood to 27 now living recipients, of whom 13(48%) were viremic, 6 (22%) RIBA-2 positive but HCV-RNA negative, 4(15%) RIBA-2 indeterminate and HCV-RNA negative, 2(7%) negative in all tests, in 2 (7%) patients data were missing. In viremic individuals the HCV genotype was identical between donor and recipient, spanning from 1a, 1b, 2b to 3a. Four HCV-RNA negative donors, one positive and three indeterminate in RIBA-2, did not transmit HCV infection. Conclusion: In this look-back study HCV-RNA positive blood donors transmitted HCV infection to at least 76% of the recipients. About half of the recipients were still viremic.

0200

HCV RNA AND LIVER HISTOLOGY IN ANTI-HCV RIBA2 INDETERMINATE BLOOD DONORS.

D.Prati, A. Zanella, D. Conte*, C. Capelli, M. Fraquelli*, P. Bosoni, F. Mozzi, L. Calcagno, G. Sirchia. Centro Trasfusionale e di Immunologia dei Trapianti, Ospedale Maggiore and *Cattedra di Gastroenterologia, Ospedale Maggiore, Milano, Italy.

Background: The clinical significance of anti-HCV RIBA2 indeterminate pattern is still unclear. Therefore, liver histology was evaluated and serum and hepatic HCV RNA determined in a large series of RIBA2 indeterminate blood donors. Subjects and Methods: Since the introduction of anti-HCV testing in our center, 112 subjects were found to be RIBA2 indeterminate (M/F 60/52, age 19-65, mean follow-up 12 mo, 104 reactive to c22). All were symptomless and ALT pattern was normal in all but 5 (1 persistently, 4 intermittently altered). 68 of them were eligible for and 40 agreed to undergo liver biopsy (M/F 24/16, age 20-63, 1 with persistently altered ALT). Serum and hepatic HCV RNA were determined by RT-PCR. Results: 10/40 subjects were HCV RNA positive (25%, CI 12-38); one of them had HCV RNA in the liver, but not in the serum. Chronic active hepatitis was found in one and chronic persistent hepatitis in two HCV RNA positive subjects. None of the HCV RNA negative blood donors had histologic evidence of major liver damage. Comments: HCV RNA positive, RIBA2 indeterminate blood donors should be considered for liver biopsy independently of ALT profile, as 30% of our series has chronic hepatitis. The finding that HCV RNA was confined to the liver in one case is consistent with a status of low viral replication carrier.

0201

LOOK-BACK ON HCV-INFECTED BLOOD DONORS.

H. Vrielink[1], C.L. van der Poel[1], H.W. Reesink[1], E. Scholten[1], D. Bresters[1], H.L. Zaaijer[2], H.T.M. Cuypers[2], P.N. Lelie[2]. 1)Red Cross Blood Bank Amsterdam, 2) Central Laboratory Blood Transfusion Service Amsterdam, The Netherlands.

Aim: To establish: 1) the duration of HCV infection in blood donors who recently were found HCV infected, 2) the number of implicated blood products transfused to patients, 3) the number of infected recipients.

Methods: Since May 1990 all blood donations are screened for anti-HCV antibodies. From 1986 serum samples of all donations are stored and all blood products delivered to hospitals are registered in a computer.

Results: 32 ELISA repeatedly reactive donors (10 first time and 22 repeat donors) were HCV infected, confirmed by RIBA-2 (Ortho) and/or cDNA-PCR. From the 22 repeat donors, 213 implicated blood products were issued for transfusion in hospitals and 68 plasma units were used for fractionation. All repeat donors were anti-HCV ELISA (Ortho 2.0) reactive at any time that they had given blood in the past (mean follow up: 39 months, range 4 - 64 months). No seroconversion for HCV was observed in any of the donors. Information was received of 95/213 (45%) recipients. Of these 95 patients, 32 (34%) had died, 47 (49%) were not traced back and 16 (17%) could be tested. Of these recipients, 15/16 (94%) were RIBA-3 and/or cDNA-PCR positive, and 1 (6%) was negative in all tests (EIA-3, RIBA-3 and cDNA-PCR).

Conclusion: All repeat HCV +ve donors were found to be infected with HCV during a mean follow up period of more than 3 years. This implicates that a very high proportion of blood donations, given in the past, from HCV infected donors probably was infectious. Of recipients of HCV infected blood products in the past, 94% became HCV-positive.

0202

EVALUATING APPARENT HAV SEROCONVERSION ASSOCIATED WITH CLOTTING FACTOR CONCENTRATES

Transfusion Safety Study Group[1] represented by J.W.Mosley[2]
1Participating institutions, 2Univ. So. Calif., Los Angeles, CA, USA.

Background: Recent European clusters indicate that HAV can be transmitted by some clotting factor concentrates. Our initial conclusion (*Vox Sang*, in press) that there were no identifiable cases in the Transfusion Safety Study requires further evaluation.
Aim: To define criteria for evaluating apparent HAV seroconversion in concentrate recipients.
Method: A serum repository collected over 8 years identified 34 (4.7%) among 719 persons with congenital clotting disorders who were initially anti-HAV (-) and became (+) by the last specimen. Their serial specimens were tested quantitatively (WHO standard) for anti-HAV-IgG and for anti-IgM (Abbott Laboratories, North Chicago, IL).
Results: 14/34 (41%) did not have the high, sustained anti-HAV-IgG response expected from infection. 13 (38%) others had anti-HAV-IgG positivity coinciding with beginning IVIG therapy for HIV-1 infection, and were IgM (-). The last 7 (21%) persons were IgM (-), but infection by HAV in concentrate is not excluded by present data.
Discussion: Criteria for concentrate-associated HAV infection include a sustained, quantitatively appropriate IgG response beyond the level and duration of sources for passive antibody. Lack of an IgM response does not exclude a new, asymptomatic infection among persons who have lost IgG after a previous infection (*Am J Epidemiol* 1982;115:577). Neither the absence of a known cluster, nor other possible exposures of the individual (*e.g.*, raw clams and oysters) necessarily preclude concentrate as a possible source. (NHLBI Contracts No. NO1-HB-4-7003 and 9-7074.)

0203

POTENTIAL FOR HEV TRANSMISSION BY BLOOD

Transfusion Safety Study Group[1] represented by M.J.Nowicki[2], P.Yarbough[3]
1Participating institutions, 2Univ. So. Calif.,Los Angeles, 3Genelabs Inc., Redwood City, CA, USA.

Background: Like HAV, there is potential for a donor in an endemic/epidemic area to transmit HEV to a susceptible blood recipient. Pooled plasma has a broader potential if S/D inactivation is used alone, particularly if exported from endemic to non-endemic areas for use in populations of the latter.
Aim: To evaluate HEV prevalence among US residents.
Method: Among all study subjects, we selected: 1) persons born, or with one or both parents born, in an endemic country; 2) US-born hemophiliacs (US parents) treated with concentrates; 3) random US donors (controls). Anti-HEV was by EIA (Genelabs).
Results: The table gives the prevalences.

Donor place of birth	No.	(+)
Born in endemic area	97	11 (11%)
Both parents endemic area	62	6 (10%)
1 parent endemic area	36	1 (3%)
US hemophiliacs	276	9 (3%)
US donors (controls)	90	2 (2%)

Chi-square for trend in association with endemic area, 2p<0.001. There were no seroconversions between 1st and last serum in follow-up.
Conclusions: Anti-HEV in the US is strongly associated with endemic/epidemic area background. US plasma concentrates appear safe but plasma derivatives from endemic/epidemic areas may have same potential for transmission as does HAV if S/D inactivation is used alone. (NHLBI Contracts No. NO1-HB-4-7003 and 9-7074.)

0204

PHARMACOKÍNETIC EVALUATION OF A NEW HIGHLY PURIFIED DOUBLE INACTIVATED F.VIII CONCENTRATE

U. Martinowitz, S. Schulman and D. Varon
The National Hemophilia Center, Sheba Medical Center, Tel-Hashomer, Israel.

Several recent reports aroused suspicion that factor concentrates treated with solvent detergent alone may still transmit non lipid coded viruses (such as hepatitis A). Octavi SD Plus® (Octapharma) is a new factor VIII concentrate in which a heat inactivation step was added to reduce this risk. An open, non randomized, cross over pharmacokinetic evaluation was conducted to compare the characteristics of the new product to that of the currently used, Octavi SD. Single doses of 50 IU/kg (based on declared potency) were given to 8 severe hemophilia A patients. Blood samples were drawn according to ISTH recommendation. All calculations using a model independent method were based on the measured potency. No differences were found between Octavi SD and Octavi SD Plus in terms of recovery (1.92±0.41 vs. 1.83±1.59 %/IU/kg), clearance (3.99±1.3 vs. 4.25±1.56 ml/kg/h), terminal half-life (10.2±2.7 vs. 10.8±3.2 h) and volume of distribution (56.2±13.3 vs. 60.9±11.6 mg/kg). We conclude that the addition of heating process does not change the pharmacokinetic characteristics of this factor VIII concentrate.

0205

Inactivation of high titered HIV-1 in single donor preparations of human fresh frozen plasma by methylene blue/light treatment

Bernd Lambrecht[1], Stephen G. Norley[2], Reinhard Kurth[2] and Harald Mohr[1]

[1]German Red Cross, Niedersachsen, Oldenburg and Bremen, Postfach 100109, 31830 Springe, Germany
[2]Paul-Ehrlich-Institut, 63225 Langen, Germany

HIV-1 infectivity in human fresh frozen plasma (FFP), which is collected during the "window period" between infection of the donor and the subsequent seroconversion, cannot be detected by antibody screening tests. In Germany the risk for transfusion associated infection is estimated approx. 1:1,000,000 for HIV-1. The risk may be reduced by quarantine storage in combination with retesting after several months or applying virus inactivation procedures to the plasma. We therefore tested the efficacy of photodynamic virus inactivation by methylene blue (MB)/light treatment. FFP was spiked with highly titered HIV-1 and illuminated with visible light in the presence of 1 μM MB. The infectivity of the virus containing plasma was rapidly lost during illumination (≥ 6.32 log_{10} $TCID_{50}$ after 10 min). Thus our data indicate that the MB/light treatment is an effective method to eliminate the transfusion associated risk of HIV-1 infection through use of photodynamically inactivated FFP.

0206

IMPORTANCE OF TYPE I AND TYPE II REACTIONS IN THE PHOTODYNAMIC INACTIVATION OF VIRUSES WITH METHYLENE BLUE

K. Müller-Breitkreutz, H. Mohr
DRK-Blutspendedienst Niedersachsen, Springe, FRG

We investigated the relative importance of type I and type II mechanisms in the photoinactivation of suid-herpes-virus type 1 (SHV-1) in human plasma and PBS with methylene blue using several quenchers and solvents.

Plasma had an inhibiting effect on virus kill compared with PBS: Treatment of human plasma with 1 μM methylene blue and 15 min illumination with red light (LED_{660}) resulted in 2 log_{10} inactivation of SHV-1 compared with >4.5 log_{10} in PBS.

Quenchers of type I photoreactants such as mannitol (up to 100 mM), katalase and superoxide dismutase (up to 300 U/ml) had no significant effect on the virus inactivation kinetics in PBS and human plasma. In case of the type II (singlet oxygen) quenchers imidazol and histidin, the rate of SHV-1 kill was inhibited, if the quenchers were used in high concentrations (10 - 50 mM). Additionaly, the inactivation of SHV-1 in PBS was enhanced if water was replaced by deuterium oxide (known to prolong the life time of singlet oxygen) and reduced if oxygen was displaced by argon.

Taken together, these results demonstrate that singlet oxygen is one, but probably not the only mediator of the antiviral effects of methylene blue, as there is some virus inactivation even in the absence of molecular oxygen.

0207

EXTENDED INVESTIGATION OF VIRUS INACTIVATION IN PLASMA PRODUCTS BY PASTEURIZATION

J. Hilfenhaus[1], T. Nowak[1], T. Weimer[1], B. Cummins[2]
1 Research Laboratories Behringwerke, Marburg, Germany,
2 White Sands Research Center, Alamogordo, USA

Pasteurization (= 10 hour heat treatment of a stabilized, aqueous plasma protein solution at 60°C) is a method that efficiently inactivates different viruses, e.g. HIV, HSV, poliovirus, HAV. In a recent series of experiments, we investigated whether

- hepatitis C virus (HCV) is inactivated by pasteurization
- a small fraction of heat stable human immunodeficiency virions (HIV) exist in a HIV-preparation
- pasteurization inactivates in addition to infectious viruses also viral genomes, particularly of RNA-viruses, resulting in a negative polymerase chain reaction (PCR).

We were able to show that HCV was efficiently inactivated by pasteurization, because a HCV-spiked stabilized factor VIII sample which was infectious in a chimpanzee, whereas all infectivity was lost after a 6 hour heat treatment at 60°C. When subjecting a number of RNA-viruses to pasteurization, we were able to show that the infectivity of these viruses was destroyed, but the determination of viral genomes by PCR was not influenced. When studying the inactivation kinetics of HIV using stabilized plasma protein samples containing increasing amounts of HIV, we did not find any delay of HIV-inactivation due to more heat stable variants of HIV. From these results we conclude (i) that pasteurization is a method that excellently inactivates HCV, (ii) that a positive PCR for viral genoms in a pasteurized plasma protein sample does not indicate the presence of infectious virus, (iii) that heat-resistant variants of HIV may not occur in high titer HIV-preparations.

0210

CONTROLLED TRIAL OF THE USE OF CYTOMEGALOVIRUS (CMV) - SERONEGATIVE BLOOD PRODUCTS IN PEDIATRIC ONCOLOGY PATIENTS.
S. Desai, J.K. Preiksaitis, S. Roberts, W. Vaudry, J. Akabutu, P. Grundy, B. Wilson, M. Joffre, University of Alberta, Edmonton, Alberta, T6G 2R7, Canada.

Cytomegalovirus (CMV) is known to be transmitted by blood transfusion. It has been suggested that transfused CMV-seronegative oncology patients who may require bone marrow transplantation in the future should receive CMV-"safe" blood to prevent transfusion-acquired CMV infection. In order to validate this recommendation a randomized study was done of 71 CMV seronegative pediatric oncology patients (25 with solid tumor; 45 with lymphoid malignancy). Patients were followed monthly with throat swabs and urine for CMV isolation and serology (IgG and IgM) by EIA for one year after their last transfusion and six monthly thereafter. The mean length of follow-up is 20.7 months with a range of 1 to 47 months. Patients were randomized to receive unscreened (32) or CMV-seronegative (30) cellular blood products (cbp) (platelets and rbc). The patients received a total of 729 rbc units, mean 10.3 ± 10.6 units, range 0-39 units and a total of 1,184 platelet units, mean 16.7 ± 21.9 units, range 0-123 units. 34.5% of all cbp received by patients given unscreened blood were anti-CMV IgG positive, 0.4% of all cbp were anti-CMV IgM positive. Two patients developed asymptomatic CMV infection, one in each study arm. CMV infection occurred 10 and 12 months after transfusion suggesting a community-acquired rather than transfusion-acquired infection in both cases. Transfusion-acquired CMV infection is uncommon in pediatric oncology patients and the use of CMV-seronegative blood to prevent this complication cannot be justified.

0211

INTRAUTERINE TRANSFUSION FOR TREATMENT OF HYDROPS FETALIS CAUSED BY PARVOVIRUS INFECTION
A.A. Konugres, V.C. Smith
Brigham & Women's Hospital and Harvard Medical School, Boston, USA

A high proportion of the nonimmune hydropic fetuses have hematologic changes suggestive of fetal infection. Profound anemia in cases of nonimmune hydrops has been caused by B-19 parvovirus. The increased capabilities of transfusing fetal patients enables us to treat hydrops fetalis due to anemia.

A 30-year-old woman, with 4 previous uncomplicated term pregnancies, at 16 weeks gestation showed fetal ascites on ultrasound, which increased on follow-up scans. The patient had undocumented exposure to a parvovirus infection 3-4 weeks earlier. Antibody screen, VDRL, TORCH titers and the Kleihauer Betke were negative; karyotype was normal (46 XX). The fetal blood was positive for B-19 parvovirus. On percutaneous blood sampling (PUBS) at 19 weeks, fetal Hct was 3. The patient underwent an uncomplicated 30 cc intra-abdominoperitoneal transfusion. At 19.5 weeks, the fetus remained hydropic, Hct 15. A 25 cc intravascular blood transfusion (IVTR) was given. At 20.3 weeks, the fetus had continued ascites and scalp edema, Hct 41. A 15 cc IVTR was given. The fetus had a total of 3 blood transfusions. Subsequently, the fetus did well with a gradual resolution of ascites. At term, the patient delivered a healthy female. All reported untreated cases of nonimmune hydrops caused by parvovirus B-19 resulted in fetal or neonatal death. The etiology of hydrops in parvovirus infection is probably an inhibition of fetal erythropoiesis resulting in severe anemia.

0213

SIGNIFICANCE OF ANTI-HBc SCREENING OF BLOOD DONORS IN AN EPIDEMIOLOGICALLY LOW RISK POPULATION
Susanna Wessberg, Ruth Naukkarinen, Tom Krusius: Finnish Red Cross Blood Transfusion Service, Helsinki, Finland
HBV infections are rare in Finland. During the last three years 0.07 % of new blood donors have been HBsAg positive. The annual seroconversion rate among known donors has been 0.01 %. About 360.000 blood components are transfused annually in Finland and on the average only 1 case of PTHB can be confirmed. To reduce the risk of PTHB blood donors are tested in many countries in addition to HBsAg for anti-HBc. In populations with high prevalence of HBV serologic markers increased infectivity has been found to be associated with donors with a high titer anti-HBc. We have analyzed 14.970 consecutive blood donors in Finland for anti-HBc and correlated the results with those of anti-HBs, ALT and HBV PCR. 188 (1.26 %) of the donors were repeatedly anti-HBc positive. None of the donors was positive for HBsAg or IgM class anti-HBc. Out of the 188 donors 76 (40 %) had no detectable anti-HBs and 74 of these 76 donors were anti-HBc negative after reduction (microparticle based anti-HBc method) suggesting a false positive anti-HBc result by the EIA method used for screening. 32 out of the 188 anti-HBc positive donors were also positive in 1:60 dilution and 1 of them was anti-HBs negative. All the strongly anti-HBc positive donors were HBV DNA negative by PCR. The results suggest that a conventional anti-HBc screening EIA is nonspecific and that anti-HBc is an inefficient method for screening of potential HBV infectivity in an epidemiologically low risk population.

0214

TRANSMISSION OF HEPATITIS B VIRUS BY HBV-DNA PCR NEGATIVE BLOOD TRANSFUSION.
C.L. van der Poel[1], J.H. ten Veen[2], H.W. Reesink[1], H.T.M. Cuypers[3], P.N. Lelie[3], 1) Red Cross Blood Bank Amsterdam, 2) Prinsengracht Hospital, Amsterdam, 3) Central Lab RC Blood Transfusion Service Amsterdam, The Netherlands.

Background: Blood donations collected during the open window (HBsAg -ve) period of an Hepatitis B Virus (HBV) infection may transmit HBV to recipients. In such cases HBV-DNA PCR may detect HBV below the detection limits of serological tests.

Case report: A case of acute post-transfusion hepatitis B was reported to the Blood Bank. A recipient received 4 red cell transfusions, and developed acute hepatitis B 15 weeks after transfusion (HBsAg +ve, HBeAg +ve, ALT elevated). Implicated blood donations were traced by automated blood bank registration system. In our Blood Bank a serum sample from every blood donation is kept frozen since 1984; stored sera from implicated donations (all negative by HBsAg ELISA) were re-tested by HBV-DNA PCR and HBsAg RIA. All implicated donations were PCR and RIA negative. Independently, 2 months after the implicated transfusion, one of the implicated blood donors reported to have had an icteric period 4-5 weeks after the implicated donation, later diagnosed as acute hepatitis B (HBsAg positive, anti-HBc positive, anti-HBs negative).

Conclusion: This is the first reported case of HBV transmission by a blood product donated during a HBV-DNA PCR negative period of the open window phase of the donor. HBV-DNA PCR negative blood may contain infectious HBV in levels below the detection limits.

0215

ACUTE HEPATITIS B INFECTION IN A MULTI-TRANSFUSED PATIENT PROVEN UNRELATED TO TRANSFUSIONS BY HBV-DNA SEQUENCING.

B. Ekermo[1], H.Norder[2], J.O Hildén[1], L. Magnius[2],
1Blood Centre, University Hospital, Linköping, 2Swedish Institute for Infectious Disease Control, Sweden.

A 9-yr-old boy with congenital pure red cell aplasia (PRCA) and chronically dependant on transfusion therapy, developed acute hepatitis B infection. The transfusions were given during 2-3 days at hospital every two to three weeks.
Samples from implicated donors were negative in HBV serology including anti-HBc.
However a 10-yr-old immigrant child from Kosovo in Jugoslavia, chronic carrier of hepatitis B surface antigen (HBsAg) and e antigen, was treated at the same nursing ward during several months before the outbreak of hepatitis in the first patient. HBV-DNA from blood samples of both patients were amplified by polymerase chain reaction (PCR) and part of the S gene was sequenced. An hitherto unique nucleotide sequence leading to an amino acid substitution was found in both samples, linking the two patients to each other. Sequence data from 183 other patients or HBV carriers differed from our two patients.
We conclude that results from sequencing of PCR amplificates are of great value in establishing routes of HBV transmission.

0216

DETECTION OF HBsAg VARIANTS IN HEPANOSTIKA HBsAg MONOCLONAL, HEPANOSTIKA HBsAg UNI-FORM I AND HEPANOSTIKA HBsAg UNI-FORM II SCREENING AND CONFIRMATORY TEST

I. de Boer[1], J.J. Gray[2], J.A. Hellings[1]
[1] Organon Teknika B.V., Boxtel, The Netherlands
[2] Addenbrooke's Hospital, Cambridge, England

Purpose of the evaluation
Recently, a number of HBsAg variants have been reported which have point mutations causing amino acid substitutions in the "a" determinant. The point mutations which have been described most frequently result in a substitution of arginine for glycine at amino acid 145. Arginine 145 variants have been reported from all over the world. These variants have been detected, for instance, in transplant patients whose grafts became re-infected despite treatment with monoclonal anti-HBs.

Materials/Methods
A large panel from a Japanese patient consisting of 1 pre-transplant (wild-type) and 16 post-transplant (145 mutant) follow-up samples has been studied in our assays. The anti-HBs mouse monoclonals used for coating in the Hepanostika HBsAg Monoclonal and the Hepanostika HBsAg Uni-Form I are different from the ones that are used in the Hepanostika HBsAg Uni-Form II. Therefore the mutant sera were evaluated in all three HBsAg screening assays. They all contain polyclonal sheep anti-HBs HRP conjugate. Four 145-mutant sera were tested in the Hepanostika HBsAg Uni-Form II confirmatory assay.

Results
The pre-transplant sample from the Japanese patient contains the wild-type HBsAg and reacts positive in all HBsAg assays. The first four post-transplant samples react negative in all HBsAg assays because in that period the patient was given human monoclonal anti-HBs, that neutralizes the wild-type HBsAg. In accordance with the results found with PCR, after the monoclonal antibody administration the HBsAg Monoclonal, the HBsAg Uni-Form I and the HBsAg Uni-Form II assay detect the 145-mutant and give high S/COV ratios. The four samples, that were all taken after the monoclonal antibody administration, are correctly neutralized by the polyclonal macaque anti-HBs and give correct strong positive results in the control wells.

Conclusion
Hepanostika HBsAg Monoclonal, Hepanostika HBsAg Uni-Form I and Hepanostika HBsAg Uni-Form II screening and confirmatory test correctly detect the arginine 145 HBsAg variant.

0218

STORAGE OF RED CELLS AND PLATELETS FOLLOWING GAMMA IRRADIATION.

G. Moroff[1], S. Holme[2], J. AuBuchon[3], A. Heaton[2], J. Sweeney[2]
1American Red Cross, Rockville, MD, 2Mid Atlantic Region, Norfolk, VA, 3Dartmouth-Hitchcock Medical Center, Lebanon, NH, USA.

Gamma irradiation(γ) is being used extensively to prevent transfusion-associated graft-versus-host disease. A paired study approach with post-treatment storage of non-irradiated(NI) and irradiated(I) [2500 cGy, Cs-137] red cells and platelet units was utilized to assess the retention of in vivo viability and in vitro properties. Mean in vivo 24-hour recovery and survival time (T 1/2 - ^{51}Cr loss, no correction for elution) for ADSOL-preserved red cells stored in PL 2209 containers were as follows:

Day of γ	Total Storage (Days)	Recovery(%) NI	Recovery(%) I	Survival(Days) NI	Survival(Days) I	n
1	28	84.2	78.6	28.0	26.0	16
14	42	76.3	69.5	26.4	25.4	16
14	28	85.2	82.3	26.3	26.4	8
26	28	82.1	81.7	27.7	26.8	5

Although extracellular K^+ was substantially increased by γ, other in vitro red cell properties were comparable. Viability and in vitro properties of CS-3000 (TNX-6) platelets after 5 days of storage were not influenced by γ on day 1 (n=4) or day 3 (n=4). With day 1 γ, the mean recovery of NI and I platelets was 52 and 51 %; platelet survivals were 6.1 and 6.1 days. These studies define acceptable storage conditions after γ.

0219

ASSESSMENT OF LIPID PEROXIDATION IN STORED RED CELLS BY MR-RELAXATION MEASUREMENTS

H.P.Benn[1], C.Bleckmann[1], B.Dresow[2], R.Engelhardt[2], R.Fischer[2], R.Maas[3], P.Kuehnl[1]. [1]Transfusionsmedizin, [2]Med. Biochemie, [3]Radiologie, Universitätsklinik Eppendorf, Hamburg, FRG.

Introduction and Methods: During long-time storage membrane compounds of red cell concentrates (RBC) are affected by lipid peroxidation (LPO). High oxygen tension, and large amounts of hemoglobin iron generate free radicals known as initiators of LPO which was assessed by magnetic resonance measurements (MR). MR proton relaxation times (T_1 and T_2) of the RBC were obtained on the day of blood donation and weekly thereafter, with a mixed sequence (Gyroscan S15, at 20 °C).

Results: T_1 was nearly constant within the first 3 weeks of storage (1084 ± 44 ms), but decreased continuously during the following time (1004 ± 49 ms between week 3 and 5, 900 ± 60 ms afterwards). T_2 was roughly stable over the entire time interval (139 ±10 ms). In the fast exchange two-state model (FETS), T_1 is determined predominantly by interactions between macromolecules and single bound hydration layers, whereas T_2 is dominated by exchange diffusion of water between bound and free water phases and by the paramagnetic dipole-dipole interaction of hemoglobin.

Conclusion: Due to LPO, macromolecular changes and alterations of the red cell membrane, occur after 3 weeks storage. This early impairment during storage was detected by non-destructive MR-relaxation measurements, which may be an additional tool for quality assessment of storage solutions.

0220

BIOTIN LABELING OF RED CELLS FOR IN VIVO SURVIVAL STUDIES

F. Rossi, A. Guffanti, S. Fumagalli, P. Rebulla, G. Sirchia. Centro Trasfusionale e di Immunologia dei Trapianti, Ospedale Maggiore Policlinico, Milano, Italy.

Red cells labeled with water-soluble long-chain biotin and detected by fluorescent (FITC) streptavidin and flow-cytometric analysis have been used for determination of red cell survival in animals and measurement of red cell mass in man. To assess optimal biotinylation of human red cells, 1 ml of biotin solution at concentration ranging from 1 to 6 mg/mL was used to label 0.5 mL of red cell suspensions with concentration ranging from 1 to 6 $x10^6$/µL; the amount of biotin per red cell ranged from 0.4 to 12 pg. One pg of biotin per cell was sufficient to label more than 99% of red cells. Hemolysis was not observed at any tested biotin concentration. The best labeling was obtained by using 4 mg/mL biotin solution for $4x10^6$ red cells/µL. Biotinylated red cells were detected by adding 10 µL of streptavidin-FITC (1 mg/mL) to 10^7 red cells suspended in 1 mL of PBS. Fresh red cells collected in ACD and EDTA, and donor red cells stored in SAGM up to 42 days took up the same amount of biotin uniformly. No biotin elution was demonstrated during 4 week storage at 4° C in PBS. A mixture of 0.3% labeled and 99.7% unlabeled red cells was prepared to simulate the dilution of 15 mL of labeled cells (Hct 0.5) in 4,500 mL of blood volume. The coefficient of variation of the assay, assessed by counting 10^6 cells for 6 times, was <5%. A volunteer healthy subject was injected with 15 mL of autologous biotinylated red cells; a distinct peak of labeled cells was detected up to 30 days after infusion. These preliminary results support the opportunity of further investigating biotin labeling as a possible alternative to the use of radionuclides in red cell survival studies.

0221

IMPROVED VIABILITY OF RED CELLS STORED IN AN ADDITIVE SOLUTION CONTAINING GLYCEROL

U.J. Dumaswala, N. Rugg, C.M. Allen, T.J.Greenwalt
Hoxworth Blood Center, University of Cincinnati Medical Center, Cincinnati, Ohio, USA.

The purpose of this research was to establish whether a hypoosmolar additive solution containing glycerol (EAS-25) would improve the preservation of red blood cells (RBCs). The ingredients of EAS-25/Adsol® in mM were: adenine 2/2, dextrose 110/122, mannitol 55/42, NaCl 50/154, glycerol 150/0; mosm/kg of non-penetrating components 109/196. Packed RBCs from citrate-phosphate-dextrose units of blood were divided by weight into two aliquots. One aliquot was stored with an equal volume of EAS-25; the other with Adsol®. The research protocol was approved by our Institutional Review Board. The salient data after nine weeks of storage are in the table. Supernatant K^+ and shed vesicle

	ATP µmol/gHb	24h ^{51}Cr Recovery	% Hemolysis
EAS-25	2.15±0.58	73.0±4.2	0.52±0.20
Adsol®	1.87±0.29	60.9±7.1	1.18±0.54
P	0.11	0.01	0.001

n=7;mean±SD; initial ATP=4.48±0.30;P by student's t-test.

membrane proteins were significantly less in EAS-25 and the MCVs were significantly larger. These data indicate that RBCs stored in a hypoosmolar solution with glycerol are better preserved than in Adsol®.

0223

SMALL POOL HEAT-TREATED INTERMEDIATE-PURITY FACTOR VIII CONCENTRATE : A STRATEGY FOR DEVELOPING COUNTRIES

I Petersen, A Bird

Western Province BTS, Cape Town

We report a 2-year experience with the production of a small pool, heat-treated intermediate purity Factor VIII (FVIII) concentrate. The method involves pooling of 7-8 cryoprecipitate units and modification of a glycine/sodium chloride precipitation procedure to yield intermediate purity FVIII. The recovered FVIII is resuspended in buffer, lyophilised and then subjected to heating at 80°C for 72 hours. The mean yield of FVIII is 4µ/mg protein indicative of a consistent intermediate purity product. Recovery studies were performed on 3 severe haemophiliacs: mean FVIII recovery was 94% and mean biological half-life was 8.3 hours. To date we have produced 11 680 bottles of FVIII with a mean yield of 618 units per bottle, based on random testing. This converts to ± 316 µ/ℓ plasma processed. Although we have no data on previously untested patients, there have been no HIV seroconversions in the haemophiliacs treated with this product and few reactions have been reported. We believe that this product has potential for production in developing countries unable to afford more highly-purified products since it does not require a sophisticated manufacturing plant.

0224

DEVELOPING UGANDA BLOOD TRANSFUSION SERVICE

E.J.Watson-Williams,P.Kataaha,J.Goddard
Nakasero Blood Bank, MOH, Kampala, Uganda.

Purpose. In 1987 the AIDS TASK FORCE of the E.E.C. funded the rehabilitation of Nakasero Blood Bank as the headquarters of the UBTS. Additional funding in 1991 provided four regional blood centres and 'safe' blood for all 92 hospitals in Uganda. We analyse the first five years of this programme.

Results. As the programme developed numbers of donors and percent of voluntary donors increased, whilst frequency of anti-HIV and other causes of discard and outdating, and cost of each unit transfused, decreased.

Table 1. Units of blood collected, discarded and used 1989-1993

Year	Donors	%Vols.	HIV+ve	HBsAg	Other	Outdate	%used	$/unit
1989	6588	53.3	956	.-.	103	58	83.0	53.8
1990	13806	47.7	1910	769	149	984	72.4	53.1
1991	18392	51.6	1612	920	610	936	77.8	47.8
1992	29104	64.6	1867	1880	870	1086	80.4	39.5
1993*	32100	65.4	1782	2025	962	1129	81.6	35.5

*1993 figures are provisional.

Table 2. Annual expenditures for UBTS 1989-1993 US$ X 1000

Year	Build.	Equip.	Suppls.	Staff	Transpt	Other	Training	Total
1989	4.0	12.0	116	32.1	24.5	5.1	90	294.5
1990	38.3	55.8	273	51.1	40.8	21.2	90	570.2
1991	38.3	55.8	325	79.8	46.2	24.9	112	684.0
1992	42.5	87.8	375	123.5	104.5	25.9	164	923.2
1993	42.5	93.2	355	199.6	102.6	32.0	105	929.9

The capital cost of buildings is spread over fourteen years and that of vehicles and equipment is spread over four years.

Conclusion. 1. The funding from ATF has made 'safe' blood transfusion in Uganda possible. 2. International aid for blood transfusion in developing countries should be increased.

0225

BLOOD COLLECTION SYSTEM AT THE K.E.M.HOSPITAL, BOMBAY.

DR.MAYA PARIHAR & DR V.RAY.

Dept.of Transfusion Medicine
K.E.M.Hospital,Parel,Bombay-12 (INDIA)

Commercial blood banks have been an integral part of the blood donor system in India. Professional paid donors still meet 29% of the requirement. (Range 0-96%, Bombay 15%).

We have reviewed the blood collection system at our centre, which is the largest hospital-based blood bank in Bombay. Paid donors were banned since 1976 and the voluntary donor system encouraged. Presently our collection is 19 units /bed/yr and the acute shortages felt in the begining of the programme are uncommon. From 1976 -1993 about 4,61,309 blood units have been collected, with 1% repeat donors. (Voluntary-60%; Relative replacement-40%; M:F = 8:1). A reverse situation is observed in a highly motivated and captive donor population like an industry, where 36% of the donors were retained with 7.4% having donated more than 5 times.

Now ,our donor motivation programme is geared to increase donor retention through education at outdoor camps and adoption of patients requiring regular transfusions, eg.Thalassaemics. This interaction between donors and patients enhances commitment to the donor programme.

0226

BLOOD DONATION IN VIETNAM

Nguyen Chi Tuyen, et al. National Institute of Haematology and Blood Transfusion, Bach Mai Hospital, Hanoi, Vietnam.

Up to 1992 every donation is paid, the price of 100ml being fixed by both the Ministry of Health and the Ministry of Finance. Only people of low socio-economic background give their blood. In effect they sell their blood to satisfy their needs to some extent. As giving blood for money is considered as a shameful action, everybody tries to keep it secret when doing so. The healthy economical secure people fear the consequence of the venepunctures, thinking that with each drop of blood lost they will lose part of their lives.

- Population of Vietnam: 71,061,053
- Number of patient beds: 221,224
- Theoretical need of blood: 888,000 litres = 3.5 million units (1 unit = 250ml)
- Collected blood in 1992: 34,152 litres = 136,608 units (representing only 3.84 percent)
- Blood donors registered (paid donors): 87.6 percent
(family and replacement donors, unpaid): 12.4 percent
- Percentage of blood donations on the total population: 0.19 percent
- Number of blood units per patient bed: 0.61

0227

THERAPEUTIC DOSE OF PERIPHERAL BLOOD PROGENITOR CELLS (PBP)

Reich L, Raptis G, Vahdat L, Fennelly D, Schneider J, Shapiro F, Gulati S, Norton L, Bengala C, Crown J. Memorial Sloan-Kettering Cancer Center, New York, NY, U.S.A.

PBP have been recognized as being instrumental in shortening the nadir cytopenia that follows high dose chemotherapy. The lower threshold of PBP necessary for this autograft is still unclear. It has been reported that the number of CD34+ cells in the product correlates with the speed of recovery. We have treated 60 stage IV breast cancer patients with 116 cycles of PBP. Flow cytometry was utilized for quantification of the total CD34+ cells. The patients were peripheralized with G-CSF, CTX $3gm/M^2$ + G-CSF and CTX $5gm/M^2$ + G-CSF. The harvests were performed at the time that patients peripheral white cells count was ≥ $1.0x10^9$. Patients who received G-CSF only yielded one tenth of the $CD34^+$ cells that were harvested when they were recovering from CTX $5mg/M^2$ + G-CSF.
All the patients who received more than $1.0xE^6$ CD34+ cells/kg/cycle had an ANC ≥ 500 in 13 days or less and 90% had platelets ≥ 20 in 15 days or less. Clearly more CD34+ cells were harvested with CTX $5g/m^2$ + G-CSF, however, 76% of these patients had to be admitted for nadir fever whereas only 29% needed admission after CTX $3gm/M^2$ + G-CSF. Since reinfusing more than 1.0 x E^6 CD34+ cells did not significantly shorten cytopenia, we conclude that it is unnecessary to peripheralize patients with CTX at higher doses than $3gm/M^2$ since 1.0 x E^6/kg CD34+ cells can be collected easily after this peripheralization regime.

0228

HAEMOTHERAPY AND HAEMATOLOGICAL RECONSTITUTION AFTER PERIPHERAL BLOOD STEM CELL (PBSC) TRANSPLANTATION

K.P.Krause, M.John[1], W.Schultze[1], M.Straube[1], G.Matthes
Department of Transfusion Medicine, [1]Bone Marrow Transplantation Unit, University Hospital (Charité), Humboldt University Berlin, Germany

PBSC transplantation became a new and widening field in transfusion medicine. Recently, peripheral blood has been used as a source of human haematopoietic progenitor cells for autologous and in near future allogeneic transplantation. The transfusion of these cells enables the physician to increase the doses of chemotherapy in the treatment of haematological malignancies and solid tumours.
After ultra-highdose chemotherapy (and TBI) 30 patients with haematological malignancies (9 LG, 5 NHL, 4 MM, 2 CML) or solid tumours (6 Mamma tumours, 2 testicular tumours, 1 sarcoma, 1 neuroblastoma) were transfused with $7.7*10^8$ MNC/kg bw. ($1*10^8$-$4*10^9$), $5.3*10^5$ CFU-C/kg bw. ($6*10^4$-$2*10^6$) and $10*10^6$ CD34 positive cells/kg bw. ($1*10^5$-$2*10^7$).
In every case an engraftment occurred. The nadir of granulocyte and platelet count occurred on day 6 and 7, respectively. Granulocytes reached again 500/µl on day 13 (9-23), platelets reached 20.000/µl on day 10 (5-16) and patients could be dismissed from the ward 23 (18-35) days after starting with ultra-highdose chemotherapy, e.g. 15 days after transplantation.
During their stay at the ward the patients were transfused at average with 7 erythrocyte and 7 single donor platelet concentrates. After dismissal their blood cell count recovered during the next 2 to 6 month and reached normal values after 2 month regarding platelets and granulocytes and 6 month regarding erythrocytes. In contrary to the cell count there was a sustaining lack in the patients immune system also after 12 month. The CD4/CD8 ratio, the absolute CD3- and CD4-count were significantly lower in comparison to the normal population as a sign of impaired immune system.

0229

PERIPHERAL BLOOD STEM CELL VERSUS BONE MARROW TRANSPLANTATION. HAEMATOLOGICAL RECOVERY AND MANAGEMENT.

M Torrabadella, L Massuet, A Cabanillas, E Argelagués and C Martín-Vega
Banc de Sang de l'ICS. Barcelona. Spain.

Peripheral blood stem cells (PBSC) are an alternative to bone marrow stem cells (BMSC) when used for bone marrow rescue. The aim of our study is to compare these methods. Between January 1993 and November 1993, 16 leukaphereses were performed in our Centre to obtain PBSC in 14 neoplasic patients. Chemotherapy and G-CSF was used for mobilization. This data were compared with those obtained from 16 BMSC over a similar period of time. The mean-in hospital time was 19 days (range 13-28) and 29 days (range 12-45) for PBSC and BMSC-transplanted patients, respectively (P=0.05).The granulocyte count (GC) reached $0.5x10^9/L$ in 12 days(range 6-28) in PBSC-transplanted patients and in 24 days (range 10-60) for those BMSC-transplanted patients (P=0.001). Platelet count (PC) reached $20x10^9/L$ in 16 days (range 9-49) in PBSC-transplanted patients, and 32 days (range 11-91) in those who were BMSC-transplanted (P<0.001). We found no statistically significant differences in the number of packed red cells transfused to both groups of patients. The average number of platelet transfusions was 3 (range 1-8) and 11 (range 1-25) in PBSC and BMSC-transplantated patients, respectively (P=0.003). **Conclusions:** 1. In-hospital time is shorter in PBSC than it is in BMSC-transplanted patients. 2. GC and PC recovered more quickly in patients transplanted with PBSC than in those with BMSC. 3. PBSC-transplanted group received fewer platelet transfusions.

0230

PERIPHERAL BLOOD HEMATOPOIETIC STEM CELLS KINETICS FOLLOWING CHEMOTHERAPY: CORRELATION WITH RETICULOCYTE MATURATION.

B. Houwen, L. K. Lebeck, L. Chang, E. Choo, A. A. Bedros, Loma Linda University Medical School, Loma Linda, USA.

Peripheral blood from 10 consecutive, mainly pediatric patients, suffering from various forms of cancer, were analyzed for changes in reticulocyte maturation index (RMI), as an early indicator for bone marrow recovery after cytotoxic chemo-therapy. RMI was determined as the fraction of highly and medium fluorescent reticulocytes on a Sysmex reticulocyte analyzer (R-1000). The presence of circulating hematopoietic stem cells (characterized by $CD34^+/CD38^-$) and progenitor cells ($CD34^+/CD38^+$) was determined by flow cytometry (Facscan, Becton Dickinson). In addition, routine hematologic parameters were determined on a new hematology analyzer, the Sysmex SE-9000.
We found that changes in RMI coincided with, or preceded (by 1 to 2 days) a significant increase of stem cells and progenitor cells in the peripheral blood. The range for stem cells was 0.02 - 10.81 %, for progenitor cells 0.05 - 3.99 % of white blood cells. Also we observed that stem cells and progenitor cells could be identified as separate entities on the SE-9000. Often stem cells could be detected for a single day only, but as a relatively high proportion of the WBC population. These findings may have implications for determining the timing for peripheral blood stem cell harvests as well as for the scheduling of different types of chemotherapy.

0231

PERIPHERAL BLOOD STEM CELL COLLECTION FROM HEALTHY VOLUNTEER DONORS MOBILIZED BY RECOMBINANT HUMAN GRANULOCYTE COLONY-STIMULATING FACTOR

T.A. Takahashi[1], Y. Mogi[1], T. Nakase[1], K. Sawada[2], N. Sato[2], T. Koike[2], K. Ozawa[3], S. Asano[3], S. Sekiguchi[1]
[1]Hokkaido Red Cross Blood Center, Sapporo, [2]Hokkaido University, Sapporo, [3]The Institute of Medical Science, The University of Tokyo, Tokyo, Japan.

To investigate the feasibility of collecting a sufficient number of peripheral blood stem cells from healthy volunteer donors for use in allogeneic transplantation as a substitute for bone marrow transplantation, we examined the optimal dose of recombinant human granulocyte colony-stimulating factor (rhG-CSF), the administration period necessary to mobilize stem cells to peripheral blood, the timing for stem cell collection by apheresis and the side effects of rhG-CSF.

Stem cells and progenitor cells were mobilized from bone marrow to peripheral blood by subcutaneous injection of rhG-CSF at the dose of 2 µg/kg/day for longer than 3 days. The number of granulocyte-macrophage colony-forming units (GM-CFU) in peripheral blood increased 15 fold (n=12), after injection of rhG-CSF (2 µg/kg) for 5 days, and had increased 20-fold at 24 hours after the last injection. Six thousand milliliters of blood was processed with a Fenwal CS 3000 Plus on the day after the last injection of rhG-CSF and about 150×10^5 GM-CFU were collected from the donors injected at the dose of 2 µg/kg for 5 days. No severe side effects were observed among donors injected with rhG-CSF.

0232

HÜFFNER MEMORIAL SYMPOSIUM: ANALYTICAL AND PHYSIOLOGICAL ASPECTS OF 100 YEARS OF HEMOGLOBIN RESEARCH

ICSH, the International Council for Standardization in Haematology (organizer)
ICSH Secretariat, Haematology Dept., Western Infirmary, Dumbarton Rd., Glasgow G11 6NT, UK

100 Years ago G. Hüffner published his definitive paper in which the oxygen (O_2) capacity of hemoglobin (Hb) is given as 1.34 ml O_2 per g, and the relative molecular mass, derived from the iron content of the Hb monomer as 16 622 (Arch. Anat. Physiol., physiol. Abt., 130, 1894). The corrected value of 16 114.5 for the relative molecular mass was determined in the early 1960ties (G. Braunitzer, Bibl. Haemat. 18, 59, 1964). With a Hb iron content of 0.347%, the theoretical O_2 capacity should thus be 1.39 ml O_2 per g Hb. Careful measurements, however, have shown that there are always 1-2% dyshemoglobins present (P. Dijkhuizen et al., Pflügers Arch. 369, 223, 1977) and that the total Hb concentration must be corrected for these before the value of 1.39 per g Hb can be applied.

This commemorative symposium will highlight advances in the spectrophotometric determination of Hb and Hb derivatives, and, using dedicated photometers, the measurement of Hb O_2 saturation in the laboratory and in alternate sites; will discuss clinical and therapeutic considerations surrounding hemoglobin variants; and will summarize advances in the search for (synthetic) blood substitutes and how these could affect routine or acute-care hematological measurements Speakers include O.W. van Assendelft, B. Houwen, A.L. van Kessel, R.M. Winslow, A. Zwart, W.G. Zijlstra, and others. Further particulars will be available at the Congress venue.

0234

PASSIVE IMMUNOTHERAPY IN AIDS : A DOUBLE BLIND RANDOMISED PHASE II STUDY

Lefrère JJ*, Vittecoq D** and the French Passive Immunotherapy Collaborative Study Group.
*INTS, hôpital Saint-Antoine, Paris
**Hôpital Paul-Brousse, Villejuif, France.

The aim of this study was to determine the long term efficacy of passive immunotherapy in the treatment of symptomatic HIV infection. The phase I was published in 1992 in the *JID.* The present study was a prospective double blind phase II trial and started in June 1990); the trial was attended to include 180 CDC IV patients randomized in 2 groups : plasma rich in anti-p24 antibody (HIV+P), standard seronegative plasma (HIV-P). Each patient received infusion of HIV+P or HIV-P every 14 days over a one-year period, in addition to zidovudine and other prophylactic treatments. To obtain HIV+P, donors were selected among symptomless anti-HIV+ individuals with CD4>400, absence of hepatitis C and B markers, normal transaminase concentration, high concentration of anti-p24 antibody (Abbott). HIV+P and HIV-P were heated at 56°C before infusion. According to the request of the steering committee, the inclusion of patients ceased in July 1993. At this time, 86 patients were included. A significant difference was observed between both groups in the delay of appearance of the onset of first AIDS defining event (p<0.009, log-rank) and in the cumulative number of events (p<0.0008, Wilcoxon) over the study period ; 7 deaths occured in the treated group within the study period, versus 11 in the control group.

0235

RECONSTITUTED HIGH DENSITY LIPOPROTEIN (RHDL): PREPARATION AND PHYSIOLOGICAL PROPERTIES.

Lerch PG, Doran JE, Hubsch AP, Casas AT, Moudry R, Amstutz HP, Omar A, Morgenthaler JJ
ZLB Central Laboratory SRC, Bern, Switzerland

We have isolated apolipoprotein A-I (apoA-I) from precipitates obtained by cold-ethanol fractionation of human plasma by methods suitable for large-scale production. Reconstituted high density lipoproteins (rHDL) were then prepared from apoA-I and lipids (molar ratios 1:150) by cholate dialysis. The physicochemical properties of the particles obtained were investigated by electrophoresis, gel chromatography, electron microscopy, and CD spectral analysis. At this protein to lipid ratio, a discrete pattern of particle sizes was obtained. The preparation supplied as a lyophilized powder is stable, virus safe, and pyrogen free.

Since HDL is known to be involved in the removal of excess cholesterol from tissues, as well as to interact with lipopolysaccharides (LPS), we tested rHDL for its ability to modulate cholesterol transport and for its anti-LPS properties. rHDL induced a dose-dependent efflux of cholesterol from LDL-loaded cells (J774 and endothelial cells); it dose-dependently decreased LPS-induced production of tumor necrosis factor (TNF; protein and mRNA) by mononuclear cells as well as LPS-induced expression of endothelial cell adhesion molecules. In a rabbit endotoxemia model, rHDL reduced LPS-induced TNF production and significantly decreased the severity of shock.

In summary, we have prepared a product suitable for intravenous infusion which may be useful in the treatment or prevention of septic shock and may have a potential use in atherosclerosis.

0236

Direct Capture of Cryosupernatant Plasma FVIII:C by Anion-exchange Chromatography.

D G Woodfield, L C Teh.
Auckland Regional Blood Services, Auckland, New Zealand

Recent studies* indicate that FVIII:C can be directly captured from fresh plasma by ion-exchange chromatography. This results in substantial improvements in the yield of FVIII:C/kg plasma.

The most common method of extracting Factor VIII:C from plasma is by cryoprecipitation. However, only about 40% of the Factor VIII:C is recovered, with the remainder left in the cryosupernatant plasma.

To recover the Factor VIII:C from cryosupernatant, an ion-exchange method has been used, similar to that used for plasma. Frozen cryosupernatant was thawed, and batch stirred with DEAE-Sephadex A50. After filtration and dilution, it was loaded onto a column packed with DEAE-Fractogel TSK 650 M. Unwanted proteins were largely not absorbed and the bound FVIII:C was eluted by increasing the ionic strength of the buffer. An overall yield of 200 IU Factor VIII:C/kg of plasma was obtained, equivalent to a 60% recovery of FVIII:C present in the cryosupernatant. The enriched FVIII:C eluate contained traces of albumin, ceruloplasmin, fibrinogen, fibronectin and prothrombinex complex factors.

This technique, by permitting a yield of FVIII:C from cryosupernatant and thus increasing the total amount of FVIII:C available from a given volume of whole plasma, may prove useful in FVIII:C processing methods. Further developmental studies are now required to extend these observations and to assess the potential of the methodology.

*. Teh LC, Froger H, Vox Sanguinis 1994. In press.

0237

A NEW LIQUID ANTI-D IGG FOR I.V. USE

M. Stucki, P.G. Lerch, J.-J. Morgenthaler

ZLB Central Laboratory, Swiss Red Cross
Blood Transfusion Service, Bern, Switzerland

A chromatographic fractionation method has been developed for the production of a virus safe, stable, liquid anti-D IgG preparation for intravenous use. Source plasma containing anti-D immunoglobulin was obtained by plasmapheresis of Rh-immunized volunteers. Pooled, cryoprecipitate depleted plasma was incubated with Triton®X-100 and tri-n-butylphosphate in order to inactivate enveloped viruses. The solvent-detergent treated plasma was then fractionated by cation exchange chromatography on a MacroPrep® 50 CM column. An IgG-fraction enriched in anti-D was eluted and further purified first by anion exchange chromatography and thereafter by incubation with aluminiumhydroxide gel. Finally, the anti-D IgG fraction was concentrated by a second cation exchange chromatography. The specific activity of the purified anti-D IgG-fraction was increased five- to ten-fold during the purification procedure with an overall yield of about 60%; IgA and other undesirable plasma components were depleted concomitantly. The final product was stabilized by the addition of human albumin. Doses of 200 µg of anti-D IgG in 2 ml of solution were filled in ready-to-use syringes. The anti-D product was shown to be stable for at least 6 months at storage temperatures of 4° and 26° C.

0244

IMPLEMENTATION OF BLOOD SCREENING IN INDONESIA

Melani Wikanta, Indonesian Red Cross Central Blood Transfusion Service.

Effort and Implementation a safe and sustainable blood supply in developing countries have been facing much more problems to be struggled and solved, due to various obstacles such as financial limitation.

Geographical situation of widely strectched out archipelago with 138 chapters of Blood Transfusion Service have made another difficult handling to conduct the uniform screening policy, otherwise it is supported by the government.

Implementation of blood screening against transmissible diseases has been carried out :

- VDRL : 36 BTS Chapters (26,66% of total BTS chapters)
- HBsAg : 105 BTS Chapters (77,77% of total BTS chapters)
- HIV : 131 BTS Chapters (97,04% of total BTS chapters)
- HCV : has not yet been done.

VDRL and HBsAg have to finance by BTS itself by charging Service cost from patient, while HIV screening was supported by the government through Department of Health.

National prevalence of the various examinations would be presented.

Informed Consent was conducted in big BTS, passive informed consent by listing the examinations would be performed in the billboard had been performed in most BTS, and no informed consent at all in very small BTS.

0245

SCREENING FOR MALARIA ANTIBODY AMONG SAUDI ARABIAN BLOOD DONORS IN THE RIYADH REGION.

S.S. Bernvil, V. Andrews.
Blood Bank, Department of Pathology and Laboratory Medicine, King Faisal Specialist Hospital and Research Centre, Riyadh, Saudi Arabia.

Although malaria is not endemic in the City of Riyadh due to high altitude and dryness of climate, malaria remains endemic in larger parts of the country with more than ten thousand cases reported annually. Over 90% of cases are due to *P. falciparum* but *P. malariae* and *P. vivax* are found as well. Transfusion transmitted malaria remains a sizeable risk and blood donor history should be supplemented by a screening test for these agents. Tradionally, a thick smear has been used as a screening test, requiring considerable technologist time with very limited sensitivity due to the paucity of parasites in asymptomatic carriers. We tested a commercial ELISA kit on serum from 346 consecutive Saudi national donors and found 20(5.8%) positive for antibodies to malaria. The average sample to cut off ratio was 1.7 (range 1.1-2.9). Six sera had absorbances just above the cut off value, which could indicate cross reactivity to plasmodia other than falciparum. Donor sero-positivity would call for temporary deferral in case of past infection with *P. falciparum* and permanent deferral in case of *P. malariae.*

0249

P-SELECTIN AND GPIb AS PREDICTORS OF LOSS OF PLATELET VIABILITY DURING STORAGE. S.Holme, J.Sweeney, S.Sawyer. American Red Cross, Norfolk,VA,USA.

Expression of p-selectin and loss of GPIb on the surface of stored platelets has been related to with loss of viability (Transfusion 1991;31:409, J LAB CLIN MED 1992;119:144). In this study, the applicability of these two measures as predictors of viability was systematically investigated using various adverse storage (2-3 days) conditions previously linked to loss of viability (in vitro studies only, n = 21), and current standard storage conditions in CPD-plasma at 22°C using PL-732 bags. GPIb and p-selectin expression was determined by flow cytometry and expressed as % positive platelets. Post-transfusion viability was determined after isotope labeling and reinfusion into the donor. Use of EDTA as anticoagulant (n=7), exposure to 4°C (n=5), or to pH below 6.2 (as caused by storage in bags with low gas diffusion, n=9) resulted in increased expression of p-selectin: 50 ± 17%, 65 ± 18%, 83 ± 6%, respectively, as compared to standard conditions: 22 ± 9%. These adverse conditions also caused loss of discoid shape (ESC) and hypotonic shock response (HSR) as measured photometrically, and increased lactate production (LACT), while GPIb remained unaltered at levels above 90 %. With storage at current standard conditions, the following correlations between in vivo and vitro variables were observed at day 5 of storage (n=63, *p < 0.05):

	p-selectin	GPIb	ESC	HSR	LACT
% Recovery	-0.25	0.08	0.40*	0.39*	-0.41*
Survival	-0.42*	0.19	0.50*	0.40*	-0.38*

In conclusion, p-selectin expression, but not loss of GPIb, on the surface of stored platelets is a predictor of loss of viability, although to a lesser extent than loss of discoid shape.

0250

APPR. DOUBLED SHELF-LIFE OF APHERESIS PLATELETS OBTAINED WITH ACETATE IN THE ANTICOAGULANT ACD-A

[1]S. Jonsson and T. Ahlgren[2]

[1]Transfusion Medicine, [2]Haematology/Dpt.Medicine, MAS University Hospital, Lund University, Malmö, Sweden.

NaAc (25 mL 2.5M, pH 6.0) was injected through the port of 500 mL ACD bags. Ac-APCs and proper controls (C-APCs) were procured with V50/PCSPlus/Spectra, then stored at RT for up to 15 days. *Inter alia*, their pH, pO_2, pCO_2, Ac and swirling were monitored. Each APC intended for transfusion beyond day +5 was sampled on day (+2) +3 or +4 for aerobic blood culture (Bactec™ or BactAlert™), issue stopped at 1st sign of growth. $^{51}Cr/^{111}In$ double labelled 5 day pairs of Ac-APC and C-APC platelets/labelled 12 day Ac-APC platelets were reinjected for survival studies, and appr. 900 plate let aphereses/750 transfusions have been monitored. Results: Ac is gradually consumed while pH remains at appr. 7.0 for >12days. Recovery of $^{51}Cr/^{111}In$ platelets: mean at 55% on day +5 for Ac and C alike, at 45% on day +12 (Ac platelets only!). No neg reactions related to Ac have been reported by donors/patients, nor appeared in lab tests. Up to 5 day old Ac-APCs giving satisfactory clinical effects, outdating has been delayed stepwise up to day +10 (+11). In 9 of appr. 400 Ac-APCs bacterial growth was reported but only in 2 cases confirmed with growth of *Staph.albus* from the storage bags at +3/+4 days.

CCIs in patients responding to acetate apheresis PCs

days of storage	0-1	2-3	4-5	6-7	8-11
n	17	25	19	21	20
CCI-1h (a)	17.8	19.4	11.8	16.8	16.7
CCI-18h (b)	12.7	11.6	7.2	10.5	7.3

Ac plus bact control allows for 10-11 day shelf-life.

0251

PLATELET MORPHOLOGY DURING STORAGE IN PVC AND POLYOLEFINE CONTAINERS.

M.N. Boomgaard[1], I. Steneker[2], R.N.I. Pietersz[2], D. de Korte[1].1Central Laboratory of the Netherlands Red Cross Blood Transfusion Service, Amsterdam. 2Red Cross Blood Bank Amsterdam, The Netherlands.

Morphology scores according to Kunicki i.e. disc = 4, sphere = 2, dendrite = 1 or balloon = 0 are used to judge shape changes of platelets. It was observed with light microscopy (LM) that during storage bizarre platelet shapes appeared.

Aim: To study platelet morphology in platelet concentrates (PC) during storage in either polyvinylchloride (PVC) or polyolefine (PO) containers by LM.

Method: Two PC derived from buffy coats were pooled and split up into a PVC and PO container, respectively. Samples were taken at day 0, 1, 3 and 6 of storage at 20-24°C and fixed with 0.5% glutaraldehyde (n = 6 experiments).

Result:

storage time (after collection)	PVC % discs	PO % discs
day 0 (24 hr)	56 ± 7.4	57 ± 6.7
day 1 (36 hr)	48 ± 3.8	36 ± 4.6
day 3 (84 hr)	36 ± 8.7	17 ± 7.1
day 6 (156 hr)	19 ± 5.0	3 ± 2.4

Already on day 0, 28% of the platelets in both containers could not be classified according to Kunicki i.e. disc-like (14%) or sphere-like (10%) platelets with protrusions and bizarre shapes(rings, crescents and elongated forms) (4%). Despite well maintained pH, bizarre shapes increased in PO to 15% at day 6, whereas in PVC it remains 4% throughout storage. Moreover, 80% of the platelets in PO at day 6 were spheres with dendrites compared to 68% of the platelets in PVC.

Conclusion: The above findings indicate that the morphology score according to Kunicki should be reconsidered. It is unclear whether the bizarre shapes correlates with impaired survival in vivo.

0252

PREPARATION OF COMPONENTS FROM UNITS OF WHOLE BLOOD HELD FOR 24 HOURS AT 20-24°C.

G. Moroff[1], J. AuBuchon[2], A. Heaton[3], S. Holme[3], 1American Red Cross, Jerome H. Holland Laboratory, Rockville, MD, 2Dartmouth-Hitchcock Medical Center, Lebanon, NH, 3Mid Atlantic Region, Norfolk, VA, USA.

In the United States, units of whole blood can be held for up to 8 hours at 20-24°C before preparation of platelets. Extending the hold time to 24 hours will provide additional logistical flexibility. A paired study approach was used to evaluate the in vivo viability and in vitro properties of ADSOL-red cells (PL 2209 containers) and platelets prepared from platelet-rich plasma and stored (PL 732 containers)after hold periods of 8 and 24 hours. Mean in vivo 24 hour red cell recovery (% 24-Hr recov) after 35 and 42 days of storage and mean in vivo platelet recovery after 5 days of storage with 8 and 24 hour holding times were as follows:

Red Cell Storage	n	% 24-Hr Recov 8 Hr	24 Hr	Platelet Storage	n	Recovery(%) 8 Hr	24 Hr
35 days	10	79.0	79.4	5 days	18	54.5	57.1
42 days	18	76.2	73.0				

Mean red cell survival (T 1/2 - ^{51}Cr loss, no correction for elution) values were 25.7 and 26.7 days; platelet survivals were 6.6 and 5.8 days, respectively. In vitro properties, including red cell ATP, extent of hemolysis, platelet morphology and response to hypotonic stress, were comparable with 8 and 24 hour hold periods. These data show that a 24 hour hold period does not have a deleterious influence on red cell and platelet properties.

0253

HTLV IN THE NETHERLANDS: RESULTS OF DONOR SCREENING AND CONFIRMATION.

H.Zaaijer[1], C.Dudok de Wit[2], H.Cuypers[1], I.Winkel[1], P.Lelie[1].
1 Central Lab Netherlands Red Cross Bloodtransfusion Service;
2 Red Cross Blood Transfusion Council; Amsterdam, Netherlands.

Aim: To determine the prevalence of HTLV-I among Dutch donors and to optimize confirmatory testing.

Method: In 1993, the screening of Dutch donors for presence of HTLV-I antibodies was introduced. From jan-sept.'93, Dutch blood banks screened approximately 550.000 donors; 718 EIA positive donors (0.13%) were submitted for confirmation (171 samples were suitable for PCR on HTLV-I/II DNA: CLB or Roche assay).

Results-1: Western blot (WB, Diagnostic Biotech. HTLV 2.3) on 718 samples confirmed HTLV-I infection in 14 donors (1:39.000); of which 12 were available for PCR and tested positive for HTLV-I DNA.

Results-2: We interpreted WB patterns in 158 donor samples (10 PCR+, 148 PCR-) following the manufacturers guidelines (1) and following a modified algorithm (2):

(p19/p24)+(gp46/rgp21)	= HTLV-I/II pos.(1) / indet.(2)
(p19/p24)+(gp46/rgp46-I)+rgp21	= HTLV-I positive (1,2)
p24+rgp46-II+rgp21	= HTLV-II positive (1,2)
no reactivity	= HTLV-I/II negative (1,2)
other patterns	= HTLV-I/II indeterminate (1,2)

The 10 PCR+ samples were blot-positive in both algorithms. 38/148 PCR- samples tested WB-positive following the manufacturers guidelines; only 3/148 tested positive following the modified algorithm. Cluster analysis revealed the existence of 2 groups with different WB patterns: the majority of 148 PCR- samples either showed reactivity against rgp21/p24 or against p19/p26/p28/p32/p36.

Conclusion: in this low risk population (HTLV-I 1:39.000; no HTLV-II), modified WB pattern interpretation improves WB specificity, without damaging sensitivity. Among EIA+, PCR- donors, we observed two distinct types of indeterminate WB patterns, with unknown origin.

We gratefully thank all Dutch blood banks for their co-operation.

0254

PERFORMANCE OF AN IMMUNOASSAY FOR SIMULTANEOUS DETECTION OF ANTIBODIES TO HTLV-I AND HTLV-II

E. Robertson, J. Stephens, E. Chan, C. Motley, M. Buytendorp, J. Johnson, and B. Phelps
Abbott Laboratories, Abbott Park, Illinois U.S.A.

An HTLV-I/II enzyme immunoassay was developed using HTLV-I and HTLV-II antigens in a single test. The purpose of this study was to compare performance of the HTLV-I/II EIA to an HTLV-I EIA with enhanced sensitivity. Specificity performance was evaluated with blood donor and plasmapheresis sample populations (n=1428) obtained from geographically diverse regions. The combined population reactive rate was 0.21% (3/1428) for the HTLV-I/II EIA compared with 0.14% (2/1428) for the HTLV-I EIA. A panel of potentially interfering substance samples (n=149) was tested and none (0/149) were reactive by the HTLV-I/II EIA compared to 2.01% (3/149) falsely reactive in the HTLV-I EIA. Assay sensitivity was evaluated with a panel of HTLV-I, HTLV-II, and HTLV-I/II confirmed positive samples (n=96). The HTLV-I/II EIA detected 100% (96/96) compared to 92.7% (89/96) detected by the HTLV-I EIA. The HTLV-I/II EIA detected 5 HTLV-II samples which were non-reactive by the HTLV-I EIA. HTLV-I and HTLV-II dilution panels were also tested and the HTLV-I/II EIA detected 9/12 HTLV-I dilutions and 10/12 HTLV-II dilutions, compared to 8/12 HTLV-I dilutions and 9/12 HTLV-II dilutions for the HTLV-I EIA. These data demonstrate that the HTLV-I/II EIA benefits from increased HTLV-II sensitivity, due to the addition of HTLV-II viral lysate, without compromising assay specificity.

0255

PREVALENCE OF ANTI-HTLV-I/II ANTIBODIES IN ETHIOPIA.

H. Vrielink[1], C.L. van der Poel [1], H.W. Reesink[1], Y. Sisay[2]. 1)Red Cross Blood Bank Amsterdam, The Netherlands, 2)Blood Transfusion Service, Ethiopian Red Cross Society, Addis Abeba, Ethiopia.

Objective: The prevalence of anti-HTLV-I/II antibodies in Ethiopia was established by testing serum samples (n=2,533) of different population subsets.

Methods/serum panels:

A.Serum samples (n=1,600) from voluntary non-remunerated blood donors.

B.Serum samples (n=933) from different population subsets i.e., representatives of urban and rural communities and putative risk groups (male and female STD clinic attendees).

All samples were screened with HTLV-I/II ELISA (Murex Diagnostics). ELISA repeatedly reactive samples were confirmed by Western Blot (Diagnostic Biotechnology).

Results:

Panel		ELISA +ve	Western Blot results			
			HTLV-I +ve	HTLV-II +ve	HTLV-I/II +ve*	ind
	n	n (%)	n (%)	n (%)	n (%)	n (%)
A	1,600	29 (1.8)	3 (0.2)	4 (0.3)	0	18 (1.1)
B	933	17 (1.8)	5 (0.5)	7 (0.8)	1 (0.1)	4 (0.4)
ALL	2,533	46 (1.8)	8 (0.3)	11 (0.4)	1 (0.04)	23 (0.9)

*]Samples double reactive for HTLV-I and HTLV-II.

Conclusion: In Ethiopia 0.4% of blood donors were anti-HTLV-I/II confirmed positive of whom 57% were exclusively infected with HTLV-II.

0256

DISTRIBUTION OF ANTI-HTLV-I ENV/GAG ANTIBODY TITERS IN JAPANESE HTLV-I CARRYING HEALTHY DONOR PLASMA.

T.Suzuki[1], K.Ikeda[1], R.Ametani[1], T.Ohori[1], T.Tomono[1], H.Itoh[1], M.Ikeda[2], R.Fujino[2], K.Higashimoto[2], H.Hoshino[3], and I.Miyoshi[4]

[1]Japanese Red Cross Plasma Fractionation Center, Tokyo, JAPAN, [2]Fujirebio Inc., Tokyo, JAPAN, [3]Dept. of Hygiene, Gunma University School of Medicine, Gunma, JAPAN, [4]Dept. of Medicine, Kochi Medical School, Kochi, JAPAN

Recently it was found by rabbit infection experiments that a human immune globulin product prepared from HTLV-I carrier plasma successfully prevented vertical or horizontal transmission of HTLV-I. In order to elucidate the availability of Japanese HTLV-I carrying donor plasma as a source material, we determined Ab titers against four species of HTLV-I antigens, i.e., anti-gp46(SU), anti-gp21(TM), anti-p19(MA), and anti-p24(CA), by using agglutination tests of gelatin particles conjugating corresponding isolated antigens from HTLV-I producing TCL-Kan cells. The tested donor plasma showed relatively good correlations between anti-gp46 and anti-gp21 titers and also between anti-p19 and anti-p24 titers, but not between anti-env and anti-gag titers. Anti-HTLV-I titers estimated by a commercially available anti-HTLV-I Ab test (SERODIA-HTLV-I) had especially a good correlation with anti-gp21 titers, indicating a predominant occupation of SERODIA particle surface by gp21 antigen. The anti-HTLV-I titer of donors showed a nearly normal distribution with a peak at 2^{11}x. The higher titer plasma ($\geq 2^{14}$x) was only 6% of Ab positive plasma. The higher titer of pooled plasma also showed a higher neutralizing activity against VSV(HTLV-I) pseudotype virus.

In conclusion, we could select a high neutralizing activity of plasma by the SERODIA assay in order to obtain starting materials for an efficacious anti-HTLV-I Ig product.

0257

HTLV-I IN A LOW RISK POPULATION: COMPARISON OF AN AGGLUTINATION AND TWO EIA ANTI-HTLV I SCREENING TESTS.

RL McShine[1], AH de Vries[1], GHJ Alderkamp[2], J de Wildt-Eggen[3];

[1] RC Blood Bank Groningen-Drenthe, NL, [2] RC Blood Bank Friesland, NL, [3] RC Blood Bank Zwolle, NL.

In the blood banks of 3 provinces in the Netherlands repeatedly reactive (RR) samples in the anti-HTLV I screening test were exchanged for comparitive testing (specificity). One centre uses the Fujirebio (F) Serodia agglutination test and the other two, EIAs, Abbott (A) and Ortho (O).

RESULTS:

Test	Total nr.	Nr. (%) pos	Ratios EIA pos	nr. pos. other tests O	A	F
A	25,191	16 (0.064)	1.0-1.5	2		0
		9 (0.036)	1.6-2.0	3		0
		1 (0.004)	>2.0	0		0
O	24,240	12 (0.049)	1.0-1.5		2	0
		9 (0.037)	1.6-2.0		3	0
		4 (0.017)	>2.0		0	0
F	28,002	10 (0.036)		1*	1*	

* ratios >4.5

Only the 1 sample strongly reactive in all 3 tests (see table) was confirmed anti-HTLV I pos. Specificities: F=99.96%, A=99.90%, O=99.90%

CONCLUSION: The F (agglutination) test shows less false-positivity and seems to be more specific compared to both EIAs.

0258

EFFICACY OF SELECTED, VERSUS RANDOM BLOOD DONOR SCREENING FOR ANTI-HTLV-1/2 ANTIBODY.

C.L. van der Poel, H. Vrielink, H.W. Reesink. Red Cross Blood Bank Amsterdam, The Netherlands.

Objective: To establish the efficacy of anti-HTLV-1/2 screening among blood donors native of endemic areas compared to routine screening of all blood donations.

Methods: From 1/12/91 to 14/1/93, (period A) all blood donors from HTLV-1/2 endemic countries were tested once for anti-HTLV-1/2 by ELISA (Wellcozyme). Since 14/1/93 to 31/12/93 (period B) all blood donations to are routinely tested for anti-HTLV-1/2. ELISA positive donors were confirmed by Western Blot (DBL) and HTLV-1/2 DNA-PCR.

Results: In period A, 1 / 371 (0.27%) tested donors was found confirmed HTLV-1 positive, this donor was native from Surinam (S-America). In period B, 2 / 85,000 (0.002%) donations were found confirmed HTLV-1 positive. These 2 latter donors were women with sexual contact with natives from endemic areas (Caribbean basin) and would have been missed by the selected anti-HTLV-1/2 screening.

Conclusion: Selected screening of blood donors for anti-HTLV-1/2 antibody detected only a minority of the HTLV-1/2 infected donors in Amsterdam.

0259

TEN YEARS' EXPERIENCE WITH A NATIONAL PROFICIENCY CONTROL PROGRAMME IN BLOOD GROUP SEROLOGY

Hans Erik Heier*, Leif Kornstad**
* Ullevaal Hospital Blood Bank, Oslo, **National Institute of Public Health (NIPH), Oslo, Norway.

A programme for external quality control of immunohaematological procedures in the 68 Norwegian hospital blood banks has been run by the NIPH since 1983. Uncomplicated ABO and Rh(D) grouping has been performed satisfactorily. Testing of cells with weak D antigen ("intermediate or low grade D^u") in direct agglutination tests has given relatively many false negative results. However, the laboratories normally testing blood donors have detected the D antigen by an antiglobulin reaction.- False positive results in typing presensitized D neg. cells with IgG anti-D in colloid media has been a problem, which has been reduced by stressing the importance of using appropriate control sera containing the same colloids. The introduction of monoclonal IgM anti-D sera may be valuable in this connection. - More than 40 sera with clinically significant antibodies have been dispatched. Indirect antiglobulin tests have given about 15 % false negative results, mostly with weak antibodies (titre 4 or lower). - Direct antiglobulin tests have been performed with cells sensitized with various alloantibodies giving a reaction strength from (+) to +++. Again, about 15 % of the reactions were false negative, mostly with weakly sensitized cells. It seems that the main sources of error are found in the terminal part of the antiglobulin test, i.a. poor training of technicians in reading weak agglutination reactions. The results show the need for good training programmes for the blood bank staff.

0260

SURVEY OF BLOOD GROUP DISTRIBUTION AMONG CHINESE BLOOD DONORS IN HONG KONG - AN UPDATE

K.H.Mak,S.Cheng,C.Yuen,E.Chua,C.K.Lin,S.Leong.
Hong Kong Red Cross Blood Transfusion Service

Purpose and Method: Further to our previous poster[1] presented in ISBT 1986, additional data were obtained by mass screening, using microplate technique(56,161 donors)and by MG 80 and Olympus PK 7100(459,839 donors)from 1987 to 1993,and the results therefrom are listed below:

A	B	O	AB	RhD(+)	D^u	D_{el}	D(-)
25.77%	26.8%	40.77%	6.66%	99.715%	0.016%	0.079%	0.19%

Le(a+b-):0%	SS: 0.16%	Di^a :2.99%
Le(a+b+):26.59%	Ss: 5.78%	Mi.III :6.28%
Le(a-b+):61.97%	ss:94.06%	CAD :0.305%
Le(a-b-):11.44%	KK: 0%	
Lu(a+b-):0%	Kk: 0.06%	Jk(a-b-):0.021%
Lu(a+b+): 0.018%	kk:99.94%	(1 in 4,771)
Lu(a-b+):99.982%	Fy(a+b-):91.02%	
	Fy(a+b+): 8.78%	C^w: 0.0067%
	Fy(a-b+): 0.2%	(1 in 14,925)

Conclusion: Results obtained were,by and large, similar to those reported among Taiwan Chinese[2,3] except that we have determined the incidence of the following phenotypes among Hong Kong Chinese: D^u, D_{el}, K, CAD, Mi.III, Lu(a+b+), Jk(a-b-). H-deficient phenotype is slightly less frequent: 1 in 17,031 vs 1 in 12,000.

Ref:
1.Poster TH-311.XIX Congress of ISBT,Sydney,1986.
2.Lin-Chu et al,Transfusion.1988;28:350-352.
3.Lin-Chu et al,Transfusion.1987;27:388-390.

0261

SCREENING OF RARE RED BLOOD CELLS AND ANTIBODIES OUTSIDE THE Rh SYSTEM IN BRAZIL

Wendel, S.[1,2]; Fontão, R.C.L.[1,2]; Pizzigatti, M.V.[2]; Takaoka, D.T.[2]; Nakabayashi, S.[2]
1- Hospital Sírio-Libanês Blood Bank - São Paulo, Brazil
2- Centro de Imunologia e Imunogenética - São Paulo, Brazil

In Brazil, there are a few data about the existence of blood donors with rare blood cell antigens or antibodies outside the Rh system. In this study, we report our first results from a screening program aiming to find rare blood donors.

MATERIAL: Red blood cell antigens (RBC An) were screened by microplate assays using: the urea lysis test for Jk:-3, *Glycin soya* lectin (RBC with low levels of sialic acid), or specific antibodies (in-house preparation or by SCARF donation), whereas antibodies against low frequency antigens (LFA) were screened against cells from our donor population or through a SCARF donation. In addition, IgA deficient blood donors were screened with IgA paraprotein sensitized red cells, and confirmed by single (radial) immunodiffusion (sensitivity= 700mg/L).

RESULTS: They are shown in the table below.

		Tested (n)	Found (%)
R	Jk: -3 (urea lysis)	40075	0
B	Low levels of sialic acid	39342	0
C	M^g (+) 002.011 *	40022	0
An	Di (a+) 010.001	2578	13 (0,5%)
	Anti-Di^a 010.001	2561	1 (0,04%)
	Anti-Wr^a 211.001	2468	5 (0,20%)
	Anti-V^w 002.009	1244	1 (0,08%)
L	Anti-M^g 002.011	520	5 (0,96%)
F	Anti-Lu14 005.014	513	0
A	Anti-Js^a 006.006	738	0
	Anti-Ri^a 002.016	511	0
	Anti-Mt^a 002.014	836	0
	Anti-Sci2 013.002	836	0
	IgA deficient	5747	12 (0,21%)

(*) ISBT Terminology on RBC Antigens

CONCLUSION: In this study, we were able to find a somewhat high number of Di(a+) cells, one of them Di(a+ b-). Among the LFA screened, an Anti-M^g became an important issue, since 5 samples could be found (4 of them apparently without other associated LFA). In addition, the prevalence of IgA deficient donors (1:500) is of great importance to supply our local demand.

0262

THE Di^a ANTIGEN IN SPAIN. A LOW FREQUENCY ANTIGEN?.

E. Muñiz-Diaz, P. Madoz, P. Santodomingo, N. Boto, C. Pastoret, R. Martino, A. Altés, LL. Puig.
Hemotherapy Service. Hospital de Sant Pau. Barcelona (Spain).

The presence of Di^a in Caucasians is an unusual observation because it is practically confined to people of Mongolian extraction. Population studies in white European people are scant. In England no Di(a+) individuals have been found and in Poland 0.5% of Poles are Di(a+) probably due to the admixture of Mongol genes. The aim of this study is to describe the prevalence of the Di^a antigen in the Spanish population.

The anti Di^a employed for typing was casually detected during the routine antibody screening performed in the serum of a female blood donor from Puerto Rico. The serum was reactive in the indirect antiglobulin test with 1 out of the 3 cells used in the screening. The phenotype of this cell from a Spanish donor resulted Di(a+b+) and the antibody specificity was confirmed. Out of the 3000 blood donor samples tested with the anti Di^a, 5 (0.16%) gave positive reactions. The 2 families studied did not have any Mongoloid or American ancestors in the most recent generations. Otherwise, another anti Di^a was detected in a Spanish woman during the study period.

In conclusion, although it has been claimed that the Di^a antigen is a low frequency antigen in Caucasians our results indicate that its incidence in Spain is higher than might be expected and that Di(a+) donors should be included in our panel cells. Owing to the close historical link between Spain and South America it is to be expected that the Di^a gene has found its way into the Spanish population.

0263

THE GLYCOSYLATION OF IgG RED CELL AUTOANTIBODIES AFFECTS FcγRECEPTOR III-MEDIATED FUNCTIONAL ACTIVITY

A.G. Hadley[1], B. Zupanska[2], B.M. Kumpel[1], K. Leader[3], J. Jones[1], D.J. Booker[4], R.T. Stamps[4], R. J. Sokol[4].
[1]IBGRL, Bristol, UK, [2]Institute of Haematology and Blood Transfusion, Warsaw, Poland, [3]University of Bristol, UK, [4]Regional Transfusion Centre, Sheffield, UK.

The aim of the current study was to assess the FcγRIII-mediated functional activity of IgG autoantibodies and the extent to which differences in activity may be due to qualitative variations in Fc region glycosylation reflected by galactose content. IgG was eluted from red cells of 25 patients with autoantibodies, and depleted of serum IgG by readsorption on red cells and elution after extensive washing. IgG anti-D from 11 alloimmunized women, and IgG1 (BRAD-5) and IgG3 (BRAD-3) monoclonal anti-D were similarly affinity-purified. Mabs high or low in galactose were produced by culturing cell lines at low or high cell density respectively. The % agalactosyl (G0) IgG of antibodies and serum IgG was determined by ELISA using a Mab (GN7) to terminal N-acetylglucosamine. Functional activity was assessed by measuring the K cell-mediated lysis of red cells in eluates diluted to achieve comparable levels of red cell sensitization (1000 IgG molecules/cell) estimated by FACS analysis. The % G0 IgG of autoantibodies ranged from 0 - >41% and showed no relationship with the % G0 of serum IgG from the same patients. Eluates containing polyclonal anti-D were all lytic (range 57 - 90%) while lysis by autoantibodies varied from 0 - 75% and correlated inversely with % G0 ($r = -0.78$, $p < 0.002$). Also, anti-D Mabs low in galactose were less lytic than the same antibodies containing more galactose. These data suggest that IgG red cell autoantibodies are functionally heterogeneous and that this is due, at least in part, to qualitative differences in Fc glycosylation.

0264

IDENTIFICATION OF A SEQUENCE HOMOLOGOUS TO THE H-GENE

P.H. Johnson, M.R.C. Blood Group Unit, London, UK.

During the course of experiments to detect variants of the blood group H-gene associated with the H-deficient phenotypes (Johnson et al., this meeting), non-allelic PCR products were detected. These bands were excised from denaturing gradient electrophoresis (DGGE) gels, re-amplified and sequenced. The bands were shown to have 70-80% identity with corresponding regions of the published H-gene sequence (Larson et al. Proc.Natl.Acad.Sci. U.S.A. 1990; 87:6674-6678). Several DGGE, SSCA (single stranded conformational analysis) and amplification polymorphisms have been observed and one may be associated with the non-secretor (Le(a+b-)) phenotype in a limited number of Caucasian individuals examined.

Whereas a PCR amplification of the 3'-end of the published H-sequence gave product only with anthropoid ape (gorilla, chimpanzee and orangutan) DNA, primers specific for the H-like sequence amplified target DNA from throughout the mammalian lineage. This finding reflects the known evolution of H antigenic determinants in haemopoietic and endothelial tissues. The evidence suggests that the homologous sequence represents part of a structural secretor gene.

The characterised homologous sequence is being extended by PCR and with the use of existing PCR products to screen a gut cDNA library from a blood group A secretor donor (Johnson and Edwards, unpublished).

0265

COMPARISON OF ACTIVITY OF PERIPHERAL MONOCYTES AND SPLENIC MACROPHAGES IN THE MONOCYTE MONOLAYER ASSAY

B.Żupańska, A.Gronkowska, M.Ziemski
Institute of Haematology and Blood Transfusion, Warsaw, Poland

Assays which try to reflect the haemolysis in vivo have been performed with peripheral mononuclear cells (mostly monocytes), sometimes only with peritoneal macrophages or monocyte-like cell lines. The immune destruction of red cells however takes place mainly in the spleen with the involvement of macrophages.The aim of the present study was to compare the interaction of peripheral monocytes and spleen macrophages with red cells sensitized in vitro with anti-D antibody using one of the functional test,monocyte monolayer assay (MMA).Fresh mononuclear cells were harvested from the same person on the same day from peripheral blood and excised spleen.Fourteen patients with different haematological diseases were investigated.Our study shows that in most patients macrophages do not show higher activity in the MMA as compared to peripheral monocytes.

0266

BLOOD GROUPING Rh(D) WITHOUT HUMAN ANTI-D REAGENT

L. MANNESSIER, C. HORBEZ, A. DELSALLE
Centre Regional de transfusion Sanguine de Lille - 21 rue Camille Guérin 59000 LILLE.

From 1986 to 1991 we used one monoclonal IgM anti-D [BROLY, 1986] and one polyclonal IgG anti-D for Rh (D) blood grouping. More than 218 000 determinations of patients, pregnant women and newborn were realized with no discrepancy in regard to normal D antigen and weak D. The only expected discrepancies concern the 57 D variant and the 29 R°Har phenotype. Among the 218 000 determinations, more than 153 000 have been performed on microplates [MANNESSIER, 1992]. Then in 1991, we decided to use two monoclonal anti-D for Rh (D) blood grouping : one IgM and a blend of two IgG and to another IgM anti-D. The combination of these 4 monoclonal anti-D produces a potent reagent "Totem" (Diagast laboratoires), that reacts with all cells tested: D positive cells, weak D and all D variant, the same as a human polyclonal reagent [MANNESSIER, 1992]. Since March 1992, we no longer use polyclonal anti-D. More than 58 000 determinations of sample patients were realized : 49 300 Rh positif, 8 243 Rh negatif, 437 weak D and 20 D variant were identified. All these data proves the efficacity of monoclonal anti-D. We no longer have the right to use human anti-D for Rh(D) blood grouping. Human anti-D is now reserved for the fractionation of anti-Rh immunoglobulin which allows the prevention of the haemolytic disease of the newborn.

0267

AN IgM MONOCLONAL ANTI-D THAT DETECTS LOW GRADE D^u AND ALL CATEGORIES/VARIANTS TESTED EXCEPT D^{vi} - A SUPERIOR TYPING REAGENT.

M.L. Scott[1], D. Voak[2], J. Jones[1], R.E. Mushens[1], C. Carter[2], and N.C. Hughes-Jones[2]. [1]IBGRL, Bristol, UK and [2]East Anglian BTS and Division of Transfusion Medicine, Univ. of Cambridge, UK.

RUM-1 is a human-mouse heterohybridoma cell line that produces human monoclonal IgM anti-D.

The antibody reacted strongly with untreated red cells of D categories II, IIIc, IVa, IVb, Va and VII. It also reacted with Ro^{Har} cells. It did not react with category D^{VI} cells. RUM 1 was the only one of 13 IgM monoclonal anti-D's tested to react with each of seven non-category D variants.

RUM-1 was compared to two other IgM monoclonal anti-D reagents for detection of a panel of 82 low grade D^u cells. The other reagents detected 5 and 6 respectively; RUM-1 detected 77 of the 82. Four of the five it did not detect were D^B. Further tests showed that RUM-1 in saline agglutination tests had almost equivalent sensitivity for the detection of low grade D^u cells as a classical antiglobulin test using polyclonal IgG anti-D.

RUM-1 thus appears to have the potential to be an ideal direct saline reactive typing reagent - it reliably detects low grade D^u cells, and all category/variant cells tested except D^{VI}.

0268

RhD GENOTYPING IN DVI INDIVIDUALS

E.A.M.Beckers[1], S.Simsek[2], B.H.W.Faas[2], H.Th.M.Cuijpers[2] M.A.M.Overbeeke[2], C.E. van der Schoot[2,3], A.E.G.Kr. von dem Borne[2,3], D.J. van Rhenen[1,4].
1Red Cross Bloodbank Rotterdam; 2Central Laboratory of the Netherlands Red Cross Blood Transfusion Service, Amsterdam; 3Academic Medical Centre Amsterdam; 4Dept.Haematology, University Hospital Rotterdam.

The validity of recently described methods of RhD genotyping was questioned in DVI individuals. Two different genomic rearrangements of the RhD-gene resulting in the DVI-phenotype, either deletion or conversion of D-exons 4, 5 and 6, have been described. We have evaluated RhD genotyping in 21 (19 converted type, 2 deleted type) individuals expressing the DVI-phenotype, applying three different PCR assays: I. primers were used to amplify the introns between exon 4 and exon 5 of both Rh-genes; II. primers amplifying a 136 bp consensus fragment and a 186 bp D-specific fragment were applied; III. a primerset was selected to specifically amplify exon-7 of the D-gene. In assay I. all DVI-samples showed only one band specific of the CcEe-intron: 1200 bp. The D-specific band of 600 bp was missing, suggesting a D-negative status. In assay II. both the consensus- as well as the D-fragment were found, determining DVI as D-positive. Assay III. showed that exon D-7 was present in all DVI-samples.
We conclude that in genotyping individuals for RhD, DVI may be overlooked due to false-negative results. Discrepancies between the methods, described above, are indicative for DVI.

0269

A NEW STRATEGY FOR D PHENOTYPING WITH TOTEM®: Multi monoclonal anti-D reagent.

Auteurs : C. BETREMIEUX[2], M .BEOLET[1], L. KEYSER[2].

1 Centre Régional de Transfusion Sanguine de Lille, FRANCE
2 DIAGAST Laboratoires , Lille FRANCE.

The necessity for replacing polyclonal anti-D antibodies is becoming a more and more topical subject for different reasons :
- The need of human anti-D antibodies for therapeutic use and the problems linked to immunization of volontary donors (ethical viewpoint).
- Limits of polyclonal anti-D reagents (albumin, sensitivity, virology safety...).

Anti-D monoclonal antibodies, IgM and IgG classes, are well known now for their efficiency in phenotyping, and the blend of IgM and IgG anti-D antibodies into one reagent was an important advance.

However, are these new reagents capable of replacing the wide specifity of polyclonal antibodies ?

The aim of this study was to confirm the capability for Totem® to detect all D red cells, including weak D and partial D categories. Four monoclonal anti-D antibodies (2 IgG + 2 IgM classes) were chosen for their respective performances. The 2 IgM anti-D antibodies were able to detect all normal D and a large part of weak D in saline tests, the two IgG anti-D were added to complete the detection of very weak D and partial D red cells by Indirect Antiglobulin Test.

Among an extensive study of routine samples from blood donors, more than 400 weak D red cells were tested, among them, partial D red cells were identified - some of those partial D are curently being classified.

All this data proves the efficiency of the multi monoclonal anti-D - Totem® to replace conventional poylclonal anti-D reagents.

0270

A NEW IgM HUMAN MOUSE HYBRIDOMA ANTI-D DETECTING WEAK D AND VARIANTS EXCEPT D^{VI}

M. MARTIN[1],J. ANDRE[1],P.Y. LEPENNEC[2]
1 SANOFI DIAGNOSTICS PASTEUR, Marnes (FRANCE)
2 CNRGS, Paris (FRANCE)

A new human monoclonal IgM anti-D B9A4B2 was produced by EBV transformation of peripheral blood lymphocytes and subsequent fusion with a mouse myeloma.

The heterohybridoma obtained was stabilised by repeated cloning. The antibody B9A4B2 reacted strongly in saline at room temperature (using both slide and tube methods) with all D + untreated RBC of any Rh phenotype.

It also reacted strongly with untreated cells of D categories III, IVa, (IVb, Vc), Va and VII, in saline method. It did not react with category D^{VI} cells.
B9A4B2 was also tested along a panel* of 39 weak D cells. 95 % of weak D cells were detected in saline.

These results illustrate the efficacy of this IgM antibody used in direct saline techniques for detection of weak D cells and variant cells except D^{VI}.

(* Quality Assurance Programme of the Dutch Federation of Red Cross Blood banks).

0271

BLEND OF MONOCLONAL ANTI-D'S AS SUPERIOR TYPING REAGENT

H.-H. Sonneborn, M. Ernst, M.-T. Weber-Muscan, V. Lenhard
Biotest AG, Dreieich, FRG

Using EBV transformation and fusion with heterohybridomas several stable anti-D secreting human cellines could be established. These monoclonal antibodies were tested in many laboratories; some of them were additionally evaluated in national and international workshops.

BS 226 has been selected as substitute for a saline anti-D reagent, showing strong reaction with D+ cells, good reactivity with weak D's, but is negative with D^{VI}.

To develop a reagent which is positive with all D category cells, usable in all techniques including IAT for the detection of very weak D's, a blend of three monoclonal antibodies was prepared to fulfil these requirements.

BS 221 (IgG1), an improved subclone of H41 11B7[1] (IgG1), and BS 232 (IgM) were selected according to their reactivity with D category cells. The clones were produced in large scale tissue culture and blended for a typing reagent. This reagent can be used in slide tests (rapid on box and incubation test), tube tests (immediate spin, incubation at 37°C, IAT), and also in automated blood grouping systems, showing good reactivity and specificity. It reacts positive with all tested D categories and weak D's at least in the IAT.

The combined testing with Seraclone Anti-D (BS 226) and Seraclone Anti-D Blend (BS 221, H41, BS 232) allows the detection of D^{VI} category cells.

[1]A. Rapaille et al., Vox Sang. 1993,64:161-166.

0272

AMINO ACID VARIATION IN HUMAN MONOCLONAL ANTI-D ANTIBODIES WITH DIFFERENT FUNCTIONAL ACTIVITIES.

J.E.M.Gilmour and B.M.Kumpel
IBGRL, Bristol, U.K.

Two human IgG1 monoclonal anti-D's, BRAD-5 and JAC10, show marked differences in their FcR-mediated functional activities. In order to investigate the structure of the antibodies in detail, cDNA spanning the hinge region was isolated from both cell lines, amplified using polymerase chain reaction and sequenced.

The results showed that the amino acid sequence from BRAD-5 matched published sequence for the hinge of IgG1. However, two alterations in the sequence, at positions 233(Glu to Gly) and 239(Ser to Leu), were noted in JAC10. The significance of the changes lies not only in the alterations in the nature of the amino acids but also in their position which flank the FcRI receptor site (amino acids 234-238). The binding site of FcRIII is also believed to be in this region. FcRI interactions(in monocyte antibody-dependent cell-mediated cytotoxicity or U937 rosette assays) were lower with JAC10 than BRAD-5, while K cell FcRIII-mediated lysis of red cells by JAC10 was markedly reduced compared to BRAD-5. The results described above suggest a possible link between the structure of the antibodies and their functional differences.

0273

A FAMILY WITH THE RARE GE:-2,3,4 RED CELL PHENOTYPE IN TWO GENERATIONS

G.L. Daniels[1], P. Johnson[1], C. Levene[2].
1 MRC Blood Group Unit, London, UK; 2 Reference Laboratory for Blood Groups, Jerusalem, Israel.

An Israeli blood donor with anti-GE2 in his serum had the rare red cell phenotype GE:-2,3,4. His son and 2 of his daughters were also GE:-2,3,4; his wife, third daughter, mother, 3 sibs, and maternal aunt had the common phenotype GE:2,3. The propositus and his wife are first cousins.

Immunoblotting with anti-GE2 demonstrated glycophorin D (GPD) in the cells of the GE:2,3,4 wife and daughter, but no band in the cells of the three GE:-2,3,4 children. In red cells of the GE:-2,3,4 children, immunoblotting with monoclonal anti-glycophorin C (GPC) revealed no GPC, but a diffuse band of higher mobility was detected. Red cells of the wife and GE:2,3,4 daughter had GPC and the diffuse band, demonstrating heterozygosity for the normal GPC gene and for the abnormal gene.

Polymerase chain reaction with primers to the intronic flanking sequences common to exons 2 and 3 of the GPC gene, followed by denaturing gradient gel electrophoresis, demonstrated presence of exon 3, but absence of exon 2 in the GE:-2,3,4 children. Both exons were present in the wife and GE:2,3,4 daughter, but comparison of staining intensity suggested heterozygosity for an exon 2 deletion.

The GE:-2,3,4 phenotype in this family appears to have the usual genetic background, with the propositus homozygous and his wife heterozygous for the mutant gene.

0274

ANTI-G ALLOANTIBODY PRODUCED BY C-POSITIVE D-POSITIVE G-NEGATIVE PATIENT

G.Kuśnierz-Alejska
Institute of Haematology and Blood Transfusion, Warsaw, Poland

Serum of 80 year old, B Rh+, A.M. woman reacted in pretransfusion testing (in the IAGT and enzyme test) with B Rh+ donors. She delivered seven children but was never transfused.Further investigations showed that IgG antibody in the patient's serum reacted with all Rh positive and Ccddee but not with ccddEe and ccddee red cells.This antibody was identified as anti-G, its titre was 32.

The patient's phenotype was CcDEe. Her red cells were investigated in the IAGT - LISS with anti-G antibodies isolated by double elution procedure from 22 out of 46 anti-C+D hyperimmunized individuals. It has been shown that although on the patient's red cells the expression of C and D antigens was normal, the G antigen was absent.

0275

Polymorphism at a Hae III site on the Rh CcEe gene and its association with Rh c/C serotypes

LC Wolter[1], CA Hyland[1], YW Liew[1], A Saul[2].
1Red Cross Blood Bank, 2Queensland Institute of Medical Research, Brisbane, Australia.

BACKGROUND: Four amino acid changes have been associated with the Rh c and C antigenic polymorphisms[1]. One, a W to C change at position 16, results from a G to C substitution which removes a *Hae III* restriction site.
AIM: To examine the association between the presence or absence of this *Hae III* RFLP site and Rh c or C serotypes among 138 blood donors.
METHOD: Genomic DNA was cut with *Hae III* for a Southern blot using a 490bp probe to the upstream and first 117 bases of the Rh CcEe and D genes.
RESULTS: RFLP analysis for c serotypes gave two bands in the range expected from sequence data. These were a >232 bp fragment (600 bases observed) and 155bp. An additional 103bp was expected but not observed under the test conditions. Two bands of 600 and 258 bases (155 + 103) were expected and observed for the C serotypes. Sequencing data showed that the designated 258bp fragment lacked the *Hae III* site (G to C). This C gene fragment was observed for 87/87 homo- or hetero-zygote C phenotypes. However, among 22 Rh ccee (rr) serotypes 3 exhibited the 258 base C fragment in addition to the expected 155bp c band.
CONCLUSION: The data suggest that the Rh c gene can lack the *Hae III* RFLP site at nucleotide position 48 and that, therefore, the W to C change may not contribute to the c/C polymorphism.

1. Mouro I, Colin Y, Cherif-Zahar B, Cartron JP, Le Van Kim C. Nature genetics 5: 62 1993

0276

SEQUENCE ANALYSIS OF cDNA's DERIVED FROM RETICULOCYTE mRNA's CODING FOR Rh POLYPEPTIDES

S. Simsek[1], C.A.M. de Jong[1], H.Th.M. Cuijpers[1], P.M.M Bleeker[1], M.A.M. Overbeeke[1], C.E. van der Schoot[1,2], A.E.G. Kr. von dem Borne[1,2]
1Central Laboratory of the Netherlands Red Cross Blood Transfusion Service; 2Academic Medical Centre, Amsterdam.

Recently, the genetic basis of the RhD polymorphism has been described using cDNA libraries. In the present study we confirm the identity of the RhD cDNA, using mRNA derived from reticulocytes of 5 phenotyped donors. Four types of cDNA's were identified, tentatively designated as RhSCI, RhSCII, RhSCIII and RhSCIV. Comparison of RhSCII with RhSCI showed a single base pair difference, resulting in the P226A amino acid (aa) polymorphism. In agreement with Mouro et al.(1993), RhSCI and RhSCII were found to be related to the presence of cE- and ce-antigen respectively. RhSCIII was a transcript derived from the RhD gene, with 35 aa substitutions as compared to RhSCI. RhSCIV was found only in RhCe-positive individuals, indicating that RhSCIV carries the mutations encoding the Ce-antigen. Six nucleotide changes, resulting in 4 aa substitutions W16C, L60I, N68S and P103S, were observed between RhSCII and RhSCIV, representing the C/c polymorphism.

0277

Rh D GENOTYPING BY PCR-BASED AMPLIFICATION OF DNA

S. Simsek[1], B.H.W. Faas[1], P.M.M. Bleeker[1], M.A.M. Overbeeke[1], H.Th.M. Cuijpers[1], C.E. van der Schoot[1,2], A.E.G. Kr. von dem Borne[1,2]
1Central Laboratory of the Netherlands Red Cross Blood Transfusion Service; 2Academic Medical Centre, Amsterdam.

We have explored the feasibility of three independent DNA typing methods based on the polymerase chain reaction (PCR), to determine the Rh D status of individuals. Genomic DNA derived from mononuclear cells of 237 Rh-phenotyped healthy donors (178 Rh D-positive and 59 Rh D-negative) was used in the three PCR assays. The Rh D genotypes, as determined by method I (N.Engl.J.Med 329: 607,1993) were not completely concordant with the serologically established phenotypes, since we have encountered 8 discrepant cases (6 false-positive and 2 false-negative). Of these 8 discrepancies one and two cases remained false-positive in method II (Blood 82:651,1193) and III (in which exon 7 of the D gene is specifically amplified), respectively. No other discrepancies were observed in the latter methods.
Thus, in order to avoid incorrect typing for Rh D, we propose to use at least two Rh D DNA typing techniques.

0278

AN EXAMPLE OF AN Rh D VARIANT WHOSE REACTION PATTERN WITH MONOCLONAL ANTIBODIES SPLITS EPITOPE D6/7 AND SUBSPLITS EPITOPE D2

M.L. Scott[1], D. Voak[2], J. Jones[1], G. Campbell[2].
[1] IBGRL, Bristol, [2]East Anglian BTS, Division of Transfusion Medicine, Univ. of Cambridge, UK.

Nine Rh(D) epitopes have been proposed by considering the reaction patterns of D category cells with monoclonal antibodies (MAbs)[1]. Epitope D 6/7 has only been split by inhibition studies.

Red cells from the propositus (Li) were tested with MAbs specific for the different epitopes. The results with papain treated cells were as follows:

epitope	antibodies	reaction
epD1	REG-A	0
epD2	GLR-04	0
epD3	HD7	+
epD4	UCHD-4	0
epD5	HAM-A	0
epD6	FOG-B	+
epD7	PAG-1	0
epD9	MS-26	+

Further MAbs previously classified as anti-epD6/7 were tested with these cells. Brad 3, Brad 5, AB5, BS226, HM10, P3X61,and HM16 were positive and therefore anti-epD6; MAD-2, BS231 and RUM-1 were negative and therefore anti-epD7.

Four further anti-epD2 MAbs were tested with these cells. BRAD 8, like GLR04 was negative, whereas BS227, P3X249 and P3X290 gave strong positive reactions. These results indicate a subsplit in epD2.

[1] Lomas et al (1993) Transfusion Med. 3, 67-69.

0279

Molecular cloning of Rh30 cDNAs from Individuals expressing different Rh phenotypes: Molecular basis of the Rh C/c and E/e polymorphisms

Avent N.D., Liu W., Jackson S., Isaac A., Anstee D.J.
International Blood Group Reference Laboratory, Bristol, UK

Rh antigen expression is associated with two groups of erythrocyte membrane proteins of M_r 30,000 (Rh30 polypeptides) and M_r 50-100,000 (Rh Glycoprotein). The Rh30 polypeptides are known to be responsible for the expression of the Rh antigens as the Rh30 genes map to chromosome 1p34-36, where the Rh polymorphisms have been localised by segregation analysis.

We have cloned three different Rh30 cDNA species by RT-PCR from reticulocytes isolated from individuals expressing Rh phenotypes: CDe, cDE, cDe and cde. Amplicons of the expected size were obtained, cloned and sequenced. Transcripts from both the Rh CcEe and D genes were analysed, and It was found that two transcripts from the Rh CcEe gene (Rh30A and Rh30C) differed by only 5 or 6 nucleotide (nt) substitutions. It was found that point mutations to nts 307 and 676 were responsible for the molecular basis of the Rh C/c (Ser/Pro_{103}) and E/e (Pro/Ala_{226}) polymorphisms respectively. Both changes represent alterations to predicted extracellular amino acids. These results largely confirm those of Mouro *et al.*[1]. However, Mouro *et al.*, suggest that 6 nt substitutions resulting in four amino acid changes are required for Rh C-positivity. We have demonstrated the presence of mRNAs in two Rh c^+C^- individuals that encode three of these four amino acid changes, implying that only the change to nt 307 ($Pro(c) / Ser(C)_{103}$) is critical for the Rh C or c polymorphism. We have demonstrated that the Rh C/c and E/e polymorphisms are carried on the same mRNA suggesting that these antigens are carried by the same polypeptide chain (Rh30A or Rh30C).

1 Mouro I *et al.*, (1993) *Nature Genetics* **5:** 62-65.

0280

THE EFFECT OF CYSTEINE MODIFICATION AND PROTEINASES ON THE Rh ANTIGENS

G. Schmitz[1], H.H. Sonneborn[2], M. Ernst[2], D. Blanchard[3], W. Gielen[1] and W. Dahr[4]

1Inst. of Pharmacology, Univ. Cologne, Germany; 2Biotest AG, Dreieich, Germany; 3Centre Regional de Transf. Sanguine, Nantes, France; 4Scientific Consultation & Translations, Berg. Gladbach, Germany.

It is assumed that Cys-285 of the Rh-D-protein represents a part of the D antigen. Our agglutination inhibition tests with 29 anti-D sera (predominantly monoclonal) confirm the inactivation of the D antigen by treatment of membranes (phenotype C+c+D+E+e+) with Cys-reagents (N-ethylmaleimide = NEM, p-chloromercuribenzene-sulfonate = PCMBS - in part reversible after DTE reduction, periodate, Hg++, Ellman reagent - reversible after DTE reduction). Iodoacetamide and -acetic acid do not react with the essential Cys residue, as shown by subsequent PCMBS treatment. These data suggest that at least the majority of the D epitopes is located in one region of the D protein. The C, c, E and e antigens (studied with at least 3 antibodies) showed the same behaviour as the D antigen. However, some of the C and c epitopes were only inactivated by high NEM concentrations or NEM/PCMBS treatment. This suggests that the C/c and E/e antigens are, at least in part, located on different molecules. Trypsin and chymotrypsin treatment of membranes led to a weakening of most of the D, C, c, E and e antigens. This suggests that the epitopes are located in proximity to proteolytic cleavage sites.

0281

AN AUTO-ANTI-e NONREACTIVE WITH OWN RED CELLS AND NEGATIVE IN DIRECT ANTIGLOBULIN TEST IN CONVENTIONAL TUBE TECHNIQUES

M.Písačka[1], M.Prosická[1], J.Tejnická[2]
Institute of Haematology and Blood Transfusion[1], Faculty Hospital Motol[2]
Prague, Czech Republic

A five-month baby developed signs of haemolytic anaemia after pneumonia caused suspectly by Mycoplasma pneunoniae. Tests for autoimmune haemolysis were negative, there was no history of immunization. Two crossmatch negative transfusions of ccddee blood were followed with increase of haemolysis. An antibody was detected in the serum, reacting in LISS-IAT with all e+ red cells except own e+ cells although the titre of diagnostic anti-e with red cells of patient did not differ from other e+ cells. Direct antiglobulin test (DAT) was negative. All tests were performed by conventional tube techniques.
The positivity of DAT (with polyspecific and anti-IgG AHG) and positive reaction of own cells in IAT were detectable only in DiaMed gel test, the specifity of the antibody remained anti-e.
This case shows that in early phases of some autoimmune haemolytic anaemia the conventional tube antiglobulin test can be insufficient and that transfusion therapy should be approached with reserve.

0282

EVALUATION OF AN ANTI-e TYPING DISCREPANCY BETWEEN MONOCLONAL AND POLYCLONAL REAGENTS

N. Seewer-Eicher[1], M. Plantos[2], B.A. Brick[3]
1 Swiss Red Cross, Berne, Switzerland, 2 Canadian Red Cross, Hamilton, Ontario, Canada, 3 Baxter Diagnostics AG, Düdingen, Switzerland

During a field trial of new monoclonal (mc) Rhesus blood grouping reagents, a red blood cell (RBC) sample showed a discrepancy in saline tube e typing between the monoclonal test reagent and the polyclonal reference reagent. The mc anti-e reacted 3+ with the cell whereas the polyclonal reference anti-e was negative.
The RBCs had been previously typed as RzR2 (CDE/cDE) using polyclonal reagents by another laboratory. Five different mc anti-e were tested by the saline tube test against this cell. All but one gave positive reactions from w+ - 3+. All polyclonal anti-e were negative after 15 minutes 37°C incubation but were weakly positive in the antiglobulin phase. All results were confirmed by a second laboratory. The cells were also tested in the DiaMed Micro Typing System which uses bromelin treated RBCs and polyclonal anti.e. Six different lots of cartridges showed weak to moderate reactions (± - 2+).
The reaction of the polyclonal anti-e's in the Diamed system and in the indirect antiglobulin test seem to indicate that the RBCs from this donor do possess the e antigen but in a greatly reduced amount. The monoclonal reagents that were positive must be directed to an epitope not generally recognized by polyclonal reagents. Additional testing with this cell and possible family studies may illuminate the genotype of this donor and the molecular basis for this serological discrepancy.

0283

INHERITANCE OF ABNORMAL GLYCOPHORIN C GENES IN A FRENCH FAMILY

M.J. Loirat[1], F. Pineau[2], C. Schiffer[2], J.Y. Muller[1], D. Blanchard[1].
1CRTS, Nantes, 2 CRTS, Le Mans, France.

The discovery of an anti-Ge:2 in the serum of the propositus (Lal. A.) prompted us to study its RBCs by using mAbs directed to the Gerbich (Ge) antigens. MAb NaM10-7G11 (anti-Ge:4) agglutinated both untreated and trypsin-treated cells whereas mAb NaM19-3C4 (anti-Ge:3) only agglutinated untreated cells. These data indicated that the Ge3 and Ge4 antigens are located on different molecules, one of which has characteristics of the abnormal GPC^{Ge} (Ge-type) molecule. Immunoblotting analysis performed with a mAb directed to aa residues 106-121 of GPC showed that the variant RBCs do not contain normal GPC and GPD but a diffuse band of strong intensity that may contains both GPC^{Ge} and GPC^{Yus} (Yus-type) molecules.

The inheritance of both the GPC^{Ge} and GPC^{Yus} abnormal molecules was demonstrated by studying the family. The parents carry one dose of either the $GYPC^{Yus}$ or the $GYPC^{Ge}$ abnormal genes whereas two sisters were also identified as heterozygotes for both the $GYPC^{Yus}$ and $GYPC^{Ge}$ genes. The third sister inherited the normal GYPC gene from both parents whereas the child of the propositus inherited the $GYPC^{Ge}$ gene.

Of interest, "natural" anti-Ge:2 were identified in the serum of the three Ge-negative individuals.

0284

AN ALLELIC RHESUS SUB-SYSTEM INCLUDING C^W (RH8), C^X (RH9) AND MAR, A NOVEL HIGH INCIDENCE RH ANTIGEN.

Hannele Sareneva, Pertti Sistonen
Finnish Red Cross Blood Transfusion Service, Helsinki, Finland

We present new genetic evidence obtained from population studies on Finns and from the studies on 10,045 Finnish blood donors as well as 8 of their selected families. An antibody detected after the delivery of her 2nd child in the serum of a 39-year-old Finnish female with a rare Rh phenotype C^W+C^X+ defines a novel high incidence Rh antigen MAR. The finding of the new antibody is apparently correlated with the fact that the Rh antigens C^W (RH8) and, more strikingly, C^X (RH9) have each an exceptionally high phenotype frequency in Finns, 4.0% and 3.5%, respectively. Anti-MAR antibody shows an antithetical relationship to both anti-C^W and anti-C^X. Thus, both data on Finnish blood donors and studies on 8 families of MAR-negative and C^W+ or C^X+ propositi reveal that MAR-negative individuals are either homozygous for C^W or C^X or heterozygous C^WC^X. Highest logarithm of odds (Lod) score of 10.76 between Rh and MAR was obtained at zero recombination fraction when the allelic relationship suggested by the segregation and population data between C^W, C^X and *MAR* was allowed for.

Our studies on their genetic relationship indicate that the three antigens C^W, C^X and MAR behave as if being determined by alleles of the same Rh sub-system. Furthermore, we conclude that this sub-system manifests an inheritance pattern that is distinct from but analogous to that of the two well-known allelic sub-systems of C/c and E/e antigens.

0285

EXPRESSION OF LEWIS ANTIGENS IN Le(a-b-) INDIVIDUALS

Henry S[2], Breimer ME[1], Oriol R[3], Woodfield, G[2], Samuelsson BE[1], .

[1]Dep. of Clinical Chemistry and Transfusion Medicine, Sahlgren's Hospital, Gothenburg, Sweden. [2]Auckland Regional Blood Centre, Auckland, New Zealand. [3]Unité de recherches sur la differenciation cellulaire intestinale, INSERM, Villejuif Cedex, France.

Objective: To investigate the expression of Lewis histo-blood group antigens in individuals of Lewis negative phenotypes.

Methods

Total non-acid glycosphingolipids were isolated from plasma and small intestine of Lewis negative individuals of various secretor phenotypes. The glycolipids were separated by thin-layer chromatography and immunostained with radio labelled Lewis antibodies. Histological paraffin embedded sections of small intestine from Lewis negative individuals were also fluorescently stained with Lewis antibodies.

Results

Trace amounts of Lewis glycolipids were identified in Lewis negative non secretor and secretor plasma and small intestinal samples. Immunohistologically Lewis activity was absent, or poorly expressed, at the intestinal brush border but Lewis activity was clearly demonstrated in the Golgi apparatus of the deep areas of the Lieberkühn's crypts.

Conclusion

These results clearly demonstrate that although the Lewis negative phenotype exists at the crude serological level, this phenotype is not an "all-or-nothing" phenomenon at the chemical level. The results obtained may explain the observed influence of the secretor system on the type of Lewis antibodies a Lewis negative individual will make.

0286

Sugars Block Binding of Anti-NB2 to Neutrophils

RM Minchinton, T Johnson, P Shariff.
Red Cross Blood Transfusion Service Queensland, Brisbane, 4000, Australia.

The NB1 antigen has been located on a 58-64 kDa glycoprotein, however, the molecular nature of NB2 is still a mystery.

We examined the ability of simple sugars bound in vitro to neutrophils, to block the binding of anti-NB2 and anti-NB1 antibodies. Granulocyte immuno-fluorescence (flow cytometric) was used to demonstrate binding and blocking of saturating quantities of antibody to NB1NB2 and NB2NB2 neutrophils. Solutions of 0.5M, 0.25M, 0.1M glucose, galactose, maltose, mannose, lactose, galNAC, glcNAC and fucose were used.

Pre-incubation of neutrophils with all 0.5M sugars resulted in efficient blocking of anti-NB2 antibodies. Variables affecting percent blocking included donor NB phenotype, fixation (blocking reduced by 10%) and sugar concentration. 0.25M maltose, mannose, lactose and GalNAC consistently blocked anti-NB2 binding. Variation in percent blocking was seen amongst different NB1NB2 donors. An anti-NB1 anti-body was not blocked by 0.5M glucose or galactose but was 70-99% blocked with all other 0.5M sugars.

Blocking of a neutrophil site rather than an anti-NB2 antigen binding site was suggested by 30% more blocking when neutrophils were pre-incubated with sugar compared with incubation of sugar, antibody and cells together. Although simple stearic hinderance at higher (0.5M) sugar concentrations may be the explanation, these data raise the possibility that NB2 and NB1 antigenic epitopes could be closely associated with a lectin like (sugar binding) molecule on the neutrophil surface.

0287

HLA haplotype frequencies in Taiwan

M. Lin, T.F. Yang, S.L. Chang

National Health Research Institute Transfusion Medicine Laboratory, Mackay Memorial Hospital, Taiwan, ROC

Among 169 cases of paternity testing investigated during 1988-1993 a total of 432 HLA haplotypes were eligible for use in calculating haplotype frequencies in our population. The Terasaki Oriental tray was used in this study. Frequencies of the most common haplotypes together with the most common HLA antigen gene frequencies are listed in the tables below.

Haplotype	No.	%
A2B46Cw11	27	6.3
A11B60Cw7	20	4.6
A33B58Cw3	15	3.5
A11B60Cw3	11	2.5
A2B60Blank	9	2.1
A11B46Cw11	9	2.1
A2B46Cw1	7	1.6
A2B60Cw7	7	1.6
A11B58Cw3	7	1.6
A2B13Cw3	6	1.4
A2B51Blank	6	1.4
A11B27Blank	6	1.4
A11B75Blank	6	1.4
A2B38Cw7	5	1.2
A2B38Blank	5	1.2
A11B13Cw3	5	1.2
A11B60Blank	5	1.2
A24B60Cw3	5	1.2
A24B60Cw9	5	1.2
A33B58Cw9	5	1.2
A30B13Cw6	5	1.2

HLA-A	Gf
A11	0.336
A2	0.257
A24	0.167
A33	0.083
A26	0.037
A31	0.032
A30	0.019

HLA-C	Gf
Cw3	0.215
Cw7	0.164
Blank	0.153
Cw1	0.148
Cw9	0.122
Cw11	0.100
Cw4	0.053
Cw6	0.044

HLA-B	Gf
B60	0.250
B46	0.134
B58	0.104
B13	0.081
B51	0.049
B62	0.044
B38	0.035
B75	0.032
B27	0.028
B35	0.028
B54	0.028
B52	0.023
B55	0.021
B57	0.019
B56	0.016
B48	0.016
B64	0.014

Linkage disequilibrium was most often observed in the haplotypes A2B46Cw11, A33B58Cw3 and A30B13Cw6.

0288

MONOCYTE CROSS-MATCH IN RENAL TRANSPLANT.

N. Puig[1], L. Pallardó[2], I. Gomez[1], Gimeno M[1], C. Marín[1], F. Carbonell[1], J. Villalba[1] and JA. Montoro[1].
1 C.de Transfusión de la C. Valenciana.
2 Serv Nefrología HG La Fé, Valencia, Spain.

In order to know if monocytes antibodies are relevant or not in renal transplantation, we made a donor specific monocyte cross-match (MNCM) in 76 patients who received a kidney allograft (lymphocytotoxicity CM test negative). The MNCM was made by fluorescence using the donors' peripheral white cells and the patients' current sera. FITC sheep anti-human IgG F(ab)'2 was used. The monocytes reactivity was analyzed by flow cytometry (FC), using a gate to select the monocytes by Facs-can. The FC, MNCM was considered positive when the mean of the fluorescence values were higher (mean+3SD) than negative controls (AB sera). In 74 patients CM by FC was also made with other cells. Eigtheen of the patients had positive MNCM (23,6%). This reactivity was correlated with the granulocyte CM, p=0,0000; B lymphocyte CM, p=0,06; but not to T lymphocyte CM, p=0,5. The positive MNCM was more frequent in patients with previous allografts, p= 0,01; A blood group, p=0,02; and patients with less than 12 months on dialysis treatment, p=0,008. We did not find any correlation between the MNCM and the allografts evolution after a mean follow-up of 18,3±5,3 months.

0289

GRANULOCYTE ANTIBODIES IN CORD SERA FROM PREMATURE TWINS.

Prema Madyastha and Linda Tribble. Med Univ of South Carolina, Charleston, SC., USA.

We have utilized umbilical cord sera to detect granulocyte antibodies (GrAb) in 8 sets of twins (ST) with gestational age ranging from 28-36 wks. Sera were tested against Gr from 10 normal donors(dr) by Gr agglutination (GA) and flow cytometry (FCy). Sera with fluorescent positive cells (FPC) ≥14% were considered positive in FCy, as established previously. Negative (0-13%) or weak (14-19%) reactivity was observed with one dr in 3 ST and stronger with 1-7 drs in 3 other ST (14-78%), which was lost after 3 months of storage at -80°C. However, 4 sera from 2 ST, continue to show 15-95% reactivity with 4-9 drs without any known Gr antibody specificity and were negative with dr lymphocytes. One serum was positive with 1 dr in GA(3+). In 3 ST, the serum from one of each ST showed consistently greater reactivity with dr Gr as compared to its counterpart:

%FPC With Reactive Donors (Dr)

ST	Dr1	Dr2	Dr3	Dr4	Dr5	Dr6	Dr7	Dr8	Dr9	Dr10	Dr11	Dr12
A♀	94	73	47	90	56	50	74	95	50	-	-	-
B♀	79	0	34	57	29	22	66	50	20	-	-	-
A♀	48	15	-	43	24	-	38	23	14	-	-	-
B♀	34	12	-	24	12	-	14	5	10	-	-	-
A♀	15	-	-	-	-	-	-	-	83	18	74	20
B♀	13	-	-	-	-	-	-	-	76	16	33	15

Although the implications of these GrAb currently are unknown due to non-availability of complete blood and differential counts, these results suggest the possibility of differential placental passage of maternal GrAb.

0290

NON HODGKIN'S LYMPHOMA ASSOCIATED WITH A MONOCLONAL ANTI-i ANTIBODY.

J.Cartron[1], P.Gane[2], J.F.Delfraissy[1], G.Tertian[1], R.Oriol[3] and J.P.Cartron[2].
[1]Hôpital Kremlin-Bicêtre, Paris, [2]INTS and INSERM U76, Paris, [3]INSERM U178, Paris

Mrs VI, a sixty years old female was referred to the hematology unit for the treatment of a diffuse high-grade non Hodgkin's lymphoma. She presented episodes of fever in a contex of neutropenia (neutrophils $0.1x10^9/L$ from $0.7x10^9/L$ white blood cells). Hb level was 7.2g/dl; and platelets $146x10^9/L$.A monoclonal IgM-K protein (48 g/L) was present in her serum.
The direct antiglobulin test on red cells was positive with anti-C3 (not with anti-IgG) due to the presence of a cold antibody with a serological anti-i specificity.The IgM antibody recognized all neutrophils tested, whatever their phenotypes in systems NA, NB, and 5 as tested by microgranuloagglutination and indirect immunofluorescence with an anti-IgM antiglobulin.Flow cytometry analysis showed the anti-i antibody to bind strongly to neutrophils, lymphocytes and monocytes. Binding to neutrophils was inhibited by oligosaccharides (Synsorb[R] Chembiomed) with anti-i specificity, suggesting that it may be responsible for the neutropenia.

0291

CD11a, CD11b, CD11c, CD18 EXPRESSION IN B-CELLS CHRONIC LYMPHOCYTIC LEUKEMIA.

C.Cacciapuoti, E.Cosentini, M.Cavalcanti, D.Graziano, F.Chiurazzi°, S. Formisano
Immunohematology-Medical School University "Federico II" Naples
° Hematology-Medical School University "Federico II". Naples Italy

Aim of our study was to investigate possible correlation between the expression of leucocyte adhesion molecules on B- CLL lymphocytes and the clinical stage of the disease.

Materials and methods. The immunological phenotype of 27 patients affected by B-CLL, at various clinical stages (Rai and Binet clinical staging systems were used) was CD5+ / CD19+ in 77% of cases and CD5- / CD19+ in the remaining 23%. The leukemic cells showed kappa or lambda light chains. The determination of leucocyte markers was made in peripheral blood using FITC or PE monoclonal antibodies: anti-CD18, -CD11a, -CD11b, -CD11c purchased from B.D. Fluorescent cells were analysed by flow cytometer. As normal control, 50 healthy subjects were examined.

Results. The expression of CD18, CD11a, CD11b on patients lymphocytes was considerably decreased. The expression of CD11c was increased (see Table)

Table

	CD11a	CD11b	CD11c	CD18
Patient (n.27)	16 ± 4 %	1,5 ± 1 %	35 ± 14 %	17 ± 3 %
Control (n.50)	72 ± 11 %	10 ± 5 %	7 ± 4 %	81 ± 14 %

Any significant correlations was found between the adhesive molecules expression and the clinical parameters considered (peripheral lymphocytosis, splenomegalia, medullary infiltration, auto-immunitary and/or infectious pathologies). In 10 patients the determination of leucoyte adhesion glycoproteins were repeated during the course of disease: no variations occurred, not even in patients showing an evolution of disease.

Conclusion. Any correlation between the expression of these molecules and the clinical stage of disease emerged from our research.

0292

PECULIARITIES OF T-LYMPHOCYTES IN PATIENTS WITH HEREDITARY GLUCOSE-6-PHOSPHATE DEHYDROGENASE DEFICIENGY

A.A.Umnyashkin[I], F.M.Abdullayev[2]
Institute of Pulmonary Diseases & TB, Baku, Azerbaijan.

Hereditary Glucose-6-Phosphate Dehydrogenase (G-6-PD) deficiency in blood white cells is the reason of primary immunodeficiency. I72 persons (I group) with zero and II5 persons (II group) with normal G-6-PD activity in blood white cells were examined in order to define the level of enzyme defect manifestation in matured T-lymphocytes and to study macroorganism's compensator mechanisms. T-lymphocytes differentiation antigens study was undertaken with the help of OKT monoclonal antibodies of different specification in order to analyse cell maturation processes. The investigation detected a sharp increase of "early" thymic lymphoid cells (OKT IO) in the first group. Spectrophotometric study of G-6-PD activity in "early" thymocytes detected its zero activity. The level of OKT3 cells was equal for both groups, whereas the number of cells with T4TII phenotype in the first group was smaller. Thus, enzyme defect of immunocompetent cells will bring to compensator ejection in peripheral blood of "early" thymocytes.

0293

INVESTIGATING THE VALUES OF THE IgG,IgA,AND IgM IN ACUTE LYMPHOBLASTIC LEUKEMIA (ALL) IN CHILDREN

Tarabadi F,A. Vossough,P.Doostar,S.Lotfi,H.
iranian blood transfusion service Tehran Iran

In the past years the rate of mortality was veryhigh among children and adults but in the recent yearsdue to eariy diagnosis of the different kinds of leukemias the rate of mortality has come down.

The study of cellular and humoral defence mechanism is ofgreat help for the diagnostic and treatment of - children with ALL. we have quantified the levels of IgA,IgG and IgMby the SRID method. In this work 200 ALL patients have been studied,all of which were under 14 years of age. The percentage of this disorder is higher in male patients and in patients between 2 to 10 years of age. we have observed a lower level of IgG and a higner level of IgM in these patients , when compared to healthy children of the same age group . These differences predict a higher suscebility to the infection and such patients have a higher mortality rate The IgM level in sepsis during the period of different treatments is compared with international reports.
in our patients the difference of IgA level was not - signicent

0294

NEUTROPHIL FUNCTION IN CML

L. Hamidpour, S. Ajdary, T. Zandieh,
Dr B. Shafaiian
Immunology laboratory of Iraian Blood Transfusion Service and Tehran University, Iran

In chronic myeloid leukemia the mature granulocytes are produced from a stem cell line containing and abnormal chromosome.
It is therefore possible that metabolic-functional abnormalities might appear in the mature fully differentiated cells. In the presented study the phagocytic activity in CML patients was studied. NBT reduction ingestion in 37 patients with CML and 37 normal controls. Patient's granulocytes display significantly lower ingestion, NBT reduction and intracellular killing than normals.
There is no significant difference in opsonization between CML and normal controls. Analysis of results showed an inverse correlation between phagocytc activity and WBC count, percentage of immature cells. Results suggested that neutrophils of CML patients have impaired phagocytic activity. This defect correlates with WBC count and percentage of immature cells.

0295

CHRONIC GRANULOMATOUS DISEASE: A FLOW CYTOMETRIC STUDY.

C.Cacciapuoti, E.Cosentini, M.Cavalcanti, U.Scognamiglio, V.Poggi,° S.Formisano.
Immunohematology-Medical School University of Naples "Federico II"
° Pausillipon Hospital Naples

CGD is a heterogeneous disorder inherited as an X-chromosome linked trait or as an autosomal recessive form. Using flow cytometry, phagocytosis, oxidative burst and adhesive glycoproteins of polimorphonuclear leucocytes were studied in a 5 years old boy and in his family. In the child severe clinical picture suggested CGD; moreover his early history showed recurrent infections, lymphadenitis, dermatitis.

Methods.

Phagocytosis : 100 ul whole blood were incubated at 37° C with 20ul of fluorescent E.Coli suspension for 10' and 20'. Measurement of oxidative metabolism: 100 ul whole blood were preincubated with 1ng/ml PMA for 10' at 37°C, then 15 ug/ml Dihydrorhodamine 123 was added. Adhesive glycoproteins were determinated with monoclonal antibodies. The fluorescence in all the methods were analysed by flow cytometry.

Results.

In the patient, the ingestion of fluorescent bacteria was increased: 97% phagocytizing cells showed 3623 mean fluorescence intensity (n.v. 1124± 286). Respiratory burst was absent after stimula. In the peripheral blood of the mother, two PMN populations with different response were detectable after PMA stimulus, while all PMN of the father responded to the PMA. In one of the patient's brother respiratory burst was absent and in his early history there were cutaneous infections. The older brother's PMNs responded to PMA.

Conclusion.

Detection of granulocyte reactive oxygen species formation in whole blood , using flow cytometry, is a very sensitive test and an alternative to the clinically used NBT test in the diagnosis of CGD.

0296

HUMAN PLATELET-SPECIFIC ALLOANTIGENS,PHENOTYPE FREQUENCY IN THAI BLOOD DONORS ; PRELIMINARY REPORT

R. O-Charoen, P. Kuptawintu, N. Jitjak.
National Blood Centre, Thai Red Cross Society, Bangkok, Thailand

The most common immunological cause of patients who develope platelet refractoriness is most likely due to HLA alloimmunigation. However, more and more cases due to platelet-specific alloantibodies are recovered and more recognition of it's clinically significant. Platelet antigens not only consist of blood group ABO antigens.HLA class I antigens but also platelet-specific alloantigens Since in thailand no report about the platelet-specific antigens in thai population, so the National Blood Centre, Thai Red Cross Society conducted a preliminary study on phenotye of platelet-specific alloantigen in Thai plasmapheresis donors, by the mixed passive hemagglutination technique (MPHA) developed by Dr.Shibata, Tokyo,Japan. One hundred and eighty nine group O plasmapheresis donors of age between 27-46 year old were included in the study. The phenotype frequency are as followed : HPA-1a (Pl^{A1}) 100%, HPA-2b (Sib^a) 21.4%, HPA-3a (Bak^a) 74%, HPA-4b (Yuk^a) 4%, HPA-4a (Yuk^b) 100% and Nak^a 71.6%. The result is quite comparable to the phenotype frequency reported in Japanese and Korean population.

0297

FREQUENCY OF HUMAN PLATELET ANTIGENS AMONG NORTHEASTERN-THAI BLOOD DONORS

Y. Urwijitaroon, S. Barusruk,
A. Romphryk, C. Puapairoj
Blood Transfusion Centre, Faculty of Medicine,
Khon Kaen University, Khon Kaen, Thailand 40002

Human platelet antigens (HPA) were studied for the phenotype in unrelated Northeastern-Thai blood donors using Professor Shibata's improved mixed passive hemagglutination (MPHA) technique.

The phenotyping was done in 483 blood donors including 358 males and 125 females. There were 298 group O, 65 group A, 102 group B and 18 of group AB. The results demonstrated 100% frequency of HPA-1a (Pl^{A1}), 15.94% of HPA-2b (Sib^a), 60.25% of HPA-3a (Bak^a), 98.76% of HPA-4a (Yuk^b), 1.86% of HPA-4b (Yuk^a), 5.38% of HPA-5b (Br^a) and 97.72% of NaK^a. There is no statistically significant difference according to sex.

0298

BLOOD GROUP A AND B ANTIGEN EXPRESSION IN PLATELETS IS ASSOCIATED WITH GLYCOPROTEIN Ib AND IIb. EVIDENCE FOR AN A_1/A_2 DIFFERENCE.

H. Wadenvik[1], D. Stockelberg[1], S. Jacobsson[2], L. Rydberg[2], J Kutti[1].
From the Department of Medicine, Hematology Section[1] and the Department of Clinical Chemistry and Transfusion Medicine[2], Sahlgrenska Hospital, Göteborg, Sweden.

Blood group ABH antigens are associated with platelets as intrinsic determinants and extrinsically adsorbed antigens, and exist both on glycosphingolipids and glycoproteins (GP). We now provide direct evidence that blood group ABH antigens are associated with GPIb and GPIIb. By immunoprecipitation, a murine monoclonal anti-A antibody precipitated surface-biotin-labeled blood group A_1 platelet membrane proteins with electrophoretic characteristics identical to those of GPIb/IX and GPIIb/IIIa. By immunoblotting of SDS-PAGE separated blood group A_1 platelet proteins the monoclonal anti-A antibody bound to proteins with electrophoretic characteristics identical to those of GPIb and GPIIb; GPIIIa did not display any significant staining By ELISA wherein monoclonal antibodies specific for GPIb (AP1) and the GPIIb/IIIa complex (AP2) were used to capture and hold antigens from platelet lysate, human anti-A antibodies reacted with these proteins derived from A_1 platelets; proteins from blood group A_2, O, and B platelets showed no reactivity. These results indicate that blood group A antigen is associated with GPIb and GPIIb derived from blood group A_1 but not A_2 platelets. The same result was found for B antigens, i.e. an association with GPIb and GPIIb.

0299

GENOTYPIC ANALYSIS OF HUMAN PLATELET ANTIGENS - COMPARISON WITH THE MIXED PASSIVE HEMAGGLUTINATION (MPHA) METHOD.

N.H.Tsuno[1)], M.Miyamoto[1)], K.Shimada[2)], M.Hashiguchi [2)], Y.Shibata[1)]
1) The Department of Transfusion Medicine and Immunohematology, University of Tokyo, Tokyo and 2) The Diagnostic Section, Sumitomo Metal Industries, Ltd., Ibaragi, Japan

Human platelet alloantigens (HPA) are of importance in neonatal alloimmune thrombocytopenia (NAITP), refractoriness to platelet transfusion therapy, and post transfusion purpura (PTP). Five distinct biallelic platelet "specific" alloantigen systems have been identified to be involved in these pathological processes. The HPA-1 to -5 systems have been found to be associated with point mutations leading to single amino acid substitutions. Platelets from 35 normal volunteers were typed for HPA-1 to -4 by the PCR amplification method, using type-specific primers recognizing the single point mutations. For DNA extraction and PCR amplification, kits were used. The results of the DNA typing were compared with that of the phenotypic analysis by the MPHA. The results obtained by both methods were strictly concordant, demonstrating that the phenotypic analysis of HPA by the high-sensitive MPHA method is of high reliability. Moreover, the simple method for DNA typing using these kits may be of great value in typing for alleles that encode platelet alloantigens when no platelets are available.

0301

SCREENING FOR THE ANTI-HUMAN PLATELET ALLOANTIGENS (HPA) BY MIXED PASSIVE HEMAGGLUTINATION (MPHA) TEST.

S.Morita[1)], K.Hando[1)], M.Hattori[1)], A.Ishijima[2)], N.Kozaki[2)], N.Kim[3)], K.Takahashi[3)], M.Miyamoto[4)], Y.Shibata[4)]
1) Ina Red Cross Center, Saitama 2) Saitama Red Cross Center, Saitama 3) Dept. of Transfusion, Toranomon Hospital, Tokyo 4) Dept. of Transfusion Medicine and Immunohematology, University of Tokyo, Tokyo, Japan

Antibody to the human platelet alloantigens (HPA) in the plasma of 15,000 inpatients was investigated by the mixed passive hemagglutination (MPHA) test. From the 15,000 samples examined, anti-HPA2b antibody was found in 9 (0.06%), anti-HPA3a in 2 (0.01%), anti-HPA4b in 3 (0.02%), and anti-HPA5b in 5 cases (0.03%). Moreover, antibodies with undetermined specificity were found in 6 cases. All the patients with antibodies to HPA2b and 3a had a positive transfusional history. As these antibodies are extremely rare in the normal population, it is suggested that their production is a consequence of the blood transfusion. From the patients with antibodies to HPA4b and 5b, the majority were women with past history of pregnancy. These antibodies, contrary to the previous ones, are very frequent in the normal population, suggesting that they are produced during normal pregnancy.

0302

EVALUATION OF THE READER FOR ORTHO BIOVUE SYSTEM CASSETTES

C. Cherby, M.P. Barriau
Regional Blood Bank, Clermont-Ferrand, France.

Purpose : BIOVUE reader is composed by a CCD camera. The reading consists in picture analysis with interferential filters. The cassettes are read on each face.
Methods : Ortho Biovue system cassettes used for antibody screening and identification in indirect Coombs method and enzyme method are read on Biovue reader. First time : Biovue reader reads each well of the cassettes. Second time : on the computer we indicate the visual results for each well. Finally : the computer compares the two results and indicates the differences. The validation consists to identify the differences and to class them in a "no important difference" category (different interpretation of the reaction intensity between the two readers) or in a "mistake" category.

Results :

	Coombs method 4782 wells	Enzyme method 2940 wells
Identical results	4716 (98.6 %)	2904 (98.8 %)
Mistake	66 (1.4 %)	36 (1.2 %)
False negative	17 (0.4 %)	24 (0.8 %)
False positive	49 (1.0 %)	12 (0.4 %)

Conclusion : With this study, we obtain good results for specificity and sensitivity. Biovue reader represents an attractive evolution for Ortho Biovue system cassettes automatisation.

0303

EVALUATION OF IMAGE ANALYSIS READER FOR GEL TEST

S. Ciaffoni, A. Franchetti, S. Migliozzi.
Blood Transfusion Service, Bussolengo
ITALY

Objective. The gel test(GT) has standardized the obtention of agglutination and provided a simple reliable way to read it. Although visual inspection can determine whether agglutination has taken place, the computer is able to give quantitative data and extend the range and precision of the assay.We present the results of our approach toward an instrument to evaluate immunohaematologic test based upon image analysis of gel test.
Methods.The Liss/AHG microtyping system was obtained by Diamed and all AHG-GT were performed in accordance with the manifacturer's instructions.The image analysis reader (IAR) is based on the interpretation of the slide image obtained by mechanical sliding on high linear CCD element. A decisional fuzzy process classifies reactions in four levels of positivity, one level of negativity and different critical situations can be solved on the base of visive evaluation by operator.
Results. We tested 2500 patient sera submitted to our laboratory for antibody investigations.All Ab screening test were first evaluated in manual way, always by the same operator and then by image analysis reader. We have found no discrepancy in these ways of interpretation of GT.
Conclusions. We conclude that IAR is easy to use and offers an absolute safety about interpretation of tests' results. Finally, putting random and in rapid sequence ID-Cards containing gel suspension with barcode in the specialized board, we can read and interpret blood grouping, cross-matches and Ab screening in few seconds.

0304

THE SEROLOGIC EVALUATION OF RED BLOOD CELLS FROM PATIENTS WITH SICKLE CELL DISEASE USING THE GEL TEST

S.D. Sosler[1], M. Swain[2], P.J. DeChristopher[1], H. Malyska[2]. 1The University of Illinois, Chicago, Illinois, 2Microtyping Systems, Pompano Beach, Florida, USA.

Red blood cells (RBC) from 26 patients (14 samples drawn in EDTA, 12 clotted) with sickle cell disease (SCD) were evaluated by several serologic tests using the ID Gel Test System (MTS) versus standard test tube agglutination. Thirteen of the 26 patients had been transfused with RBCs during the prior 3 months. The serologic tests evaluated included the determination of the ABO cell group, Rh type, Rh phenotype, and direct antiglobulin test (DAT) using both anti-IgG + C3b and anti-IgG alone. There was 100% agreement between the Gel and tube technique for all of the tests described above. All 26 RBC samples had negative buffered gel test controls and Rh tube test controls even though the RBCs from 6 patients had positive DATs (+vw to 2+). The 13 transfused patients showed expected mixed-field (mf) agglutination in certain tests performed as part of the Rh phenotype by both gel and tube technique, however unlike the tube test, recognition of mf agglutination was much easier to visually observe in the Gel Test without the need of a microscope.

0305

EVALUATION OF THE BIOVUE™ TECHNOLOGY IN PRETRANSFUSIONAL CROSSMATCH AND RED CELL ANTIBODY SCREENING

M.C.Frère-Wilmotte, J.M.Loréa, D.Sondag-Thull
Transfusion Center of Liège, Red Cross of Belgium

We evaluated the Biovue™ column agglutination system (Ortho Diagnostics System), intended to detect antigen-antibody reactions on red cells.

Among 2,500 crossmatches performed simultaneously with Biovue and with conventional tube technique, 2.40 and 2.44% respectively were shown to be positive due to 46 specific antibodies, 0.80 and 2.96% due to non specific agglutinins active with enzyme-treated red cells. Thirty-eight (82.6%) of the specific antibodies were detected by both techniques. Those undetected by Biovue were all IgM while those undetected by tube agglutination were 3 IgM and 5 IgG (1-K, 2-Jka, 1-Fya, 1-S).

On 85 frozen sera with previously identified antibodies, an antibody screening was performed by Biovue, tube technique and routine microplate technique (papain and Capture R™ solid phase indirect Coombs) simultaneously. 5 among 6 undetected antibodies by Biovue were IgG, 11 among 12 undetected by tube technique were IgG and 2 among 6 undetected by microplate technique were IgG.

The comparison of techniques according to the serologic method used shows that the Biovue bromelin method, as we implemented it, is inefficient for IgG as well as IgM antibodies detection. In contrast, the Biovue indirect Coombs shows a markedly higher sensitivity than the tube technique and is equivalent to Capture R solid phase system, except for anti-Jka, which are better detected by Biovue.

In conclusion, the Biovue technology should advantageously replace the tube agglutination technique in compatibility testing, owing to its sensitivity, ease of use and objective reading. In antibody screening, the papain microplate technique associated with indirect Coombs in solid phase affords slightly better results than those obtained with Biovue.

0306

RED CELL ANTIBODIES SCREENING BY FILTRATION ON MICRO PARTICLES COLUMNS (BioVue SystemTM)

B.LAMY, C.TISSOT, C.HEYD. Régional Blood Transfusion Center, Besançon, France.

BioVue™ System has been developped in 1991 to improve red cell antibody screening. It is a plastic cassette with six columns containing filtering particles. They are prefilled with different reagents (IgG or polyspecific antiglobulin, neutral saline solution...) according to the performed test (Indirect Antiglobulin Test = IAT, enzyme tests).

After a first evaluation this system has been used for routine screening with an association of 2 techniques : polyvalent IAT, papaïn treated cells technique and the results were compared to those obtained with similar manual techniques (IAT and a two step papaïn treated cells technique).

In 1992, 21 365 samples were tested.We obtained :

		BioVue	Manual techniques
Positive sera	:	983	845
Specific antibodies	:	924	802
Auto antibodies	:	37	31
Non specific reactions	:	22	12

Among the undetected positive sera with manual technique we found 11 anti Kell, 8 anti c, 18 anti E, 4 anti Fya, 1 anti Fyb, 2 anti Jka, 1 anti S with a potential clinical risk.

The microplate size of the cassettes allows an automatic distribution of sera via the MITIS system.

BioVue™ is produced by ORTHO DIAGNOSTIC SYSTEMS

0307

EVALUATION OF ORTHO BIOVUE ABD/RH-hr/K CASSETTES

Kasulke,D.H.[1], Ellisor,S.[2] Basner,R.[3], Krause,M.[1]
1Red Cross Center, Baden-Baden, Germany, 2Ortho Diagnostic Systems Inc., Raritan, USA, 3Ortho Diagnostic Systems GmbH, Neckargemünd, Germany

107 samples were tested with the Ortho BioVue System (BVS) ABD/Rh-hr/K cassettes on selected samples: 49 transfused, 21 non-transfused patients and 37 donors. Unusual samples included 12 alloantibody positives, 1 hemolyzed and icteric, 1 hemolyzed, 3 DAT positives, and 4 with weak D antigen, 1 patient on hemodialysis, 1 with thallassaemia, and 1 bone marrow transplant. BVS was compared to manual tube tests using monoclonal reagents from various European and US manufacturers. BVS ABD cassettes contain BioClone Anti-A , Anti-B, Anti-A,B , Anti-D, Anti-CDE , and a reagent control that contains all of the ingredients of the reagent except anti-body. BVS Rh-hr/K cassettes contain BioClone Anti-C, Anti-E , Anti-c , Anti-e, Anti-K as well as a reagent control. The BVS Reverse Diluent cassettes containing macromolecules that enhance the direct agglutination of IgM and some IgG antibodies. BVS was found to be equal to or better than tube tests for antigen typing of red blood cells (RBC). Mixed field agglutination was detected as a layer of strongly positive RBC at the top of the column with negative cells at the bottom. One unusual donor sample was unable to be interpreted during routine testing on the Olympus and with Diamed gel test because of the presence of a bromelain antibody. The sample was correctly typed by BVS because no enzyme modification is necessary.

0308

CLINICAL EVALUATION OF THE ORTHO BIOVUE SYSTEM CASSETTES FOR ABO BLOOD GROUPING AND RHESUS-KELL PHENOTYPING

C. Cherby, M.P. Barriau
Regional Blood Bank, Clermont-Ferrand, France.

Purpose : In aim to obtain their qualification, we have studied in our laboratory three new cassettes for ABO blood grouping (anti-A, anti-B, anti-AB, Anti-D, anti-CDE, control), reverse ABO (neutral cassette for red cells A1, A2, B, O), Rhesus-Kell phenotyping (anti-C, anti-E, anti-c, anti-e, anti-Kell, control).
Methods : During the clinical evaluation, we have tested different patients and blood donors with normal or particular ABO-D blood group and Rh-Kell phenotype : samples with abnormal red blood cells, adult or cord samples with positive Direct Antiglobuline Test (DAT), cord sample with negative DAT, untransfused patients, transfused patients, donor segments, Weak A/B/D/C/E/c/e/K. The reactions are compared with usual methods of the laboratory.
Results : No differences are observed with ABO blood grouping and Rh - Kell phenotyping results. Weak antigens are recognized, and it's easy to distinguish two red blood cells populations.
Conclusion : These new cassettes give good results and are very easy to use : No red blood cells wash, dilution with saline, no incubation, immediate centrifugation.

0309

A COMPARISON BETWEEN THE DIAMED MICROTYPING SYSTEM AND CONVENTIONAL TUBE TEST FOR DETECTING ERYTHROCYTE AUTO-ANTIBODIES

Castilho, L.M.; Locatelli, M.F.; Violati, R.G., Bechelli, A.P.P.; Pires, C.A.; Pellegrino, Jr., J. - Hematology & Hemotherapy Center - State University of Campinas - UNICAMP - Campinas - S.P. - Brazil.

The direct antiglobulin test was performed in 760 patient samples by the ID-System and Conventional Method, using monoespecific and poliespecific antiglobulins. The eluate was performed on all patient samples. We determined the sensitivity and specificity of both methods. The results are shown in tables 1 and 2

Table 1: Conventional

DAT/ Eluate	Pos	Neg
Pos	95	13
Neg	5	647
Total	100	660

Table 2: Gel Test

DAT/ Eluate	Pos	Neg
Pos	105	0
Neg	0	655
Total	105	655

The conventional test was 95% sensitive and 98.03% specific to detect erythrocyte auto antibodies.
The gel test was 100% sensitive and 100% specific to detect these antibodies.

0310

THE GEL TEST IS MUCH MORE SENSITIVE THAN THE TUBE METHOD IN THE IDENTIFICATION OF RED CELL ANTIBODIES BY USING ENZYME TREATED CELLS.

J.G. Meerman, A.B. Scholten, H.J. Bos, G.C. van der Plas
Red Cross Blood Bank Arnhem, Arnhem, The Netherlands

The gel test is a serological technique, which allows reliable detection of immunoglobulin-mediated red cell agglutination. In the gel test, antigen-antibody reactions are observed for agglutination after centrifugation of erythrocytes through a sephadex gel in a microtube. Agglutinated red cells will stick into the gel and not-agglutinated erythrocytes will form a sediment on the bottom of the tube. Twenty patientsera containing one or a combination of the following antibodies: D, C, c, E, K, Fy^a, Le^a, M, P1 and HTLA; as detected by the tube method (albumin coombs and PEG technique) were frozen and thawn just before use.

Using untreated celpanels, the gel test showed in general a stronger reaction pattern than the albumin coombs tube method. M-antibodies, however were not very well detectable by the gel test. In one case anti-Fy^a was not clearly detectable in the gel test. In another sample an anti-Fy^a showed a stronger reaction pattern in the gel test. By using enzyme treated cells, in five patient sera the gel test was much more sensitive than the tube method. In these five sera, the following antibodies could be identified in addition to the antibodies detected by the tube method: D (2x), E, e, C (2x) and C^w. In the gel test three times less serum is needed and the test can be performed up to 50-70 % faster than the conventional tube method. Another advantage of the gel test is the standarized reading of the agglutination and the objective interpretation of weak reactions. Improvement of the gel test is needed concerning the interchangeability of red cell panels. In our lab the gel test is a usefull additional technique for the identification of irregular red cell antibodies.

0311

RED CELL ALLOANTIBODIES IN THALASSEMIC PATIENTS BY THE GEL TEST

O. Nathalang[1], S.Srichinda[2], T.Suwanasit[2], K.Torcharus[3], T.Krutvacho[2], T.Sriphaisal[1]

1 Department of Pathology, Pramongkutklao College of Medicine, 2 Blood Bank, Pramongkutklao hospital, 3 Department of Pediatrics, Pramongkutklao hospital, Bangkok, Thailand.

Abstract

The purpose of this study is to compare the Gel test (Dia Med-ID Micro Typing System, Switzerland) and the conventional tube test for antibody screening and antibody identification. A total of 63 sera from multitransfused thalassemic patients had been studied. Sera were screened for red cell antibodies by 4° - 22^oC incubation, two stage enzyme technique and indirect antiglobulin test (IAT).
The incidence of red cell alloantibodies and autoantibodies in these patients were found to be 9.5% and 20.6%, respectively by both tests. The alloantibodies were revealed to be anti Le^a 1, anti Le^a plus anti Mi^a 1, anti E 1, anti E plus anti c 1, anti Mi^a 1 and one unidentified antibody. It was found that the Gel test was more sensitive to detect anti Le^a, anti E and anti Mi^a by enzyme technique and IAT.
In conclusion, the Gel test is simple, IAT can be performed without washing red cells and the results are more objective than those with the conventional tube test.

0312

DETECTION OF RED BLOOD CELL ANTIBODIES: COMPARISON OF THREE DIFERENT TECHNIQUES

Castilho, L.M.; Locatelli, M. F.; Violati, R.G.; Bechelli, A.P.P.; Pires, C.A.; Pellegrino Jr., J. - Hematology & Hemoterapy Center-State University of Campinas - UNICAMP - Campinas - S.P. - Brazil.

We compared three techniques: a classical low ionic strength indirect antiglobulin test (LISS) using an anti-IgG reagent, an indirect anti-globulin test in polyethylene glycol using the same anti-IgG reagent, a gel test system by DIAMED using papain (GEL-PAP). We performed studies of 181 sera containing identified IgG allo antibodies. The antibodies studies by the different techniques are in table 1

Table 1 - Antibodies Specificities and Techniques

Abs /Tec	D	C	c	E	e	G	K	Fya	Fyb	Jka	Jkb	S	s
Liss	40	12	5	20	06	08	07	02	01	02	0	0	0
Peg	40	12	06	25	12	09	20	04	01	04	02	01	01
Gel -Pap	40	21	10	50	13	10	11	0	0	05	04	0	0
Total	40	21	10	50	13	10	20	04	01	06	04	01	01

The gel papain test was 100% sensitive to detect Rh antibodies. However, we didn't get a 100% sensitive technique to detect the most clinically significant antibodies, but we've considered the association PAP-GEL - PEG a good choice. These results emphasize the combination of techniques used for safely detecting irregular antibodies.

0313

APPLICATION OF COLUMN AGGLUTINATION TECHNOLOGY FOR THE DETECTION OF BLOOD CELLS ANTIBODIES.

G.Girelli , S.Pupella° , M.P.Perrone° , S.Vaglio° , A.Nicolotti°, P.De Felice°, M.Valentini°.
Exp.Medicine Dept and Hematology Institute.°Human Biopathol.Dept., Hematology Institute. University " La Sapienza " Rome, Italy.

During sep.'93-dic.'93, column agglutination technology (Ortho Biovue System) was used to detect red blood cells antibodies in 2825 patients sera sent for crossmatching. 49 from 55 Biovue-reactive sera were found to have: 37 alloantibodies, 12 autoantibodies. Specificities detected included : 4 anti-D, 2 anti-C, 3 anti-E, 1 anti-c, 10 anti-K, 1 anti-Fya, 1 anti-Kpa, 4 anti-Lea, 1 anti-Leb, 1 anti-Lex, 1 anti-N, 1 anti-Lua; 7 non-identified. 6 sera gave false-positive reactions. All sera, including those with previously detected alloantibodies, were compared to conventional Liss-Coombs technique in pretransfusion test. Never discrepant results were obteined.In conclusion, this technique can be used for antibody detection for her sensivity and specificity with the added advantages of stable results and very rapid procedure.

0314

EVALUATION OF A RED CELL SOLID-PHASE ANTIBODY SCREENING METHOD

D. Bombail-Girard, M. Girard, B. Fournier
C.D.T.S., 6, rue Emile Lesot - 80000 AMIENS - FRANCE

CAPTURE-® Ready Screen® (Pooled Cells) is a solid phase system for detection of unexpected antibodies to red cells manufactured by Immucor (Norcross, GA.). A mixture of two red cells is bound and dried to the surfaces of polystyrene microtitration strip wells. Pooled cells allow the possibility to get in a single well major red cell antigens to bind unexpected antibodies.

We investigated the quality of this reagent and its possible application to blood donations screening. This reagent was compared with our techniques routinely used in our laboratory : papaïnized red cells and Coombs' test in Liss medium. A panel of selected specificities included : 16 anti-D, 18 - E, 9 - C, 5 - c, 3 - C^w, 1 - e, 10 - K, 4 - k, 1 - Kpa, 1 - Lu^a, 11 - Fy^a, 2 - Fy^b, 2 - Jk^a, 2 - Jk^b, 2 - M, 1 - N, 2 - S, 1 - s, 7 - Le^a, 5 - Le^b, 5 - P1, 10 mixtures of antibodies and 15 auto antibodies and public antibodies. No IgG antibody was undetected.

7413 random sera from blood donors were also tested. 86 samples reacted positively (1.1%) amongst which 11 (0.14%) were false positive reactions, 21 (0.28%) were autoantibodies. 13 antibodies were only detected by this test (2 anti-D, 4 -K, 1-Fy^a, 1 -S, 1 -C^w, 1 -P1, 1 -H, 1 -M).

14 antibodies were only detected with techniques using papaïn or Liss (1 anti -D, 1 -c, 2 -E, 1 -Jk^a, 4 -P1, 2 -Le^a, 2 -Le^b, 1 -autoantibody).

This test which can be automated is a valuable addition to improve the safety of blood donation screening. However it should not be considered as a universal, stand-alone technique to detect every unexpected antibody.

0315

A SOLID PHASE TECHNIQUE VERSUS THE TUBE METHOD IN ERYTHROCYTE ANTIBODY SCREENING AND IDENTIFICATION

G.A.H. Peeters, A.B. Scholten, H.J. Bos, G.C. van der Plas
Red Cross Blood Bank, Arnhem, The Netherlands.

In the solid phase technique (SPT) reagent red cells are bound to the surface of polystyrene microtitration strip wells (Capture-R Ready-Screen and Capture-R Ready ID, Immucor). The dried membranes are suitable for use in antibody screening or antibody identification assays based on anti-IgG-coated indicator red cells. To evaluate the SPT for general use in the bloodbank we took 13 patient sera. Each of which contained one or more of the following antibodies according to the tube methode (albumin coombs and PEG technique): D, C, E, K, Fy^a, Le^b, Co^a and an unidentified cold reacting antibody.

In the SPT one sample containing an anti-E and one sample containing the cold reacting antibody were missed. Antibodies in four of the thirteen sera were further identified in both methods. In three of the four sera discrepancies were found. In two sera the SPT showed extra reactions, which could not be specified. In one sample that was missed in the screening an E-antibody could not be identified. In diluting a serum sample containing anti-K and anti-Fy^a the tube method allowed a one fold higher dilution for the detection of anti-K.

Conclusion: the SPT is less suitable for screening and identification of erythrocyte antibodies in comparison to the tube test, since in one sample a clinically relevant E-antibody was missed and extra reactions were found, which could not be further specified.

0316

AN IMMEDIATE SPIN ANTIGLOBULIN TEST?

Gopal-Patel J, Rawlings J, Barrow L, Knight R C

North London Blood Transfusion Centre, Colindale Ave, London, NW9, UK

The manual low ionic polybrene technique (LIP) is useful for quick phenotyping tests, however, some antisera (esp. anti-Fy^a, -Jk^a) give better results if taken through to an antiglobulin phase. These sera, produced in-house, were reassessed by a tube "LIM-IAT": serum, cells and low ionic medium (LIM) are incubated at room temperature for two minutes, as in LIP, but instead of adding Polybrene the tube is washed immediately, AHG added and the results read.

The LIM-IAT was assessed for phenotyping using Diamed ID "Coombs" gels, with as short an incubation time as possible. As the conventional washing and AHG addition steps are not required with gels, hands-on time is minimal. Using 25 µl antiserum plus 50 µl 1% suspension of cells in LIM, Rh antisera gave good results with a 1 min. incubation whereas other sera, anti -Jk^a -Fy^a -K, required a 5 min. incubation to achieve optimal results.

Although not strictly immediate spin IATs both the tube and gel-microtube techniques have proved to be quick and reliable for phenotyping with selected antisera.

0317

ANTIBODY DETECTION IN BLOOD DONORS. COMPARISON OF DIFFERENT TECHNIQUES.

M.MAZZUCCO,R.POMA,F.RIZZUTO,L.SALVANESCHI.

S. I. T. I.R.C.C.S San Matteo, Pavia, Italy.

AIM: Three different techniques for antibody screening are used in a parallel study on 2143 blood Donors. The aim of our study is to evaluate these methods .

METHODS AND RESULTS: Antibody screening is performed using : 1)Polybrene microplate techinque RAP-I.D. Polycation Potentiator System DADE, 2) Column agglutination technology CAT ORTHO BioVue System , 3)Gel Test DIAMED. Both indirect antiglobulin tests (AHG) and enzyme tests are performed with Ortho BioVue and Gel Test Diamed. Of the 2143 serum specimens, 2064 are negative with all techniques.The table shows positive samples obtained with the three different tests and techniques.

	BIOVUE		GEL TEST		RAP.I.D.	
	Tot.	Ab. detected	Tot.	Ab. detected	Tot.	Ab. detected
AHG	2	2	0	0		
AHG+Enz.	17	15	17	16		
Enz.only.	6	3	62	13		
Tot.Pos.	25	20	79	29	24	21

CONCLUSION:The data in the table show that the three methods are similar except for the enzyme only Gel Test Diamed. Infact, Gel Test technique shows a high percentage (63.2%) of non detected antibodies for unknown reasons (too weak to identify?, clinically irrelevant?, aspecificities?).For this reason we think this technique should not be used in the Donors' antibody screening.

0318

DETECTION OF WEAK-D USING DIFFERENT ANTI-D IN NEUTRAL GEL

C.MAZZEI,G.CAVAGNARO.G.BARBERIS, F. NOTARIS U.GIANATTI,G.IMBERCIADORI

C.Trasfusionale,Osp.S.Corona,Pietra Ligure (SV)Italia

Monoclonal anti-D and new technologies dicreased subjects previously classified D neg - Du pos.(weak-D) detected only in IAT with polyclonal sera.We studyied sensitivity of Gel-Test (DiaMed) in typing Du and the reac-tivities observed dispensing,in DiaMed neutral gel,polyclonal (Ortho,Biotest,Dr.Molter,Baxter,Menarini),IgM + IgG monoclonal (Ortho),IgM monoclonal (Biotest, Menarini, Immucor),IgG monoclonal (Immucor), and IgM monoclonal + polyclonal (Baxter,Murex,Immucor,Fresenius,GammaBilogicals) anti-D sera. We typed 36.600 subjects and demonstrated 108 Du.The ID-Mycrotyping System failed to detect 3 CC.Du.ee.,also negative with IgM or IgG monoclonal and IgM monoclonal + IgG polyclonal anti-D,reacting only by polyclonal anti-D,in tube ,with IAT.The occurrence of D-variant was confirmed by monoclonal anti-D (IgM or IgG) directed to eight different epytopes of D mosaic (Diagast). The three Du showed a low reactivity with other polyclonal anti-D dispensed in neutral gel and no reactivity with monoclonal sera.For the other 105 Du,we observed the best strenght of reaction with monoclonal IgM anti-D (4+) and Du were classified Rh pos. with these antibodies.

0319

COMPARISON OF GEL AND COLUMN AGGLUTINATION SYSTEM FOR RED CELL ANTIBODY SCREENING

C.Mazzei,G.Barberis,C.Valle,G.Imberciadori

C.Trasfusionale, USL N.2, Osp. S. Corona, PIETRA LIGURE (SV)- ITALY

New systems for screening blood have been developed in recent years.In this study we compared the sensitivity of two methods,the Gel Test (GT) (DiaMed) and the Column Agglutination Technology (CAT) (Ortho) in detecting unexpected red cell antibodies.GT uses cards with a dextran gel, CAT glass microbeads (without or incorporating anti-globulin reagents (anti-IgG + C3d + C3b). We tested,in parallel,fresh sera from 1766 patients by both methods,at 37 C and in IAT ,using the same three reagent RBC panel (Surgiscreen-) contained cells homozygous for the following antigens: C,D,E,c,e, Fya, Fyb,Jka,Jkb,K,cellano,S,s,M,N,.We found 24 clinically significant antibodies(12 anti-D ,3 anti-K,3 anti-E,2 anti-C,1 anti-c,3 anti -Jka) with some difference : the Gel Test failed to detect 1 alloantibodies (anti-K) (sensitivity = 95%), while the CAT missed 1 anti-D (weakly reacting in GEL only with group O R2R2 red cells) and 1 anti-E (sensitivity = 91 %) also after repeat testing. The two methods are very easy to use and eliminate the need to wash red cells of traditional tube test. The reactions are stable and permit multiple reviewers.We found some difficulty in interpreting weak positive results in CAT .

0320

EVALUATION OF GEL AND COLUMN AGGLUTINATION FOR ALLOANTIBODIES IN FROZEN SERA

C. Mazzei,F.Saccone,C. Durante.G. Lavagna
C. Trasfusionale, USL 2, Osp. S. Corona
PIETRA LIGURE (SV)-ITALY

Of new technologies developed for detection of unexspected antibodies,we evaluated the sensitivity of two methods,the Gel Test (GT) (DiaMed) and the Column Agglutination System (CAS) (Ortho). In both methods, agglutinates are trapped in dextran or bead matrix,respectively, after centrifugation. We tested at 37 C. and in IAT by the GT and CAS sera containing 146 red cell alloantibodies previously collected and stored at -30 C., (50 anti-D, 35 anti-K,1 anti-Cellano,30 anti-E, 1 anti-e, 6 anti-C, 5 anti-c, 3 anti-Cw, 4 anti-Fya, 1 anti-Fyb, 7 anti-Jka, 1 anti-Jkb,1 anti-S, 1 anti-s,). Tests were performed using the same panel of 3-red cells (Surgescreen-Ortho).The two methods showed good sensitivity,but while CAS failed to detect 3/146 antibodies (1 anti-D at low titer reacting in GT only with group O R2R2 cells,1 anti-E and 1 anti-Cw), GT missed only 1/146 (1 anti-Jka).In GT,we observed higher strenght of reactivity for antibodies of Rh and Kell systems ,more evident for heterozygous red cells.On the other hand ,titration studies showed that GT was less sensitive only for antibodies reacting with Kidd and Duffy antigens expressed in single dose on red cells .

0321

SCREENING FOR UNEXPECTED ANTIBODIES. COMPARATIVE STUDY OF MICROPLATE TECHNIQUE AND GEL TYPE CHROMA TEST.

T. Chabert; Mª J. Rodrigues; A.Costa; F.Nascimento
Centro Regional de Sangue de Lisboa - IPS
Lisboa - Portugal

Objective: To compare the results of screening red cells antibodies obtained by the enzyme microplate technique and results obtained by the gel test Chroma PAP papaine method and Chroma Coombs, LISS/IAT.
Methods: During 4 weeks, 650 blood donor samples were screened for the presence of irregular antibodies with both techniques. With microplate method were used 2 papainized screening cells. The Chroma PAP and Chroma Coombs are composed of columns filled with gel in neutral solution to use with 2 papainized screening cells in Chroma PAP and with a polyvalent antiglobuline in Chroma Coombs. Also 23 frozen samples with known specificities were tested.
Results: Out of 650 samples, 26 were positive with one or more methods. Of these 26, 2 samples were positive with the three methods, 1 anti-E and 1 anti-D. Both papaine methods detected 2 anti-P1 and 6 samples with non specific reactions. The Chroma PAP detected 1 anti-P1 and 11 samples with non specific reactions. 1 anti-E was detected only with Chroma PAP and Chroma Coombs, and 1 anti-M was detected only in Chroma Coombs. Out of 23 frozen samples 5 were negative with Chroma Coombs, 2 anti-E, 1 anti-Jka, 1 anti-Lea and 1 anti-P1.
Discussion: Both papaine methods are equally sensitive. There were more non specific results with Chroma PAP than with enzyme microplate. The Chroma Coombs only failed to detect 3 probably clinical significant antibodies.

0322

THE DIRECT ANTIGLOBULIN TEST: CLINICAL SIGNIFICANCE AND PROSPECTIVE COMPARISON OF COLUMN AGGLUTINATION TECHNOLOGY, GEL TEST AND TUBE TEST IN 163 PATIENTS

H. Kroll, A. Salama, H. Berghöfer, C. Mueller-Eckhardt
Institute for Clinical Immunology and Transfusion Medicine, Justus Liebig University, Giessen, Germany

In recent years washing independent technologies have been developed for the detection of red blood cell (RBC) antibodies in immune hemolytic anemias (IHA): the column agglutination technology (CAT) by which agglutinated RBC are trapped in a microcolumn consisting of glass beads, and the gel test (GT) by which trapping of agglutinates is caused by a Sephadex gel. We analysed autologous RBC from 163 patients in different clinical conditions in direct antiglobulin test using these two techniques and validated the results by conventional saline tube test (TT) and elution techniques. Polyspecific antiglobulin sera were applied, in most patients additionally anti-IgG and anti-C3d were used in GT and TT. The reaction patterns are summarized in the table.

group	CAT	GT	TT	eluate	no.*	suspected IHA*
1	+	+	+	+	60	59/59
2	+	+	+	-	5	4/4
3	+	+	-	+	4	4/4
4	+	+	-	-	19 (8)	6/17 (-/8)
5	+	-	-	-	1 (5)	-/1 (-/5)
6	-	+	-	+	1	1/1
7	-	+	-	-	12	5/10
8	-	-	-	-	13 (35)	2/12 (-/35)

* additional cases in parentheses were not tested in eluate

A contingency coefficient of 0.745 demonstrated a good correlation of reactions in CAT and GT. Comparison of discordant reactions showed that no significant differences were detected (McNemar test, $p = 0.11$).
Of special interest are 5 patients (groups 3, 6) with elutable IgG who showed negative TT but positive CAT and/or GT. Reactions in group 4 were only weakly positive (maximum 2+). 4 patients of group 7 were positive due to C3d and cold agglutinins.
In conclusion CAT and GT are valuable and sensitive contributions to the detection of RBC bound IgG. A considerable number of patients with negative TT showed positive results in GT and/or CAT, but clinical relevance in many cases with reactions of 2+ or less is doubtful. However, in some patients both techniques if supplemented by elution techniques may help to identify clinically significant cases of socalled Coombs negative IHA.

0323

EVALUATION OF COLUMN AGGLUTINATION TECHNOLOGY FOR THE ANTIBODY SCREENING

J. Skodlar, B. Golubić-Ćepulić, F. Plenković, Z. Mach
A. Srbljinović
Zagreb University Clinical Hospital, Clinical Institute of Laboratory Diagnosis, Insitute of Clinical Transfusiology, Zagreb, Croatia

A prospective comparative study of unexpected antibody detection testing was performed on 2 948 patients samples from blood grouping routine during two month period, using column agglutination technology (CAT) and the standard tube technique (TT).
Polyspecific antiglobulin (AHG) cassettes represented the CAT. Test tube methodology included a LISS aditive, at 37°C 20 minute incubation and polyspecific AHG serum.
In 99.63% of the 2 948 samples CAT gave comparable results to standard TT. In 0.24% of the samples CAT was more sensitive than tube test. In 0.14% of the samples TT was more sensitive than CAT. Discrepant results were confirmed upon repeat testing.
In all CAT+ TT- nonagreement (2 anti-D, 1 anti-CD, 1 anti-Jk^a, 1 Le^b, 2 warm Auto), the antibody reactivity was < 1+.
In all CAT- TT+ nonagreement (in further investigation resolved as 1 anti-P and 3 cold agglutinins) the antibody reactivity was ≥ 1+.
In this study, column agglutination technology was found to be comparable to standard tube testing and more sensitive for clinicaly significant antibodies (reactivity < 1+).

0324

SEPARATION OF MIXED RED CELL POPULATIONS USING A GLASS BEAD COLUMN.

L.C. Tse, U.J. Dumaswala, T.J. Greenwalt
Hoxworth Blood Center, University of Cincinnati Medical Center, Cincinnati, Ohio, USA

The purpose of this study was to evaluate the utility of glass bead columns for separating unagglutinated from agglutinated red cells (RBCs). Ten percent suspensions with 1, 5, 10, 15, 25% of A, B, M, c, S, D, Jk^a, Fy^a, and K positive RBCs mixed with cells negative for the corresponding antigens were prepared. An equal volume of the antiserum for the minor population was added to the packed RBCs of each mixture. Incubation was at room T° with anti-A, -B, and -M. The other mixtures were incubated for one hour at 37C, washed four times before adding anti-IgG. Ten percent suspensions were prepared to pass through columns of 1gm of Ortho Bio-Vue® glass beads by gravity flow, followed by saline to wash out residual unagglutinated cells. The recovery was calculated from the volume and hemoglobin concentrations of the eluents. The average recovery of unagglutinated RBCs was 83%±5 SD. No contaminating minor populations of RBCs were detectable on retesting each free cell eluent. Chi-square test showed no statistical difference between the observed and expected results (p=0.999). These data suggest that glass bead columns can be used for separating mixed RBC populations.

0325

TWO RED CELL POPULATION DETECTION BY FLUORESCENT MICROSPHERE METHOD

W. Iamsilp(1), P. Chiewsilp(1), P. Ratanasirivanich(1), S. Jootar(2).
1. Blood Banking and Immunohematology, Department of Pathology,
2. Division of Hematology, Department of Medicine, Faculty of Medicine, Mahidol University, Ramathibodi Hospital, Bangkok, Thailand.

Two red blood cell (RBC) populations are found in recipients of bone marrow transplants (BMT), homologous blood transfusions and feto-maternal transfusions. Blood group antigen difference between the two populations of RBC enables us to demonstrate the mixed chimerism. The objective of this study was to apply the fluorescent microsphere method for the detection of two RBC populations. EDTA blood samples were periodically collected from three post BMT patients. The B, A and E antigens were used as the markers of mixed chimerism for cases 1, 2 and 3 respectively. It was shown that the percentages of donor RBC repopulation in patient case 1 at the 5th, 6th and 8th months post BMT as detected by the fluorescent microsphere method were 43.7, 52.6 and 65.8 percent, respectively; case 2 at the 12th and 38th months were 48.2 and 92.0 percent, respectively; and case 3 at the 20th month was 97 percent.
The fluorescent microsphere method is the quantitative technique which is able to detect blood group positive antigen RBC at the level of as low as 0.3 percent. The fluorescent microsphere may be detected by a fluorescence microscope as well as flow cytometer. Early detection of graft rejection may be done by observing the level of recipient RBC. In conclusion, the fluorescent microsphere method can be used to establish the engraftment of donor bone marrow and mixed chimerism after allogeneic BMT.

0326

EVALUATION OF DIFFERENT RED CELL ANTIBODY SCREENING TESTS FOR BLOOD DONORS

Scharberg, E. A., Kasulke, D., Ernst, A.
Red Cross Blood Center, Baden-Baden, Germany

In the last two years the following antibody screening tests for blood donors have been performed and compared with one another at the Red Cross Blood Center in Baden-Baden (annually 160,000 blood units):

1. Olympus PK 7100 (papain treated and untreated test cells)
2. Capture-R Ready Screen (Immucor)
3. Solidscreen II (Biotest)

We tested the blood samples of 32,300 donors by using partly the above-mentioned methods. The antibody screening test was positive in 2.64% of the blood samples tested on Olympus PK 7100, in 0.88% on Capture-R and in 1.02% on Solidscreen II. The positive samples which underwent antibody identification tests (gel-centrifugation, tube tests) yielded a specific result: on Olympus 0.17%, on Capture-R 0.23%, on Solidscreen II 0.53%.

In a second series of tests on 193 blood samples containing already identified antibodies, the antibodies were revealed with following frequencies when using these three methods of testing: Olympus 61 (=32%), Capture-R 140 (=73%), Solidscreen II 161 (=81%).

The results show that most of the relevant antibodies remain undetected when using the antibody screening on Olympus PK 7100. However, Capture-R and Solidscreen II both are proved to be reliable screening tests for detecting most relevant antibodies in blood donors. When considering the costs of both testing methods (material and personnel costs of a single 2-cell test: Capture-R: 1.10 DM, Solidscreen II: 0.85 DM) we prefer the Solidscreen II test. Though more time consuming, it is more flexible in handling. Using a poll-cell instead of a 2-cell screening test the costs of the screening can be cut in half.

0327

DETECTION OF EXTREMELY LOW NUMBERS OF LEUKOCYTES IN BLOOD PRODUCTS PREPARED WITH HIGH-PERFORMANCE LEUKOCYTE REMOVAL FILTERS

H. Abe, M. Hosoda, T.A. Takahashi, S. Sekiguchi
Hokkaido Red Cross Blood Center, Sapporo, Japan.

We have developed a polymerase chain reaction (PCR) method to measure the small number of leukocytes remaining in filtered red cell concentrates (RCC) and platelet concentrates (PC) prepared with high-performance leukocyte removal filters.

The β-globin gene was chosen as the target of PCR because it has been characterized well and is considered to be a single-copy. DNA extract prepared from 1 ml of RCC and PC was used for amplification. We examined two-step PCR using nested primers.

The PCR method could detect as few as 1-2 cells in 1 ml of RCC and PC. This detection sensitivity was 10- to 100-fold higher than that obtained by the flow cytometric method (FCM). We evaluated high-performance leukocyte-removal filters for RCC and PC developed by different manufacturers. The PCR method could detect leukocytes in all the samples of filtered RCC and PC and showed that the numbers of residual leukocytes were in the range of 1 to 10 cells/ml, whereas the FCM method could not detect leukocytes in most of the samples.

These results show that PCR will be useful for the evaluation of the new generation of filters and for the quality control of leukocyte-depleted blood products.

0328

THE EFFECT OF LEUKOREDUCTION BY RED CELL FILTRATION ON THE $CD4^+/CD8^+$: A FLOW CYTOMETRIC ANALYSIS

R.R. Stromberg, R.M. Slay and L.I. Friedman
Holland Lab., American Red Cross, Rockville, MD, USA

Flow cytometry was utilized to study changes in $CD4^+$ and $CD8^+$ cell levels in Adsol® red cells after filtration. Residual leukocytes (WBC) were concentrated with dextran T-500 and assayed. Pre and post filtration cell results for 2 of 4 filters studied are shown here.

Filter Type	Sample	WBC/mL	% Lymphocytes $CD4^+$	% Lymphocytes $CD8^+$	$CD4^+/CD8^+$
Asahi: Sepa-cell® R500II (n=4)	SS/Pre	5.0×10^6	28±6	39±9	0.8±0.3
	SS/Pst	2.0×10^2	80±12	6±2	15.1±4.2
	HS/Pre	6.3×10^6	43±15	30±6	1.6±0.8
	HS/Pst	1.0×10^2	67±24	8±4	9.4±3.2
Pall: BPF4™ (n=4 or 6)	SS/Pre	5.0×10^6	33±8	39±6	0.9±0.4
	SS/Pst	2.5×10^2	76±18	5±2	18.4±6.5
	HS/Pre	4.0×10^6	33±7	42±5	0.8±0.2
	HS/Pst	6.3×10^1	46±35	8±4	6.1±2.9

SS=1,471g/5 min; HS=7,268g/10 min; Values=mean±SD

Although dextran isolation resulted in some decrease in $CD4^+/CD8^+$ (~1.0) with prefiltered WBC, post-filtered ratios were increased. The conclusions are that the increase in $CD4^+/CD8^+$, observed for all 4 filters, results from relatively larger decreases in $CD8^+$ post-filtration, as compared to $CD4^+$ cells.

0329

BED-SIDE FILTRATION OF SAG-MAN ERYTHROCYTE SUSPENSIONS IS, REGARDING LEUKODEPLETION, INFERIOR TO BLOOD BANK FILTRATION

U. Sprogøe-Jakobsen, A.M. Sætre, J. Georgsen
Department of Clinical Immunology,
Odense University Hospital, Denmark.

We compared 3 different SAG-MAN red bloodcell suspension (RBCS) leukocyte filters/ filtersystems:
(1) Baxter Triple Optipac with Sepacell R2000 filter (SC).
(2) Pall BPF4 (PB) docking filter with collection pack.
(3) Pall RC100 (PR) bed-side filter for 1-2 units of RBCS.
SC and PB were applied in the blood bank, and PR bed-side. 30 units of buffycoat depleted SAG-MAN RBCS were filtered through each filter (PR: 16 units as 1. and 14 units as 2.). RBCS units were weighed and had samples taken before and after filtration. Pre- and postfiltration samples were analysed for hemoglobin (Hb), hematocrit (EVF) and white blood cell count (WBC) on an automated counter (Sysmex). In addition post filtration sample WBCs were counted in a Nageotte chamber. Median prefiltration volume for the three filters were 259-274 ml, EVF 59-62%, total Hb 3.22-3.39 mmol, total WBC count 0.27-0.34 10^9. All leukodepleted units produced with SC and PB contained < 5×10^5 WBCs, whereas 4/30 (13%) units produced with PR contained > 3×10^6. Median WBC content were significantly (p< 0.02) lower for PB (< 45×10^3) and SC (51×10^3) compared to PR (138×10^3) (1.unit PR WBC count was significantly (p<0.02) lower than for 2. unit). Median total Hb loss ranging 0.32-0.34 mmol/ unit (about 10 % of total Hb), were the same for the three filters (p >0.5). We conclude that, to ensure adequate leukodepletion of filtered RBCS, filtration ought to be performed in the blood bank, rather than bed-side.

0331

IN-LINE FILTERED RED BLOOD CELLS IMPROVE THE EFFECTIVENESS OF TRANSFUSION

G. Matthes, K.-P. Krause, E. Richter, U. Tofoté

In preceding in-vitro investigations of in-line filtered erythrocyte concentrates we showed, that despite decreased 2,3-DPG content the p050 and the oxyhemoglobin of this blood was maintained at normal levels over the whole storage period of 42 days.
We investigated the kinetics of p050 and oxyhemoglobin changes after the transfusion of in-line filtered blood. Altogether 18 hematological patients were transfused with 2 units of either traditional stored (SAGM) or in-line filtred erythrocyte concentrates (SAGM) with different storage periods. Before as well as 20 min after the transfusion hematological parameters as well as the p050 and hemoglobin derivatives in the patient's blood were measured.
The transfusion effectiveness at all patients lay between 75 and 100 %. In the patient group, which had received the in-line filtered erythrocyte concentrates the expected effect of a maintenance or increase of p050 and oxyhemoglobin was shown while in the control group after the transfusion of more than 14 days stored blood these parameters sank significantly.

0332

A FILTER SYSTEM FOR THE PREPARATION OF LEUKOCYTE- AND PLASMA-POOR RED CELL CONCENTRATES

R. Reverberi, M. Lunghi, G. Graldi

Blood Transfusion Service, Arcispedale S. Anna, Ferrara, Italy.

About 200 thalassemic patients are regularly transfused at our institution. Among them, 14 (7%) complain or recurrent allergic reactions to bedside filtered, SAGM red cell concentrates (RCC), whilst tolerate well RCC washed after filtration. Here we describe a filter system (CELLBARRIER, B. Braun-Carex, Italy) which has been designed to facilitate and speed up this sort of preparation. The system is composed of a leukocyte filter to which two bags are attached, one empty and one containing 400 ml of saline. The RCC are filtered and collected in the empty bag, the filter is rinsed with part of the saline through a by-pass connection tubing, and the rest of saline is added directly to the RCC. This procedure typically completes in < 15'. After centrifugation, the supernatant is expressed into the saline bag and this bag is detached. Our initial experiences with a pre-market release of this product indicate that it removes >99.5% of leukocytes, >97% of platelets, >98% of plasma and <8% of red cells. Leukocyte-, platelet- and plasma-poor RCC can be prepared in a closed system with just one sterile connection.

0333

35-DAY-STORAGE OF RED BLOOD CELLS IN-LINE FILTERED WITH SEPACELL INTEGRA SYSTEM

G.Matthes[1], E.Richter[1], U.Tofoté[1], J.Kadar[2]
Institutes of Transfusion Medicine, University Hospital Charité Berlin[1], University Clinic Essen[2], Germany

In-line filtrations of erythrocyte concentrates were accomplished under routine conditions by means of Sepacell Integra Systems within 6 hours after whole blood collection. The pre-storage filtration proved itself as simply feasible and effectively as concerns the leukocyte elimination. The residual white blood cell count lay with 2.2 x 10^5 per concentrate (Nageotte chamber) in the area of the CILL dosis. The leukocyte depleted erythrocyte concentrates were stored 42 days at 4 C and analysed in intervals of 7 days.

There could be ascertained no differences to known data of the preservation of red blood cells without in-line filtration. The quality of the SAGM resuspended erythrocyte concentrates (haematological, biochemical and clinical-chemical parameters) corresponded to conventionally collected and separated blood. Noticeable and in the contrast to known preservation data is that the oxygen transport function of the red blood cells (pO50, haemoglobin derivatives) is preserved over the whole preservation time in the norm area. Furthermore in the first phase of the preservation is to be recorded a negligibly better preserved 2.3-DPG concentration in in-line filtered blood.

The Sepacell-Integra-Filter system can be recommended for application in the clinical routine by virtue of the effective leukocyte elimination, the slight erythrocyte loss and the good results of hypothermic preservation over 42 days.

0334

IN-LINE FILTRATION OF RED BLOOD CELL CONCENTRATES WITH SEPACELL INTEGRA™ SYSTEM

N. Müller[1)], E. Richter[2)], G. Matthes[2)], J.G. Kadar[1)]
Institutes of Transfusion Medicine, University Clinic Essen[1)], University Charité Berlin[2)]

Using the Sepacell Integra™ System (Diamed Transfusionstechnik) for in-line filtration of red blood cell concentrates (rbcc's) in SAG-M solution, the filtration capacity of the system was evaluated in two centres. 53 whole blood units stored for 2 - 6 hours at ambient temperature were processed for investigation as follows: Group 1 (N=24) high speed centrifugation and buffy coat removal, group 2 (N=29) high speed centrifugation only.

		Group 1(N=24) BC Removed	Group 2(N=29) BC Not Removed
WBC: Before Filtration	(10E9/l)	5,76 +/- 2,77	9,41 +/- 4,17
After Filtration	(10E5/l)	0,53 +/- 0,47	0,59 +/- 0,45
Htc After Filtration	(%)	60,63 +/- 2,48	59,38 +/- 3,09
RBC: Before Filtration	(10E12/l)	7,39 +/- 0,38	7,15 +/- 0,68
After Filtration	(10E12/l)	6,66 +/- 0,33	6,62 +/- 0,68
RBC Loss	(%)	9,98 +/- 2,44	7,19 +/- 3,55

WBC contamination (Nageotte Chamber) in rbcc's was without exception well below the level of Critical Immunogenic Load of Leukocytes. The filtered rbcc's fulfil the quality standard of the Council of Europe. The system could be readily implemented for routine use. The benefit of early leukocyte removal on the quality and clinical effectiveness of rbcc's produced according to this method will be evaluated in a prospective nation-wide study called GEMUSEF (German Multicentre Study for Erythrocyte Filtration).

0335

IN-LINE FILTRATION OF SAGM RED CELL CONCENTRATES BY OPTIPAC®LS FILTER SYSTEM

T.Hervig[1], I.Aksnes[2],A.Ryningen[3], H.Holmsen[3], V.Franck[4], A. Reppucci[4]
[1]Rogaland Central Hospital, Stavanger, [2]Haukeland Hospital, Bergen, [3]Department of Biochemistry and Cell Biology, University of Bergen, Norway, [4]Baxter R&D Europe, Nivelles, Belgium.

A new in-line filter system was tested that allows the blood bank to stock sterile, quality-controlled blood components available for transfusion at all times. 30 SAGM-concentrates were tested; 10 were filtered within 8 hours after collection (warm filtration), 10 were filtered after 66-72 hours storage at 4°C (cold filtr.), and 10 units were left unfiltered (controls). The results of the filtration were:

	Cold filtr.	Warm filtr.
Leukocytes(x10^6/unit)	0.05±0.00	0.99±0.59
Leukocyte reduction	99.99%	99.8%
Red cell loss	10.2%	10.6%

Measurements of pH,glucose,lactate,haemolysis, plasma K, plasma haemoglobin,2,3BPG and ATP showed lesser,but not statistically significant, storage lesion in the filtered units.Subsequently, autologous transfusions were performed in 8 volunteers after 35 days storage of filtered SAGM-units. The mean 24 hour recovery was 86.3% (range 73.4-92.4%).

Conclusion: The Optipac®LS filter system provides efficient leukocyte depletion and these filtered units have good transfusion qualities.

0336

EVALUATION OF A NEW PRESTORAGE WHITE CELL (WC) REMOVAL FILTER.

A.Vanhonsebrouck[1],V.Franck[2],T.Repucci[2],L.Muylle[1].
1.Blood Transfusion Center Antwerp, Red Cross, Edegem, Belgium,2.Baxter, Nivelles, Belgium.

The performance of a new filter composed of polyethylene layers (Baxter LDF-350) was evaluated for the WC depletion of red cells (RC) suspended in SAG-M. The filters were connected to the RC bags by sterile docking. The units were filtered 4 to 8 hours after blood collection. Filtration (F) was performed by gravity in the laboratory without filter priming or rinsing. WC removal and RC recovery were compared in 21 filtered RC units, divided in two groups : RC with buffy coat (BC) and BC removed RC. WC content was determined before and after filtration by an automated cell counter and by manual count with a Nageotte chamber respectively. Results expressed as means ± SD are shown in the table. At weekly intervals during 42 days of storage we measured pH, plasma Hb, ATP, 2,3-DPG, glucose, lactate, potassium and sodium contents.

	RC (n=11)	BC removed RC (n=10)
WC x10^9/unit Pre-F	2.35 ±1.29	* 0.70 ±0.31
WC x10^6/unit Post-F	1.1 ±1.8	** 0.4 ±0.2
% WC removal	99.95±0.04	** 99.93±0.05
% RC recovery	85.2 ±7.7	** 85.3 ±7.7
F time (min,sec)	17.31±7.39	* 10.49±2.51

* $p < 0.02$ ** $p > 0.05$

The filter achieves a 3 log WC reduction of RC stored for 4 to 8 hours with all units having an average of 0.75 x 10^6 WC/unit. Removal of the BC, accompanied by a considerable loss of red cells (12 %) before filtration, does not significantly change the WC removal. Filtration time was significantly higher in the RC with BC. During storage acceptable values of all the metabolic parameters were obtained. Conclusion : the new prestorage leucocyte filter allows efficient WC removal and the RC properties are maintained during storage.

0337

A NEW LEUKOCYTEFILTER FOR RED CELL CONCENTRATES: CELLSELECT FR

D.de Korte, C.H.Palfenier, I.E.Pankalla-Blandeau, J.A.Loos
Central Laboratory Netherlands Red Cross Blood Transfusion Service, Amsterdam, the Netherlands.

A new leukocyte filter for red cell concentrates without buffy coat in SAGM (RCC) from NPBI (the Netherlands), Cellselect FR, was tested. The new filter consists of a filterbed sealed in a bag of PVC, with a satellite bag attached to the filtrate bag to transfer the air originally present in the filter system, together with a test sample. About 150 filtrations with fresh RCC (haematocrit 60±2 and <15x10^9 platelets) were performed and only one filtrate contained >5 x 10^6 leukocytes (in fact 8 x 10^6). Red cell recovery was around 90 % and the filtration time about 15 min. The results for Cellselect FR are shown in table 1, in comparison with BPF4 (Pall,USA) and Bio R01* (Biofil, Italy). The collapsible filterhouse of the Cellselect FR gives spontaneously a recovery around 90 %, whereas for the other filters the air inlet was opened, to improve recovery with about 4 %. The residual leukocytes in the filtrate were counted in a Nageotte haemocytometer (lower limit < 200 leucocytes/ml). The CELLSELECT FR is suitable for unattended filtration of buffy coat depleted red cell suspensions in SAGM in a completely closed system.

Table 1	CELLSELECT FR	BPF 4	BioR 01*
volume before (ml)	293 ± 16.3	302 ± 15.1	291 ± 17.5
filtration time(sec)	730 ± 71.9	542 ± 70.6	404 ± 28.7
WBC before x 10^6	866 ± 499.7	722 ± 217.2	865 ± 253.9
WBC after x 10^6	< 0.53	< 0.13	< 0.54
% recovery red cells	91 ± 3.7	92 ± 2.4	88 ± 3.9

N = 8, data as mean ± SD

0338

EVALUATION OF THE NEW CELLSELECT-F FILTER (NPBI) FOR LEUCOCYTE DEPLETION OF RED CELL CONCENTRATES.

H.J.C. de Wit, P.Holwerda, C.Marsman, Th.Hatzmann, A.Knevelman.
Red Cross Bloodbank Friesland, Leeuwarden, The Netherlands

Introduction: The performance of a new filter Cellselect-F (CF) for leucocyte depletion of erythrocyte concentrates (EC) was studied and compared with the performance of the Cellselect Optima filter (CO) used in routine. Both filters are manufactured by NPBI.

Methods: 20 buffycoat depleted EC in SAGM (4°C) were filtered ≤72hr after donation (500 ml whole blood) through the CF filter. An additional 20 units were filtered through the CO filter. Filtration procedures were carried out according to the manufacturers specifications. Pre- and post filtration volumes were calculated from net weight. Post filtration leucocyte measurement was carried out in Nageotte- and platelet in Bürker haemocytometer; all the other haematologic parameters by Sysmex F800 cellcounter.

Results: (mean ± sd)

	CO	CF
filtration time (min)	11±2	20±4
erythrocyte recovery (%)	88.5±2.5	87.9±2.4
residual leucocytes (10E6)	0.6±1.5	0.1±0.03
residual platelets (10E6)	1.0±1.0	0.7±1.0
haematocrit (%)	49±2	60±2

Conclusions: Post filtration leucocyte contamination (p=0.12) and erythrocyte recovery (p=0.50) for both filters did not differ. The results comply with current Dutch standards (≤5x10E6 leucocytes, ≥80% recovery).The omission of a rinsing procedure for the CF filter results in a significantly higher Ht and an easier and more cost effective procedure in comparison to the CO filter. The time needed to filter one unit using the new CF filter however is nearly twice the filtration time using the CO filter.

0339

STUDY OF 5 RED BLOOD CELL CONCENTRATE (RBCC) FILTERS

A. Rapaille, D. Sondag-Thull
Blood Transfusion Centre, Liège, Belgium

The filtration efficiency of five different RBCC filters were examined. Blood samples were counted on Sysmex 5000. The number of residual leukocytes were determined with a Nageotte chamber in Plaxan dilution. A study was made with both RBCC and leukocyte-poor RBCC. The different filters were Pall RC50 and BPF4, Sepacell 4C2446, Erypur Optima A1 and Biofil BioR01.

RBCC :	RC50	BPF4	4C2446	A1	BioR01	
n	11	18	5	12	8	
n<5 10^6	5	18	5	11	4	
mean	1.62	0.43	0.08	0.9	1.40	10^6
n>5 10^6	6	0	0	1	4	
Leukocyte-poor RBCC						
n	7	7	4	5	8	
N<5 10^6	0	7	3	5	0	
mean	-	1.38	0.94	0.06	-	10^6
n>5 10^6	7	0	1	0	8	

BPF4, 4C2446 and Optima A1 have a good efficiency either in RBCC or in leukocyte-poor RBCC. RC50 and BioR01 give bad results with the two types of RBCC.

0340

WHITE CELLS REMOVAL FROM RED BLOOD CELL UNITS :A COMPARATIVE ANALYSIS OF 4 DIFFERENT FILTERS.

GUASTELLA G., BRESCIA A., TALARICO G., VERATTI M.A.

IMMUNOTRANSFUSION SERVICE. USL 7. CATANZARO,ITALY

The removal of white cells (WBCs) from red blood cells (RBCs) by filtration has been recognized as important for reducing the nonhaemolytic • febrile transfusion reactions and WBC -associated HLA immunization.With this background we prospectically evaluated the effectiveness of 4 different filters currently used in our laboratory. For this purpose we collected pre-filtration and post-filtration blood samples.Initial WBC count was carried out by means of an automated counter, while post-filtration WBC count was performed by flow cytometry (F) in order to improve the accurancy of determination.As shown in table, residual WBC count was in all instances lower than 1,7 x 10E6 while RBC recovery exceeded 88% .

Laboratory Filters	WBC x 10E6 pre	post	RBC % recov.	WBC % deplet.	Log. deplet.
Imugard Ig 500	1288	F 1.25	88.65	90.90	3.01
Erypur Optima g/2	1345	F 0.30	89.71	99.97	3.65
Leucostop 4	1373	F 1.63	88.35	99.88	2.92
Pall-BPF 4	1156	F 0.20	89.70	99.98	3.76

In our experience all filters used gave similar results in terms of WBC depletion, and a good assurance for the haemocomponent quality control.
Flow cytometry (F) is especially useful when dealing with blood samples whose WBC count is lower than 10 ul.

0342

EVALUATION OF LRF AND SEPACELL PL LEUKOCYTE REMOVAL FILTERS FOR APHERESIS COLLECTION PLATELETS.

Yoshiaki Ogawa, M Wakana, S Matsubara, H Aso, H Matsukura, Kitaosaka Red Cross Blood Center, Osaka, Japan.

We attempted leukodepletion of platelet concentrates (PC) using white cell reduction filters pre-connected in MCS (Haemonetics,MA) PLP and Autopheresis-C-2 (Baxter,IL) PRP collection kits.

Method: Group A-1 represents 42 collections made with an MCS PLP kit incorporating the LRF6H (Pall,NY) leukoreduction filter. Group A-2 represents 25 collections made with a similar kit incorporating the LRF10. Bag-to-bag filtration was employed in both groups. Group B-1 represents 20 Autopheresis-C-2 collections made with a Sepacell-PL-10-N (Asahi Medical, Tokyo) incorporated directly in the PRP collection line. Group B-2 represents 24 collections which were bag-to-bag filtered after PRP concentration into PC. All subjects were volunteer donors visiting the Kitaosaka Red Cross Blood Center in Osaka. Platelet recoveries (PR),leukocyte reduction percents (LR), and residual leukocyte counts (RLC) were compared. Post-filtration platelet function and sterility tests were performed.

Results (all averages): Group A-1: PR, 87%; LR, 99.57%; and RLC, $1.2X10^6$. Group A-2: PR, 87%; LR, 99.98%; and RLC , $0.59X10^5$. Group B-1: RLC, $7.93X10^6$. Results for PR and LR were unclear. Group B-2: PR, 86.5%;LR,99.1%; and RLC, $2.0X10^6$. All four groups resulted in residual leukocyte levels considered effective in the prevention of adverse transfusion reactions.

0343

IN VITRO EVALUATION OF A NEW FILTER FOR LEUCOCYTE DEPLETION OF PLATELETS CONCENTRATES DURING COMPONENT PREPARATION.

L.D. Christensen, E. Dickmeiss
Blood Bank, Dept. of Clinical Immunology, Rigshospitalet, University Hospital Copenhagen, Denmark.

A newly developed filter (Autostop™ BC, Pall Biomedical Limited, UK) for prestorage leucocyte depletion of platelet concentrates (PC) was studied. The filter is designed for leucocyte depletion during preparation of pool PC from platelet rich buffy coats. The filter is a polyesterfilter as automately stop the flow through the filter when leucocytes and/or erythrocytes reach the filter.
The filter gave a more than log 3 reduction in leucocyte content. 19 of 20 units of LD-PC had a leucocytes content below 3×10^5 per unit and 1 contain 8×10^5 leucocytes. The standard PC contained $2,53 \times 10^8$ ($0,87 \times 10^8$ - $15,3 \times 10^8$, n=20) leucocytes per unit (median and range are given).
The quality of the LD-PC was evaluated by measurings of platelet activation (expression of CD42b and CD62 studied by flow cytometry), platelet morphology and pH pre- and poststorage. In none of the parameters studied were found differences between LD-PC and standard PC.

0344

THE PREPARATION OF LEUCOCYTE POOR PLATELET CONCENTRATES WITH THE OPTI-SYSTEM

G.VERHOEVEN, R.C. SCHAAP, Red Cross Bloodbank Kennemerland Haarlem the Netherlands

We developed a technique for the preparation of leucocyte poor plateletconcentrates with the Opti-System. Five buffycoats and a donorunit plasma are pooled together. The plasma serves as storage medium. For all pooling and connecting procedures we use a 4R2027 coupler system (Baxter) and a Sterile Connecting Device (S.C.D. Terumo). It is neccesary to create a top/bottom configuration to use the Opti-system. This is achieved by connecting a 400 ml empty pack to the bottom of the poolpack and a 1000 ml PL 732 container (Baxter) to the top. After centrifugation (1200g, 7 minutes) the triple poolpack is placed in the Optipress which expels the platelet rich plasma (PRP) to the top pack and the layer with leucocytes and erythrocytes to the bottom pack.To avoid whirling of leucocytes in the PRP, a flow reducer has to be placed between the poolpack and the bottompack.
The following in vitro results were obtained in 872 poolproducts. The leucocytes were counted with a microscope.

	volume ml	platelets $\times 10^9$ per donorunit	leucocytes $\times 10^7$ per donorunit	pH after four days
mean	273	59	0,6	7,0
SD	21	14	0,1	0,2

Conclusion: prepared with the Opti-System we obtained leucocyte poor plateletconcentrates with good in vitro results that largely meet the criteria of the Dutch Bloodbanks.

0345

LEUKOCYTE FILTERS FOR PLATELET CONCENTRATES (PCs) OBTAINED WITH DIFFERENT BLOOD CELL SEPARATORS

R. Moog[1], N. Müller[1], J.G. Kadar[2]
1 Inst. Transfusion Medicine, University of Essen
2 Dept. Transfusion Medicine, Hannover, Germany

Apheresis machines produce PCs of different quality. White blood cell (WBC) contamination varies from the apheresis technique used.
Routine bedside filtration of PCs will be performed irrespectively on the technical circumstances of production. For this reason we recommend different filter with appropriate WBC removal capacity. The recommended Asahi filters for PCs and the corresponding inhouse evaluation data (means ± SD) of the cell separators AS 104 (dual needle [DN] and single needle [SN] technique), CS 3000 Plus, COBE Spectra and PCS Plus are shown on the table.

	AS 104 DN	AS 104 SN	CS 3000 Plus	COBE Spectra	PCS Plus
Platetet WBC	2.5	2.8	2.9	2.7	2.8
yield x1011	±0.3	±0.7	±0.8	±0.6	±0.6
WBC contamin-	2.8	20.6	1.4	0.8	185
ation x106	±3.0	±17.7-	±3.3	±0.6	±139
PC volume	250	264	208	253	231
ml	±0	±16	±2	±12	±26
recommended	PL	PL	PL	PL	PL
filter	5IIA	10IIA	5IIA	5IIA	10IIA

0346

COMPARISON OF TWO LEUCOCYTE DEPLETION FILTERS FOR PLATELET CONCENTRATES: PL50 AND PL10A.

J.de Wildt-Eggen, M. Bins
Bloodbank Zwolle, The Netherlands

Two filters for leucocyte depletion of platelet concentrates (PC) were compared: PL50 (Pall) and PL10A (Baxter).
Two PC were prepared from 5 buffycoats and 1 unit of plasma, pooled and mixed. This pool was enriched with leucocytes because in routinely prepared PCs generally the concentration of leucocytes is low. The pool was divided over 2 containers of which one was filtered using a PL50 filter and the other using a PL10A filter. Remaining leucocytes and platelets were counted in duplicate, using a Nageotte chamber and a Sysmex K1000 cell counter.

Results:	PL50 (n=10)		PL10A (n=10)	
	before	after	before	after
volume (ml)	288±19	273±17	294±14	274±19
plt x 10^9	375±56	334±44	383±53	323±43
leuco x10^7	46±27	0.08±0.15	43±27	0.03±0.04
leuco removed %		99.8±0.2		99.9±0.2
plt recovery %		87.6±3.2		84.4±3.1
flow rate		15ml/min.		20ml/min.

Conclusion: Both filters met the criterium of < 5x 10^6 leucocytes per concentrate after filtration. Less leucocytes were left after filtration by the PL10A-filter; however, a platelet recovery a little bit smaller was found using this filter.

0347

EVALUATION OF THE BAXTER CLOSED APHERESIS KIT WITH INTEGRATED FILTER (PL-5A).

E. Baudoux[(1)], A. Rapaille[(1)], E. Goossenaerts[(2)], D. Sondag[(1)].
[(1)] Blood transfusion Centre, Liège. [(2)] Baxter S.A. Belgium.

In this study we tested the efficiency of the 4R2237 kit in terms of deleucocytation rates and recovery of platelets (Plt) yields. 20 platelet donors (precounts 248.8x10E3 ± 48.34X10E3/µL) were run on the Omnix Cell Separator (endpoint volume: 5000 mL, whole blood flow rate: 50-60 mL/min, ACD-A ratio: 9 to 10:1 and interface detector offset at 8), using 1-platelet collection procedure (with TNX-6 and PLT-30 chambers). Plt and white cells (WBC) counts were performed on Celldin 3000 (Abbott) except WBC counts on the Plt concentrates by the Nageotte chamber technique, and dilution with cristal violet.

Results (N=20)	Plt Yield Prefiltration	Plt yield Postfiltration	Wbc Postfiltration	PLT % Recovery
	X10E11	X10E11	X10E6	
MEAN	**5.25**	**4.95**	**0.11**	**94.6%**
SD	1.03	1.01	0.31	8.6%
Median	**5.20**	**4.85**	**0.02**	**96.8%**
min	3.00	3.10	0.01	73.5%
MAX	7.60	7.30	1.40	112.2%

We conclude that the 4R2237 kit easily ensures the deleucocytation of Plt concentrates from apheresis donors. The loss in platelets yields has no clinical signification.

0348

A LONG STORAGE TIME BEFORE PROCESSING WHOLE BLOOD UNITS DRAMATICALLY REDUCES THE EFFICACY OF LEUKOCYTE REMOVAL BY FILTRATION

H.J. Geerligs, H.J. Bos, G.C. v.d. Plas
Red Cross Bloodbank Arnhem, The Netherlands.

After donation whole blood units were stored at a temperature of 20 °C. After a storage time of 2 - 5 h or 15 - 20 h the whole blood units were after centrifugation separated in plasma, buffy coat and red blood cell concentrate. Leukocytes were removed immediately after processing using the Cellselect Optima, Cellselect F, Sepacell RS200B or BPF4 filter. Leukocytes in the filtrated units were counted in the Nageotte chamber.

Number of leukocytes per unit filtrated red cell concentrate ($x10^6$).

Duration of	Cells. Opt.		Cells. F		Sep. RS200B		BPF4	
Storage	mean	SD	mean	SD	mean	SD	mean	SD
2 - 5 h	1.7*	1.0	1.4*	0.9	0.65*	0.28	0.46*	0.26
15 - 20 h	11.7	5.1	4.2	3.1	3.6	3.8	2.2	2.2

*P < 0.05; Wilcoxon test. For every observation 10 units were used.

As shown in the table all filtrated red cell concentrates show a significant lower leukocyte number, when processed after a short storage time. It is therefore important to keep the period between donation and filtration as short as possible.

0349

LEUKOCYTE DEPLETION CAPACITY IN RELATION TO FILTRATION TEMPERATURE.

I. Steneker, R.N.I. Pietersz and H.W. Reesink, Red Cross Blood Bank Amsterdam, Amsterdam, The Netherlands.

Aim: To establish the influence of filtration temperature on the efficiency of leukocyte depletion of red blood cell concentrates (RBC) by filtration.

Method: RBC were made by removal of plasma (= RBC) or by removal of the buffy coat (buffy coat poor = Bcp-RBC). The composition of the RBC was:

	leukocytes x 10^9	platelets x 10^9
RBC	1.5 - 5.0	55 - 180
Bcp-RBC	0.2 - 1.8	0 - 30

The RBC were stored for 4 hours at room temperature (RT) or at 4°C. Consecutively 3 units of RBC or Bcp-RBC were filtered through a polyester flat-bed filter (Erypur Optima G2) at 4°C and al RT, respectively. The leukocyte depletion capacity is defined as the number of leukocytes applied to the filter which results in < 5.0 x 10^6 leukocytes in the filtrate.

Results:

	leukocyte depletion capacity x 10^9	
	4° - 11°C	20° - 22°C
RBC	6.4 ± 2.8*	2.5 ± 0.7
Bcp-RBC	1.6 ± 0.8**	0.9 ± 0.2

All values are mean ± SD of 6 experiments.
* p = 0.004, ** p = 0.08 (NS), Mann Whitney U test.

Conclusion: The Erypur Optima G2 filter had a significantly increased leukocyte depletion capacity for RBC at 4°C, whereas the leukocyte depletion capacity for Bcp-RBC was not temperature dependent. Since RBC stored at 4°C warm up quickly during filtration, standardization of the filtration procedure is difficult to achieve.

0350

ACTIVATED PLATELETS MAY CLOG LEUKOCYTE REMOVAL FILTER.

T.Asai, M.Itoh, A.Takeshita, K.Hiruma and S.Yoshida.
Chiba University Hospital, Chiba,Japan.

During the transfusion of leukocyte depleted platelet concentrates(PCs), a rare occurrence is the clogging of the filter. While the mechanism behind this occurrence is not clear, the condition of platelets during storage may be related.

PCs($1-3x10^{11}$ platelets) were collected from volunteer donors using the Haemonetics V50 and the Fenwal CS3000 and stored in polyvinylchloride and polyolefin bags. PCs were stored at room temperature on a tumbler rotator. During and after storage, pH and blood gases were monitored. The percentage of platelets expressing alpha granule membrane protein (GMP-140) was measured by flowcytometry as an indicator of platelet activation. After storage, the trapping of platelets by the leukocyte removal filter was analyzed by determining platelet recovery after filtration.

The pH of some PCs decreased to less than 6.5 and the swirling response disappeared. The expression of GMP-140 increased as the pH decrease and there was a significant negative correlation. It was further noted that the filterability of the platelets decreased after storage and filter clogging was observed with some PCs.

The decrease in platelet filterability significantly correlated with a decrease in pH ($p<0.01$) and platelet activation as indicated by GMP-140 expression ($p<0.05$). In conclusion, platelets can become activated during storage. It has been suggested that activated platelets are unlikely to circulate in vivo. Our study further indicates that during storage platelets may also contribute to clogging leukocyte removal filters.

0351

EFFECT OF FILTRATION ON PLATELET HYPERAGGREABILITY AND CELLULAR INDICIES

Pranee Krailadsiri[1] Jerard Seghatchian[2]
1 Department of Laboratory Medicine, Chulalongkorn University Hospital, Bangkok, Thailand, 2 Quality Assurance Laboratory, North London Blood Transfusion Centre, London, England

We have studied changes in the cellular indices and aggregation states of filtered and non-filtered platelet concentrates of the same origin, using Technicon H*1. Sampling performed at day 1-2 and 5, to account for changes in post-filtration stability. On day 1 samples from both products have undergone spontaneous aggregation (Sp.Agg) as identified by the fall in platelet count (PLT) and increased disparity between leucocyte peroxidase/basophil (WBCp/WBCb). The lag phase of Sp.Agg (14 and 16 minutes respectively) was prolonged by two-fold on day 2 and completely abolished by day 5. Filtration did not induce any significant disparity in WBCp/WBCb and upon exposure to EDTA PLT increased by 16% in both products. The differences in mean platelet volume with/without EDTA ($dMPV_{EDTA}$) of day 2 products was similar but at day 5 filtered product reached quickly to a negative value (-0.4 vs 0 fL), suggesting post-filtered products do not store as well as non-filtered counterpart. Loss of large subpopulation of platelets also occurred by filtration as indicated by 0.1 fL decreased in MPV even on day 2 as compared to 0.3 fL on day 1. We conclude that filtration should be performed on day 2 to reduce loss of PLT and post-filtered products should be monitored by tests reflecting platelet functional integrities, before tranfusion.

0352

INCREASED ERYTHROCYTE p050 DESPITE 2,3-DPG DEPLETION AFTER IN-LINE FILTRATION

G. Matthes, K.-P. Krause, E. Richter, U. Tofoté

Institute for Transfusion Medicine, Humboldt-University Berlin, Germany

Altogether 52 erythrocyte concentrates were collected by means of different in-line blood bag filter systems (Leukotrap, Integra, Biofil) and analyzed over a hyptohermic storage period of 42 days. While the most investigations to in-line filtration of red blood cells are concentrated on parameters like residual WBC count and biochemical parameter, we explored in addition the p050 and hemoglobin derivatives of the preserved red blood cells.

The results of the leukocyte depletion as well as the biochemical parameters (ATP, 2,3-DPG, free potassium, free hemoglobin, glucose and lactose concentration) showed the for SAGM and AS3 stabilized erythrocytes known changes during the 4°C storage. Surprisingly, the p050 and the oxyhemoglobin remained in the normal level in all in-line filtered erythrocyte concentrates up to the end of the storage at day 42 despite falling 2,3-DPG concentrations.

These changes, which could be reproduced repeatedly, should have positive consequences on the maintainance of the p050 in patients blood after transfusions of preserved in-line filtered erythrocytes.

0353

QUALITY SURVEY OF APHERESIS PLATELETS FROM A PORTABLE COLLECTION DEVICE.

M. Girard, D. Diawara, L. Dubus, O. Leroy
C.D.T.S. - 6, rue Emile Lesot, F-80000 AMIENS - FRANCE

We investigated the quality of apheresis platelets collected with 4 MCS® blood collection systems from Haemonetics® (BRAINTREE MA 02184). The procedures were performed with the extended storage platelet and plasma set (ESP®, ref 794). After processing 2.5 liters of blood we obtained 400 ml of plasma and 250 ml of apheresis platelets per donation. 137 apheresis platelets were studied. Mean platelet content is 3.12 E 11, roughly equivalent to 6 random donor platelets units. After 5 days storage, pH ranges from 6.1 to 7.4. Results are shown in the table below.

	Machine # 1	Machine # 2
Samples	38	35
Volume (ml)	243 ± 36	269 ± 84
Platelets (E 11)	3.41 ± 0.77	3.19 ± 0.69
Red cells (E 9)	10.6 ± 4.96	9.56 ± 3.60
Leucocytes (E 6)	24.47 ± 18.34	22.20 ± 19.58

	Machine # 3	Machine # 4
Samples	30	34
Volume (ml)	223 ± 40	248 ± 43
Platelets (E 11)	3.30 ± 0.70	2.60 ± 0.64
Red cells (E 9)	11.11 ± 8.81	9.85 ± 4.68
Leucocytes (E 6)	21.26 ± 15.51	32 ± 30.2

Machine # 4, with lower platelet yield and higher leucocyte contamination, had to be calibrated before implementing it in routine use.

0354

BLOOD MIXERS FAIL TO MIX AT LOW NORMAL BLEEDING RATES.

J.A. Loos, D. de Korte, H.A. Veldman.
Central Laboratory of The Netherlands Red Cross Blood Transfusion Service, Amsterdam, the Netherlands.

Combimix-x3 (Baxter, US), Donormatic (Lifescience, US) Biomixers 314,315 (Labstatus, S) and MW 5001 (Biotrans, FRG) were compared at flowrates of 50 and 100 ml/min with manual or rotary mixing (Blood shaker, Cenco, NL). Blood as a liquid, density 1.060 g/ml, can be mimicked by a glycerol solution (25%w/v) of equal density. This glycerol solution, prewarmed to 37°C, was pumped with an even flow into a 600 ml bloodbag, with 70 ml CPDA1, stained with 0.32 mM Toluidin Blue, mounted on either mixer. After 500 ml the bag was emptied with a plasma extractor in 48 fractions of 12 ml. The colour (640 nM) of each fraction was measured, expressed as % of the mean colour of all fractions and plotted against the fraction number. At 100 ml/min all combi mixers gave a slightly rising mixing curve with the darkest colour in the top- (110%) and the lightest colour in the bottom fractions (80%). At 50 ml/min all combi mixers gave a sigmoid mixing curve sometimes starting at 10% and ending at 340%, indicating that the CPDA1 solution was lifted by the incoming glycerol solution with hardly any mixing. Manual mixing, by kneading the bag, suspended on a tripping scale, once a min or mixing a bag at a flatbed mixer at 50 cycl./min gave at all rates an almost ideal mixing curve rising from 90 to 105%.
Blood mixers which are combined with weighting devices fail to mix at low normal bleeding rates, leading to a high incidence of clotting during blood collection.

0355

ERROR REPORTING AND MANAGEMENT

I.Steneker, R.N.I.Pietersz, H.W.Reesink. Red Cross Blood Bank Amsterdam, Amsterdam The Netherlands

Since 1990 current Good Manufacturing Practice (cGMP) was introduced in our blood bank. After translation of methods and procedures into Standard Operating Procedures (SOPs), SOP related job descriptions were implemented and training was continued.

Aim: To monitor if SOPs are followed and if current procedures are adequately described in the SOPs.

Method: A SOP how to report errors (SOP violations) and complaints (donor or hospital) to the QA department was made. The staff was trained according to this SOP. It was clarified that error reporting had the aim to improve procedures and was not a tool for staff sanctions (i.e. salary).

Results: In 1993, 3,515 errors and complaints were reported to the QA department.

	errors	complaints
administrative (clerical)	530	26
technical (SOP violation)	2,831	113

84% of the reported errors and complaints were due to unfamiliarity or misinterpretation of the SOPs. The majority of errors occurred at the blood collecting teams (more than 50% parttimers). In 30 of the 153 SOPs, procedures and methods were corrected and retraining of the staff was intensified.

Conclusion: Error and complaint management is a valuable tool to evaluate if SOPs are followed or if SOPs are incomplete. Training and retraining of the personnel and the development of a climat in which personnel is reporting errors and complaints will contribute to a better quality.

0356

ACTIVATION OF THOMSEN-FRIEDENREICH ANTIGEN CAUSING FALSE POSITIVE ANTIGEN TYPING WITH MONOCLONAL ANTI-Le(a).

M.Písačka, J.Suttnar, M.Stambergová
Institute of Haematology and Blood Transfusion
Prague, Czech republic

A mouse monoclonal anti-Le^a Seraclone Ch.-B.11031 from Biotest AG was found to give false positive reactions with Le^a negative red cells after neuraminidase treatment.

Agglutination titration scores:
(Treatment: 1 - intact, 2 - neuraminidase
3 - papain after neuraminidase
4 - papain)

	1	2	3	4
O Le(a+)	48	100	110	100
O Le(a-)	0	90	2	0

Results are showing cross-reactivity of anti-Le^a with a structure exposed on red cell after neuraminidase treatment and destroyed after subsequent treatment with papain. These reactions are typical for the Thomsen-Friedenreich antigen.
Testing with neuraminidase treated red cells should be included in evaluation of blood grouping reagents.

0357

MONOCLONAL REAGENTS AND POLYCLONAL SERUM FOR THE DETERMINATION OF ABO GROUP OF RED CELLS.

N.V.Mineeva, M.A.Matveeva, A.I.Ionova, N.E.Ivanova, O.N.Kirina. Russian Research Institute of Hematology and Transfusiology, St.Petersburg, Russia

The ability of following reagents manufactured in Russia to detect A and B red cell antigens for blood grouping in 2003 hematologic patients and 1204 donors was studied: a) human blood sera manufactured in Blood Banks in Russia; b) human blood sera in which the antibodies were concentrated by polyethylene glycol fractionation; c) obtained by us blood sera of animals immunized by human A and B red cells using affinity chromatography on sorbent containing A and B substances; d) monoclonal reagents commercially available. The sera obtained from blood of immunized animals were most effective in detecting A and B antigens in donors and patients. The reagent obtained from human blood detected effectively A and B antigens only when the sera contained anti-A,B IgG antibodies. When these reagents contained only IgM anti-A, they did not detect antigen A variants. Problems were associated with use of monoclonal reagents (7.8% of cases), particularly, in typing blood of patients with blood diseases. In 5 out of 20 samples of cells A_2 antigen was not detected. Thus the improved control of typing reagents is necessary in Russia.

0358

METHYL CELLULOSE IN MANUAL Rh TYPING

G. Balatzenko, L. Ivanova
National Center of Clinical and Transfusion Haematology
Sofia, Bulgaria

Methyl cellulose (MC) is known as a medium used for dilution of diagnostic reagents in blood grouping machines. In This study we present a our data concerning availability for using MC in normal testing of Rh antigens. Anti Rh plasma containing IgG antibodies (Ab), as well as commercially available anti Rh sera (anti-C, -c -D, -E, -e) for slide and rapid tube test were diluted with 1% solution of MC and tested in order to establish the effect of MC on agglutination.
It was found out that MC had weak or no effect on agglutination with IgG Ab. At the same time, in a mixture with albumin and other colloidal media, MC expressed strong potentiated effect on Abs' activity.
The comparison on undiluted and diluted MC commercially available anti-Rh sera showed that last-mentioned gave faster stronger and more reliable reaction with antigen positive RBC. Weak aggregation of negative samples completely disappeared after addition of saline. No changes in reactivity of diluted antisera were noted during 1 year storage.
According to the above mentioned data, we consider that MC could be successfully used in order to enhance the activity of ant-Rh reagents in manual testing. The low price, strong effectiveness of the media and easy performance of the method are advantages which could be useful in practice.

0359

INSPECTION INFORMATION AS A QA TOOL

E.B. Rossiter, B. Garrison *CITINGS* INFORMATION EXCHANGE, Richmond, VA, USA

CITINGS™ provides a forum for sharing information about inspections so that professionals can learn from the experiences of each other. All major blood collectors in the US submit information about their inspections with strict measures to assure confidentiality. Deficiencies and corrective actions are compiled, categorized, and published each month without identifying the facility. This information, which is also accessible via computer modem for text-based searching and retrieval, is a critical management tool for educators, supervisors and managers. It can be used to create training materials, internal audit checklists, follow trends, and identify potential problems before they occur.

Statistics on FDA inspection duration, citations per inspection, and proportion of deficiency-free inspections are tracked by center size (annual collection volume) and geographic location. Small volume facilities (collecting 30,000 units per year or less) have the longest inspections and the highest average citations per inspection. They also have the lowest percentage of "no deficiency" inspections. *CITINGS*™ membership has grown from 60 in 1991 to over 200 today.

0360

BLOOD BANK AND GOOD MANUFACTURING PRACTICE (GMP).

W.P.A. van der Tuuk Adriani, C.Th. Smit Sibinga, RC Blood Bank Groningen-Drenthe, NL.

Implementation of the European guidelines concerning blood products has brought blood banks under the influence of the pharmaceutical legislation. The purpose is to achieve compliance and harmonisation through the introduction of GMP.
APPROACH: Introduction of a GMP-based quality assurance manual focussed on general rules, procedures and documents regarding all staff and departments: people and personnel, behavior and hygiene, goods and source materials, quarantine release, recall and complaints etc. A people oriented fit for use system of motivation, explanation and training has been instituted. Support is given to heads of departments to implement the system.
RESULTS: Following initial confusion because of the change in approach and related mentality, continuous motivation and education resulted in ready acceptance. All personnel now is pleased to work according to renewed instructions/documents resulting in an increase of quality of work.
CONCLUSION: A people oriented fit for use approach in the implementation of GMP as an essential part of quality management has increased the awareness of a need of standardised and harmonised routine practice to improve overall quality in blood banks.

0361

BALANCING PHARMACEUTICAL GOOD MANUFACTURING PRACTICES (GMP) AND BLOOD TRANSFUSION STANDARDS OF PRACTICE

L Bust, G Bowie

Western Province Blood Transfusion Service, (WPBTS) Cape Town

WPBTS is divided into two functional sections:

a. Fractionation, which falls under the jurisdiction of the Medicines Control Council and has therefore followed pharmaceutical GMP guidelines for the past 10 years, and
b. Blood Transfusion, which currently follows local Standards of Practice.

The Quality Assurance Department has the role of ensuring compliance throughout the organisation. Activities have been streamlined and clearly defined to ensure that individual requirements of these dual systems are met whilst striving to standardise the level of quality. This applies to the following activities handled in Fractionation and Blood Transfusion: raw material testing, in-process checking, environmental monitoring, final product testing, product release, audits, vendor evaluation, product registration, premises, personnel, equipment, reagents, proficiency testing, documentation, corrective action, adverse reactions, etc. Although extending pharmaceutical GMP to all aspects of Blood Transfusion will be possible should local legislation require it, the respective costs and benefits thereof will need to be considered.

0362

A COMPUTERIZED BARCODE LABELLINGSYSTEM FOR A CORRECT LINKAGE OF THE BLOODDONOR AND THE BLOOD PRODUCTS

C.M.G.A. Kortekaas-Spruit, G.H. Kerssens, Bloedbank Kennemerland, The Netherlands.

For safety, tracing and regulatory purposes a correct linkage of the donor registrationnumber (DRN) to the bloodunit identification number (BUI) is extremely critical. For each donor our automated bloodbank-administration system (BAS) generates in Codabar an unique donor number of 11 positions (year of application 2 pos, a per donor ascending number 6 pos, the serial number of blooddonations 3 pos). BAS also generates in Codabar an unique bloodunit number of 10 positions (article-code 4 pos, a serial number 6 pos).

At inviting the donor a set of 8 barcode labels is printed.
One label with general information about the donor, 3 bloodunit labels for erythrocytes, buffycoat and plasma on which the DRN, the BUI, the bloodgroup and the bloodtypes to be placed on the bloodpacks and 4 labels with the DRN to be placed on the test-tubes. The serial number of the DRN has been ascended with "1".
With this method BAS has made a direct linkage between the donor and the 3 standard bloodproducts and also with the medical examination data and the test-tubes. Exchanges cannot take place.
For preparing a secundary bloodproduct BAS generates accessory BUI's. After labelling the pack a linkage is made between primary bloodproduct and the new blood-component by laserscanner.

With this method a donor can always be traced via a bloodunit identification number; a bloodproduct always can be traced via the blooddonor number in the database of the historical donor and bloodunit data in a simple way.

Thus a complete reliable, unique and simple barcode identification-system is available that provides a positive identification.

0363

ELECTRONIC DOCUMENTATION OF PROCESS DATA IN BLOOD CENTERS AND CELL PROCESSING LABORATORIES

David Dlesk and John Zeman
Cell Processing Systems, Inc.
Arlington Heights, Illinois, USA

As regulatory bodies have imposed more stringent regulations, the documentation requirements placed upon blood and cell processors have increased significantly. Since the processing history for each unit must be documented, the volume of process control data that must be collected, checked and archived can impose a substantial burden on the organization. A solution is to implement electronic documentation systems that meet the regulatory requirements for Good Documentation Practices, while reducing the workload and eliminating opportunities for errors.

Donor and testing data are routinely documented today. However, regulators are asking that there be much more control and documentation of the actual processing steps. This becomes especially important as increasingly complex cell processing techniques are developed. Process documentation is composed of two parts: the requirements and the results. The requirements are typically standard operating procedures and specifications. The results are the data that demonstrate that all the requirements of the process have been met. Real-time electronic documentation systems reduce errors and costs by providing the technician with access to the procedures as the process is being run and checking data as it is entered. The result is a database that provides full process traceability.

0364

Migration Path towards the ISBT 128 Standard for Health Care and Blood Transfusion

Error-free data collection is essential for all movements of blood samples and products within blood transfusion from donation to destination. Standardization is necessary to enable worldwide traceability:

a) State of the art

b) Logistical chain from donation to hospital

c) Legal aspects of traceability

d) ISBT 128 pros and cons and the requirements of transfusion technology

e) Migration from CODABAR to CODABLOCK: the ISBT 128 data

f) Methodology of printing and reading of the new standard in connection with data base integration.

The abstract identifies the key issues of the highly important issue of international data communication, related to products and reliability.

0365

COMPUTER NETWORK IN THE BLOOD BANK LABORATORY

M. Girard[1], D. Bombail[1], D. Fusier[2], M. Bourlioux[2].
1 CDTS. - 6, rue Emile Lesot - F-80000 AMIENS - FRANCE
2 KERNEL - 9, rue de Chateaudun - F-75009 PARIS - FRANCE

We implemented a computer network in the laboratories to process data from the analyzers before transmission to the mainframe computer. A double level of validation through built-in algorithms, one "on the bench" for daily results, one in the mainframe involving the complete history of the blood donations and previous biological results, provides a double ckeck of every data.

The hardware includes an Ethernet® network and is driven by a Hewlett Packard 486/66 ST® file server to manage 3 stations settled in 3 laboratories. Immunohematology laboratory operates 3 Mitis® (Ortho ®) and one Groupamatic ® (Kontron®). Virology equipment consists of 2 Posid Samplers® and 2 microplate processors® (Organon®), 1 Twin reader® (Flow®), 1 plate reader and 1 IMX ® (Abbott). Quality control laboratory operates 1 Argos® cell counter (Roche), 1 Ektachem® (Kodak), 1 electrophoresis reader (Sebia®).

Expanding the network capabilities only requests to plug in the new apparatus, if it is provided with an Ethernet® board. Software from Novell® allows to connect every type of microcomputer, even to build an heterogenous network. Bidirectionnal exchange of data between the mainframe and the network is of course possible.

This system allows to track every information about the analysis performed (reagent, batch number, statistics, serum storage...) providing a real process history without overloading the mainframe. Double check of data leads to a very high level of confidence.

0366

ENHANCING CRITICAL REASONING AND DECISION MAKING SKILLS OF MEDICAL TECHNOLOGISTS

LK Alexander, University of Kentucky Center for Rural Health Hazard, Kentucky, USA

As medical laboratory technicians (MLT) advance into technologist positions or as medical technologists (MT) progress into supervisory positions, there is need for greater reasoning and decision making skills. Progressive case study paper problems are used to refine and evaluate critical thinking. The student is given the initial testing results and determine the next procedure to be performed, the reason for selecting that procedure and the expected outcome or results. The use of a simple flow chart allows the instructor to evaluate the reasoning process and suggest alternatives and improvements. students generate patient reports, which must include the information needed to efficiently and safely treat the patient.
A decision-making exercise which requires the students to research a controversial area and make a recommendation for action is designed to allow the students to experience the process of preparing a recommendation for action and defending the recommendation in front of their peers. Some topics that have been used include: lowering of the donor hemoglobin levels, use of antigen matched blood for chronic transfusion patients and the immediate spin crossmatch.
Supervisory work review is simulated using laboratory worksheets which have a variety of common errors, including results and missing reactions. The students practice reviewing the workload and documenting errors. This presentation will include samples of these exercises and recommendations for use.

0367

COMBINATION OF SEMI-AUTOMATIC CROSS-MATCHING MACHINE AND PERSONAL COMPUTER RECONFIRMATION SYSTEM CAN AVOID MISMATCHED TRANSFUSION.

S.SONE[1), K.TAKAHASHI[1),Y.SHIBATA[2), A.OKADA[3)

1) Dept. of Immunohematology & Transfusion Medicine, Toranomon Hosp, Tokyo,Japan;
2) Dept. of Immunohematology & Transfusion Medicine, the Univ. of Tokyo, Tokyo, Japan:
3) Minerva Tech Co. Ltd., Tokyo, Japan.

To prevent from iatrogenic mismatched transfusion, we have developed an experimental semi-automatic machine for blood typing and cross-match test (SAMTC) in addition to check system with personal computer system(PCS).SAMTC can perform ABO and Rh(D) blood typing and compatibility test based on red blood cell agglutination in microplate. PCS can save patients data, blood products data and previous crossmatch results. Before transfusion it is easy to perform the double check with SAMTC and PCS.
The major limitation of this technique is its long-time consumption, that if shortened to 10 minutes or less, will be of great value in the near future.

0368

AUTOMATED DONOR NOTIFICATION LETTERS. N.D.Kalmin, V.Clegg, C.Harrell and B.Janes. South Texas Regional Blood Bank, San Antonio, TX. U.S.A.

Tests performed on individual blood donations have quadrupled during the last decade, resulting in thousands of laboratory test deferrals each year. This blood center, drawing approximately 90,000 units annually, experienced difficulty in maintaining a manual system of infectious disease donor notification letters.

A computer program was developed in-house to automatically generate informative letters, with relevant laboratory test results, five days after donors test reactive for infectious disease markers (retroviruses excepted). This period allows all repeat and confirmatory testing to be completed prior to letters being generated for mailing. Reactive screening tests for retroviruses are reported on data sheets. This alerts the quality assurance office to expect Western Blot test results within three weeks, after which computer generated letters are mailed. Results of special donations (e.g. autologous) are reported immediately, without the obligatory three week reconciliation period for homologous donations.

The computer is programmed to select from 40 individualized letters (single or multiple reactive results) and can generate numerous letters/hour. These are stored on an optical disk for easy access. The program has automated 90% of this center's donor notifications (approximately 152 letters/month). Computerization of donor notification has greatly improved the efficiency of this service.

0372

THE ADVANTAGE OF FULLY AUTOMATED MICROPLATE EIA PROCESSORS

P. Bachmann, J.J. Burckhardt
ZLB Central Laboratory, Blood Transfusion Service SRC, Berne, Switzerland

Since the introduction of Anti-HIV screening in 1985 the Blood Transfusion Services have had to face a continuous expansion of the screening spectrum. The inevitable cost explosion can only be controlled with automated techniques. Whereas such techniques are already fully established in blood group serology, the breakthrough in viral marker serology came with the introduction of EIA technology. Its use directly influences the following parameters when compared to partially automated systems: number of staff (full time equivalent, FTE), laboratory surface and running costs.

No of tests	No of staff (FTE)		Lab. space (m^2)		Running costs (sFr.)	
per year	PA	FA	PA	FA	PA	FA
600'000	4.8	2.7	108	54	1'296'000	729'000
800'000	6.4	3.6	144	72	1'728'000	972'000
1'000'000	8.0	4.5	180	90	2'160'000	1'215'000
1'200'000	9.6	5.4	216	108	2'592'000	1'458'000

PA = partially automated FA = fully automated

Standardised conditions moreover reduce the number of initially reactive units lowering the running costs of infectious disease screening by both fewer repeat and confirmatory testing. This minimizes the number of units with a delayed release.

0373

SCREENING FOR PLATELET ANTIBODIES USING MAIPA

Ananieva R., Alexiev I., Shinkov D.
National Center of Clinical and Transfusion Haematology
Sofia, Bulgaria

MAIPA (Monoclonal Antibody Immobilization of Platelet Antigens) developed by Kiefel et al.1987, was applied in Bulgaria for the first time for screening and identification of platelet antibodies.
Five groups of risk patiens were tested:
1.Pregnant women
2.Leukemia
3.Autoimmune haemolytic anemia
4.Thrombocytopenia
5.Haemophilia A
The following monoclonal antibodies were used:
Gi5 - against GP IIb/IIIa
Gi14 - against GP Ia/IIa - both gift from prof. Mueller-Eckhardt- Germany.
From the tested 43 sera one was positive with Gi5 (a case with PTP); six were positive with Gi14 (four were from pregnant women, one case - with leukemia, and one - with AITP). HLA antibodies were presented in 6 of the cases and only one of them showed positive results in MAIPA.
The method is discussed as a hopeful tool for screening and identification of platelet antibodies.

0374

HLA PHENOTYPE AND SENZITISATION TO HPA AND HLA ANTIGENS

D.Paunovic, R.Simonovic, O.Popovic, G.Nikolic, B.Rodic, I.Stolic, V.Miletic
Blood Transfusion Institute, Belgrade, Yougoslavia
In our five years work we have screened sera from 430 patientes refractory to pooled random donor platelets by Western blot procedure to identify circulated antibodies (ab) that bind to platelet membrane glycoproteins. As platelets share some antigens (ag) with other blood or tissue cells, we screened sera by microlymphocitotocsic test to identify anti-HLA abs. We found 25 sera with anti platelet,66 with anti-HLA abs and 16 with both of them. 328 sera were negative. 31 of sera reacting with some of platelet membrane glycoproteins were anti-HPA-1a, and 27 of them were women. 10 of 31 had IgG ab, 9 IgM and 12 both of them. For the rest of the abs we had no possibilities to identify specificity. For most of the positive patients we performed tissue typing, and we found that all exept one of HPA-1a ab positive had DRw52 ag and 84,61% of patients with anti-HLA abs had HLA-DR2 ag. Western blot iz reliable method for detection of circulated anti platelets abs. HLA phenotype could be in correlation with senzitisation to HPA and HLA ag.

0375

POST-TRANSFUSION PURPURA ASSOCIATED WITH ANTI-HPA-3a AND A PLATELET AUTOANTIBODY REACTING BY MAIPA TECHNIQUE ONLY

J.Chapman, P.Metcalfe, M.F.Murphy, A.H.Waters
Dept. of Haematology, St Bartholomew's Hospital, London UK.

Post-transfusion purpura (PTP) is characterised by acute severe thrombocytopenia occurring about one week after blood transfusion. The thrombocytopenia is associated with the production of high titre platelet alloantibody and is the result of destruction of the patient's own platelets. The mechanism of the thrombocytopenia is controversial, however platelet autoantibodies have been reported in some cases.

This report describes PTP in an 80 year old negro woman who had a history of previous transfusions and pregnancy. She was transfused three units of blood following haematemesis and melaena. 13 days later her platelet count had fallen to 6 x 10^9/l. She was already receiving prednisolone (5 mg/d) for rheumatoid arthritis, and the dose was increased to 30mg/d. Her platelet count increased to 238 x10^9/l after 6 days.

Platelet antibody studies using the platelet immunofluorescence test (PIFT) and the patient's acute serum and cells taken as the platelet count was rising gave negative reactions; positive reactions were obtained with random donor platelets. Lymphocytotoxic antibodies were also detected.

The MAIPA technique was used for further investigations. Using a monoclonal antibody against GpIIb/IIIa, positive reactions were obtained with the patient's own cells and serum and random donor platelets. The test was repeated one month later. Negative reactions were obtained with the patient's own cells and serum and anti-HPA-3a was identified using a typed platelet panel.

This is a further report of PTP where an autoantibody was found at the time of thrombocytopenia. In this case it was only detected using the MAIPA technique.

0376

LABORATORY DIAGNOSIS OF HEPARIN-ASSOCIATED THROMBOCYTOPENIA (HAT): ASSESSMENT OF DIFFERENT IN VITRO ASSAYS.

A. Greinacher[1], J.Amiral[2], V.Dummel[1], A.M. Vissac[2], C. Mueller-Eckhardt[1]
1 Institut für Klinische Immunologie und Transfusionsmedizin, Justus-Liebig Universität Giessen, FRG, 2 Serbio Research-Laboratories, Gennevilliers, France.
As clinical diagnosis of heparin-associated thrombocytopenia (HAT) is often difficult, confirmation by sensitive laboratory assays is desirable. We prospectively compared the sensitivity of heparin induced platelet activation (HIPA) test and platelet aggregation test (PAT) using sera of 209 patients with the tentative diagnosis of HAT. Both assays were performed concomitantly with platelets of the same 4 donors who varied from day to day. In addition, all sera were assessed with a newly developed PF4/heparin ELISA. Positive results were obtained with 33 % of sera in the PF4/heparin ELISA, with 33.5 % of sera in the HIPA test, and with 11.5% of sera in the PAT. PF4/heparin ELISA and HIPA test showed no difference in sensitivity ($p = 0.27$ McNemar's test) and were more sensitive than PAT ($p < 10^{-8}$ McNemar's test). However, they recognized different patient cohorts. 9 indeterminate and 12 negative sera in the HIPA test were positive in the PF4/heparin ELISA. 8 of the 9 indeterminate sera caused platelet activation with high heparin concentrations in the HIPA test. 11 of the 12 negative sera contained no IgG but IgM (9) or IgA (2) HAT antibodies. Four indeterminate and 18 negative sera in the PF4/heparin ELISA were positive in the HIPA test. None of the sera positive in the PAT was missed in the HIPA but two of them were negative in the PF4/heparin ELISA. All sera were assessed with 4 LMWH and a LMW heparinoid (Org 10172) in the HIPA test. LMWH caused platelet activation with positive sera in 99 %, the LMW heparinoid in 10-20 %. We conclude the majority of HAT antibodies reacts with a PF4/heparin complex but in approximately 20 % another protein ist involved.

0377

PLATELET AUTOANTIBODIES IN PATIENTS WITH SYSTEMIC LUPUS ERYTHEMATOSUS (SLE)

Pujol M[1], Ribera A[2], Vilardell M[3], Ordi J[3], Feliu E[1].
1Haematology Department. Hospital Germans Trias i Pujol. Badalona. 2Blood Bank.ICS, and 3Department of Internal Medicine. Hospital General "Vall d'Hebrón". Barcelona. SPAIN.

The aim of the study was to determine the prevalence of platelet autoantibodies (PAA) in patients with SLE and its correlation with thrombocytopenia.

Patients and methods. 90 SLE patients. Thrombocytopenia ocurred in 29 of them. A total of 166 PAA determinations, using the immunofluorescence test (IFT), were performed in the 90 patients.

Results. A positive direct IFT was obtained in 93 of the 166 determinations. Of these, platelet bound IgG was detected in 79, sometimes in combination with IgM (21/79) or IgA (2/79). In all but 14 samples the immunoglobulin could be eluted. PAA were also detected to a lesser extent in the sera (58/93).

56 of the 90 patients (62%) were positive for PAA. All patients with thrombocytopenia had PAA (29/29), although some patients with PAA showed normal platelet count (27/61). In the same patient, the presence of PAA was associated with current thrombocytopenia ($p=0.0005$).

The presence of PAA was observed in 63/76 (80%) of the determinations in patients with active disease compared with 30/90 (33%) in inactive SLE patients ($p=0.000001$).

Conclusions. The prevalence of PAA in SLE is high but its presence does not imply the existence of thrombocytopenia and is related to disease activity.

0378

QUANTITATION OF ANTI-D BOUND TO D-POSITIVE RED CELLS INFUSED INTO D-NEGATIVE SUBJECTS AFTER i.m. INJECTION OF HUMAN MONOCLONAL ANTI-D

B.M. Kumpel[1], P. Judson[1] and J. Goodrick[2]
1 IBGRL, Bristol, UK
2 Regional Transfusion Centre, Bristol, UK.

A flow cytometric method was developed to quantitate the IgG bound to D positive red cells when sensitized with low plasma concentrations of IgG anti-D in the presence of an excess of D negative cells. D positive red cells were infused into D negative male volunteers 2 days after injection of 300 µg IgG1 (BRAD-5) (n = 8) or IgG3 (BRAD-3) (n = 8) monoclonal anti-D. Blood samples were taken 3 hours after infusion, incubated for 1 hour at 37°C, washed, then incubated sequentially with FITC-conjugated $F(ab')_2$ anti-IgG, IgM monoclonal anti-D, biotin-conjugated anti-IgM, and R-phycoerythrin-conjugated streptavidin. For flow cytometric analysis, the use of IgM anti-D enhanced the discrimination between D positive and D negative cells, particularly at low sensitization levels. For the standards, O R_1R_2 cells were incubated in duplicate with varying dilutions of BRAD-3 or BRAD-5, and cell-bound IgG on one set quantified by ELISA [Kumpel, Vox Sang. 1990, 59; 34]. Cells from the other set were mixed with D negative cells (1:100), analysed by flow cytometry as above, and a standard curve of mean channel (green) fluorescence vs. molecules IgG/cell constructed. The sensitization levels of the infused D positive cells were found to be in the range 1,500 - 10,000 molecules of IgG anti-D per cell for the 16 subjects.

0379

SCREENING FOR HEMOCHROMATOSIS IN PROSPECTIVE BLOOD DONORS

H.P. Benn[1], P. Nielsen[2], R. Fischer[2], R. Engelhardt[2], C. Darda[1], R. Dittmer[1], B. Knödler[1], E.E. Gabbe[2], and P. Kuehnl[1];
[1]Transfusionsmed., [2]Med. Biochemie, UKE, Hamburg, FRG.

Prospective blood donors (f=632, m=633, mean age: 26y) were routinely screened for hereditary hemochromatosis (HHC) by elevated serum iron (SI) and serum ferritin (Ftn/S). After passing this first step transferrin saturation (Tfs), erythrocyte ferritin (Ftn/E), non-invasive biomagnetic liver susceptometry (BLS), and for final diagnosis ^{59}Fe absorption were performed at different levels of the screening procedure (see table).

Screening level	n	SI µg/dl	Tfs %	Ftn /S µg/l	Ftn /E ag/RBC	BLS $\mu g/g_{liv}$	^{59}Fe %
level 1 f/m	1265	>180	-	>100/200	-	-	-
level 2	99	>180	>50	>200	>50	-	-
level 3	24	>180	>50	>200	>50	>500	-
HHC	3	>180	>50	>200	>50	>500	>50

These results (3/1265) confirm the current frequency estimation for homozygotes of HHC (0.2-0.6%) for the first time in a group of young North-Germans. Screening for HHC will improve health care for blood donors by detecting affected homozygotes in the presymptomatic state of the disease. Moreover, as iron depletion by phlebotomies is the therapy of choice in these persons suffering only from malfunction of iron regulation, one may think about engaging them as "super donors".

0380

ID-SICKLE CELL TEST : PRELIMINARY REPORT

David Bashforth

DiaMed S.A., 1785 Cressier sur Morat, Switzerland

A simple test is described which permits the easy detection of haemoglobin S (HbS).

The principle employs the shape change induced when cells containing HbS are subject to low oxygen tension in vitro.

The ensuing sickle cells, or drepanocytes, are highly rigid and will not pass a micro-sieve under centrifugation (a principle originally developed by DiaMed S.A. for the detection of red cell agglutinates).

Initial results in this laboratory show differentiation between homo and heterozygous states, the detection of low levels of HbS and the demonstration of double populations, e.g. post transfusion.

The test shows promise for screening (both donors and populations) and as a diagnostic tool.

0381

HEMORRHAGE FOLLOWING CORONARY SURGERY -- TRANSFUSION SUPPORT AND CLINICAL OUTCOME

R.L. Thurer, R.G. Johnson, F.W. Sellke, C. Sirois, R.M. Weintraub
Beth Israel Hospital and Harvard Medical School, Boston, Massachusetts, U.S.A.

Between Jan 1, 1986 and July 1, 1993, 33 (1.1%) of 3101 patients (PTN) having coronary surgery (CS) required sternal reentry for postoperative hemorrhage. In 26 PTN a mechanical source (21) or no active bleeding site (5) was identified (Group I). Seven PTN (Group II) had diffuse bleeding without a defined source.

There was a significant difference in transfusion (TX) support and clinical outcome between the groups.

TX (units)	Group I	Group II
RBC	5.6 + 4.0	11.6 + 5.0 *
FFP	2.1 + 2.6	13.6 + 13.0 **
Plt	5.9 + 6.0	38.5 + 37.0 **
cryo	0.3 + 1.8	18.0 + 19.0 **

* p<0.05 **p<0.001

In-hospital mortality was 2/26 (7.7%) for Group I PTN (stroke, bowel ischemia) while 5/7 (71.4%) Group II PTN died.

CONCLUSIONS: PTN reexplored for bleeding following CS do well if a specific site is identified or if no active bleeding is found. PTN in whom bleeding continues have coagulopathies and a poor prognosis. Earlier diagnosis, better treatment or prevention is required to improve outcomes for Group II PTN.

0382

THE INFLUENCE OF LEUCOCYTE FILTRATION ON INFECTION RATE, LYMPHOCYTE SUBPOPULATIONS AND NK-CELL FUNCTION IN PATIENTS WITH COLORECTAL CANCER.

O. Mathiesen[1,2], L. Lund[2], U. Brodthagen[1], P. Gandrup[2], I. Balslev[2], C. Jersild[1], N. Grunnet[1].
1Regional Center for Blood Transfusion and Clinical Immunology, 2Dept. of Surgical Gastroenterology, Aalborg Hospital, DK-9100 Aalborg Hospital.

To elucidate the influence of leucocytes in blood transfusion on postoperative infection rates and on lymphocyte subpopulations and natural killer cell function one-hundred and fiftythree elective patients with colo-rectal malignancies were investigated in a prospective, randomised study. If blood transfusion was indicated, the red blood cells (RBC) were given principally as SAGM-RBC either with or without a leucocyte filter. Thirty-eight were transfused perioperatively, of these 15 (39.5 %) developed infection which was a significant higher rate compared with 24 (20.5 %) of the 117 non-transfused patients (p = 0.03). Twenty-one of the transfused patients received blood with a filter, of these seven (33 %) had postoperative infection, whereas eight of the seventeen (47 %) in the non-filter group had infection. This difference was material not significant, but the trend indicates a beneficial effect of removing leucocytes also from the relative leucocyte poor SAGM-RBC. The difference in infection rates between patients who have received MAF-Sagman without filter and non-transfused patients is significant (p=0.02), whereas there was no significant difference in infection rates between non-transfused and transfused with filter.

There was no significant sustained influence on lymphocyte subpopulations and natural killer cell function in blood samples taken preoperatively and six months postoperatively estimated by comparing transfused patients with or without leucocyte removal.

0383

INFECTION RATES AFTER BLOOD TRANSFUSION IN COLORECTAL CANCER PATIENTS, "THE *CRAB* CLINICAL TRIAL"

JGA Houbiers[1,2], LMG van de Watering[1], J Hermans[3], CJH van de Velde[2] & A Brand[1]
[1]Immunohaematology & Blood Bank, [2]Surgery, University Hospital Leiden, the Netherlands, tel 31-71-264007, [3]Medical Statistics, Leiden University

In a multicentre randomized controlled trial we investigated whether perioperative blood transfusions increase postoperative infection rates. Leukocyte depleted ("filtered") blood products have been shown not to induce immunosuppressive effects in organ-transplant recipients.

Colorectal cancer patients were randomized to recieve either packed cells without buffy coat (PC) or leukocyte depleted blood (LD). From 1987 till 1991 1108 patients have been randomized by 16 participating hospitals and according to the inclusion criteria 871 appeared eligible for analysis of whom 697 had been operated upon with curative intent. No significant differences in post-operative infection rates were found between the curatively operated PC (32%, N=360) and LD (36%, N=337) patients. Transfusion of red cells itself, however, remained the major risk factor for infections: the post-operative infection rate in transfused patients (39%, N=446) differed significantly from non-transfused patients (25%, N=251, p<0.01). Multivariate statistical analysis confirmed this.

0384

CLINICAL AND IMMUNOLOGICAL CONSEQUENCES OF WHOLE VERSUS LEUCOCYTE DEPLETED BLOOD IN SURGICAL PATIENTS

L.S.Jensen
University Department of Surgical Gastroenterology L Aarhus Kommunehospital, 8000 Aarhus, Denmark.

It seems most probably that leucocytes are mediating the immunosuppressive effects of blood transfusion. Blood transfusion is also reported to be followed by an increased frequency of postoperative infectious complications.

To investigate the immunological and clinical consequences of transfusion with whole blood versus leucocyte depleted blood a prospective randomized study was carried out in patients undergoing elective colorectal surgery.

In case of blood transfusion the patients were randomized to receive either whole blood transfusion or blood depleted from leucocytes. The immunological parameters were recorded before operation and day 3, 7 and 30 postoperatively.

Postoperative infectious complications developed in 23% of patients transfused with whole blood, and in 2% of patients transfused with leucocyte-depleted blood as in non-transfused patients (p<0.01). Natural killer cell function, T-helper/T-suppressor ratio and T-cell proliferation were significantly depressed (p<0.001) during the whole observation period in patients transfused with whole blood. The same parameters were only transient and non-significantly decreased in the either groups.

It is concluded that removing leucocytes from blood products significantly reduces the immunosuppressive effect of blood transfusion as well as significantly reduces the development of postoperative infectious complications.

0385

MEDICAL AUDIT OF THE USAGE OF GROUP O RHD NEGATIVE RED CELLS IN HOSPITALS SUPPLIED BY NLBTC

Mahes de Silva, Gail Abrahamson
North London Blood Transfusion Centre, London, UK.

The national stock of group O RhD negative red cells is disproportionately low when compared to the number of group O negative donors bled (7.8%). Following an audit undertaken in 1991[1], guidelines for the use of group O negative red cells were distributed to all hospitals supplied by NLBTC. A re-audit undertaken in Nov-Dec 1992 revealed that the majority of hospitals had implemented the new policies resulting in a more appropriate use of this valuable resource.

The percentage of red cells supplied as group O negative units has decreased from a median of 10.1% during Jun-Nov 1990 to 7.7% during Jun-Nov 1992. Whereas only 8 out of 27 hospitals requested <8% of all red cell units as group O negative in 1990, 16 out of 27 hospitals did so during Jun-Nov 1992. The first audit showed that only 34% of group O negative units were being used "appropriately" and the re-audit showed that this has increased to 55%.

NLBTC Guidelines for the use of O RhD negative red cells were updated to take into account that only group O RhD negative red cells from a highly selected panel of blood donors are supplied for all neonatal "top up" transfusions.

References

1 Are only 34% of group O RhD negative red cells used appropriately?: an audit of usage in NHS Hospitals. Mattock, C, Brace W, Knowles S. North London Blood Transfusion Centre (1992) Transfusion Medicine, Vol 2, Supplement 1, BBTS X Annual Scientific Meeting.

0386

MONITORING OF POST TRANSFUSION HEMOGLOBIN TO IMPROVE TRANSFUSION PRACTICES

B.A.van Dijk, V.A.J.M.Kunst, G.W.M.Winkens-Meijs
St Radboud University Hospital, Nijmegen, The Netherlands

Usually a hospital transfusion committee decides at which hemoglobin (Hb) level blood transfusion is indicated. This gives a guideline to physicians when to transfuse a patient. Our hospital has chosen a Hb level of 6,0 mmol/l for adults, above which transfusion generally should not be given. The auditing of good transfusion practice however is done by monitoring the effect of transfusion: the post transfusion Hb level. The transfusion laboratory checks every year since 1985 during the last trimester the post transfusion Hb levels of all patients. The aim is to offer a surveillance to clinicians that the percentage of patients with higher post transfusion Hb levels will not become too large. The results are presented to all departments and physicians, and are discussed when needed.
The 1993 results were (children excluded):

	post transfusion Hb (mmol/l)	
	≥ 6,5	≥ 8,0
non-surgical departments	50%	4%
surgical departments	62%	11%
TOTAL	55%	7%

In conclusion, the post transfusion Hb levels did not exceed 6,5 mmol/l in about half the cases, which we consider an acceptable result.

0387

COST-EFFECTIVENESS OF A BARRIER SYSTEM TO PREVENT MISTRANSFUSION.

J.P. AuBuchon, B. Littenberg.
Dartmouth-Hitchcock Medical Center, Lebanon, New Hampshire, USA.

Transfusion of red cells to a patient other than the intended recipient remains a significant cause of post-transfusion morbidity and mortality. Recent analyses place the risk of mistransfusion (MT) at about 1 in 12 000 units with a fatality occurring every 600 000 transfusions. We analyzed the cost-effectiveness of BloodLoc®, a barrier system designed to prevent MT, in a model that took into account the range of incidence of morbid and fatal events, costs of patient care, and liability damage awards. In the base case analysis, with US$3.35/unit as the cost of using the BloodLoc® system, application of the system resulted in *reduced* healthcare expenditures if the average damage award for a fatality exceeded US$354 000 and the chance of MT exceeded 1 in 16 700. If no damage awards were anticipated in the analysis, use of the system cost US$69 000 per year of life saved. This value decreased to US$14 300 by applying the system only to non-Group O units. Routine use of the system extended patient life by 1 yr/22 000 units transfused. The cost-effectiveness analysis was most sensitive to the damage award estimate and was insensitive to probabilities of morbidity after an incompatible transfusion > 0.4 and fatality in the presence of morbidity > 0.1. Application of the BloodLoc® system to prevent MT and related morbidity and mortality can be cost-effective; if liability damage awards follow MT, use of the BloodLoc® system reduces total costs.

0388

BLOOD COMPONENT USE IN PATIENTS REQUIRING INTRAAORTIC BALLOON PUMP

A Bracey, R Radovancevic, B Radovancevic, P Powers.
Texas Heart Institute, Houston, Texas, USA.

*Purpose.*We reviewed blood use in the group of patients (pts) that required an intraortic balloon pump(IABP) after coronary artery bypass surgery to analyze overall blood requirements.
*Methods.*We analyzed transfusion data from 45 randomly selected IABP pts and compared results with 59 redo-CAB pts. The anticoagulation regimen for IABP pts was low-molecular-weight dextran.
*Results.*The groups were comparable for age, sex, number and type of grafts. Significantly different ($p < 0.05$) variables are presented in the table. All pts enrolled received RBCs. FFP was transfused in 73% of IABP pts vs. 25% of redo-ACB pts. Platelets accounted for 58% of all blood exposure and were transfused in 53% of IABP vs. 20% of redo-CAB pts. The nadir platelet count in 14/24 (58%) of pts receiving platelets was > 80,000/ml. Compared with pts who did not receive platelets, those who did were older, had smaller body mass, lower nadir platelet count and higher bilirubin.

	Bypass time	Transfusions(units/patient)		
(mean ± SE)	min.	RBC	PLT	FFP
IABP	98 + 5	8.2±0.7	18.2±4.1	4.8±0.8
REDO	78 ± 4	3.1±0.4	2.2± 0.6	1.2±0.3

Conclusion. Our results indicate that IABP use markedly increases the need for blood components. A reduction in donor exposure may be achieved with the use of apheresis platelets and re-evaluation of the platelet transfusion threshold.

0389

USE OF PLATELET CONCENTRATES IN BLOOD SYSTEM DISEASES

K.M.Abdulkadyrov
Institute of Hematology and Transfusiology, St.Petersburg, Russia

Platelet transfusions for blood system disorders are absolutely indicated when thrombocytopenia is less than $5 \cdot 10^9$/L, thrombocytopenia is in the range of $5-10 \cdot 10^9$/L (even if hemorrhages are minimal and/or hyperthermia is 38°C or more) or thrombocytopenia is more than $10 \cdot 10^9$/L and is accompanied by pronounced bleeding.

Thrombocytopenia in itself (however, not less than $20 \cdot 10^9$/L), being not infrequent in hematological patients, is not the reason for platelet transfusion if the hemorrhages are absent, for the multiple platelet transfusions lead to allosensitization, the patient becoming refractory to blood component therapy. Transfusions of platelet concentrates are not recommended in the hemorrhages caused by thrombocytopenias of immune genesis because in such cases hemorrhages are only more severe.

A single therapeutic dose of platelets must be equivalent to not less than 400-500 mlrd cells. Thus, from 10 to 50 or more therapeutic doses of platelets are required in bone marrow transplantation to one patient.

0390

CLINICAL FACTORS INFLUENCING THE EFFICIANCY OF SINGLE DONOR PLATELET TRANSFUSIONS

K.H. Muggenthaler[1], M. Böck[2], M.U. Heim[2], W. Mempel[1]

[1]*Transfusion Center (Dept.of Med.III).Klinikum Großhadern, University of Munich and* [2]*Dept. of Transfusion Medicine, University of Magdeburg; Germany*

Introduction:
About 40-70% of transfusions of single donor platelet concentrates do not result in a sufficient posttransfusion platelet recovery. Apart from immunologic reasons (e.g. HLA- or platelet specific antibodies) there are many clinical conditions connected to transfusion success. Aim of the present study was to determine the relative importance of clinical factors on the efficiancy of platelet transfusions.

Material and Methods:
401 single donor platelet concentrates transfused to 46 patients (most of them with hematologic-oncologic disorders) were monitored retrospectively. Characteristics of the platelet concentrates (e.g. storage time, leucocyte-contamination, AB0-compatibility etc) as well as patient - specific data (e.g. fever, antibiotics, splenomegalie etc.) were compared to the posttransfusion increment after 12 to 18 hours.. Statistical analysis was performed by the BMDP-program, a p-value < 0.05 was considered to be significant.

Results:
The following criteria could be identified to influence posttransfusion platelet recovery significantly: Splenomegaly, hepatomegaly, diagnosis, application of intravenous antibiotics and its duration, number and time of previous platelet transfusions ($p<0.001$), AB0-compatibility, pretransfusion storage time ($p=0.004$) and number of contaminating leucocytes ($p=0.022$).

Conclusions:
Beside immunologic reasons like HLA- or platelet specific antibodies many additional factors play an important role. In platelet transfusion therapie a high value should set on AB0-compatibility, brief storage time and low leucocyte contamination, since these parameters - in contrast to other influencing factors - can easily be controlled.

0391

Factors Influencing the Efficacy of Platelet Transfusion Therapy

V.A.Agranenko, A.M.Kompaniets
Institute of Pediatric Hematology, Moscow, Russia.

The influence of different factors (underlying disease, presence of HLA or platelet-specific antibody, cytostatic and antibiotic therapy, status of spleen, fever, infection, clinical bleeding grade, number of previous transfusions and other) on the efficacy of platelet transfusion therapy in chronically thrombocytopenic patients on the basis of mathematic analysis was studied. The analysis of platelet concentrate (PC) types was also included (method of preparation, storage time).

The values of corrected platelet count increment at 1 hour and 18-24 hours posttransfusion was served as quantitative characteristics of platelet transfusion response. It was demonstrated that the major reason of the unsuccessful transfusion of PC was the combined influence of two or more factors.

The following are considered to be the most significant: splenomegaly, lymfocytotoxic alloantibodies, infection, fever. We have to point out such important factor as HLA-alloimmunization which appeared in 65% cases of acute leukemia and 57% cases of aplastic anemia. However in 13% of alloimmunization cases the presense of HLA-antibodies did not effect platelet transfusion response. In 3% of cases the HLA-alloantibodies disappeared despite the massive transfusion therapy. We connect this date with transfusion of massive doses pooled random donor PC.

0392

SUBSTITUTIONAL PLATELET CONCENTRATES TREATMENT OF PATIENTS WITH ACUTE LEUKEMIA

N. Nedeljkovic[1], S. Mitrovic[1], M. Antic[1], I. Maslovaric[1], R. Tomasevic[1], G. Bogdanovic[1], N. Tijanic[1], G. Cuk[1], M. Petrovic[2], A. Bogdanovic[2], N. Suvajdzic[2], M. Colovic[2], S. Tadic[3], Z. Trajkovic[4], Z. Dragojlovic[5], D. Mitrovic[6]

1 Blood Transfusion Institute of Serbia, 2 UCC Institute of Hematology, 3 Clinical Center „Dr D. Misovic„, 4 MM Academy, 5 UCC Institute of Biochemistry, 6 Institute of Pathology University School of Medecine, Belgrade Yugoslavia

The substitutional treatment of patients suffering from acute leukemia (AL) under current conditions requires Leucocyte-Depleted Platelet Concentrates (LDPC) administration.

In our transfusion practice we have already been applyng, for five years (1988-1993), the leucodepleting method with slow pool centrifugation of Platelet Concentrates (PC) obtained from Platelet Rich Plasma and Buffy Coat. LDPC from the separator have also been applied. LDPC quality controls (N=39) performed by cytometric, cytohemical and biochemical methods have shown that the decontamination index is higher then 80.5%. There were total of 2806 AL patients who were administered LDPC prepared out of 24083 PC. The patients were given 1-19 LDPC, and the average PC pool unit number was 5.5.

By retrospective supervision in 1992 and 1993 the significant prepared LDPC number decrease was evidenced, due to the lack of triple and quadruple plastic bags. Even 50% of the overall platelets need has gone to Non-Leucodepleted Platelet Concentrates. The platelets use from separator was significantly reduced (90%:21%) in the period 1992/1993.

A significant increase ($p<0.01$) of hemorrhage incidence was registered as treatment complications (54%:20%) and fatal outcame causes (34%:9%) in the course of treatment of AL patients in the period 1992/1993 as related to the period 1988/1993.

0393

PLATELET TRANSFUSION IN THE NETHERLANDS: AN EIGHT YEARS EVALUATION.

A Westerterp[1], JThM de Wolf[2], PC Das[1], CTh Smit Sibinga[1], MR Halie[2] - [1] RC Blood Bank Groningen-Drenthe, [2]Academic Hosp. Groningen, Groningen, NL

The increasing demand of platelets has been reported. To determine cost/efficiency we investigated trends of random (RDP) and single donors (SDP) platelet transfusions and its financial consequences over the last 8 years in the country. Data were collected from the National Council of Blood Transfusion and the regional Blood Banks.
RESULTS: From 1984 to 1991 platelet transfusion has almost doubled from 100,200 to 194,000. The trend was seen in university centres (UCs) and most district hospitals (DHs). In the UCs platelet use per bed increased from 9 (range 6-12) in 1984 to 17 (range 10-23) in 1991. Patient population receiving platelet transfusion broadened from 1987 (mostly haematological) to a larger variety of clinical specialties in 1991. In the Netherlands 6% of the total platelets representing 30% of the platelet budget were transfused as SDP, where in the UCs 5-17% of the total platelets transfused were SDP, costing 27-58% of the platelet budget.
CONCLUSION: The increasing demand of platelets is mostly met by routine blood donations. Variations in the use of platelets per hospital bed might represent different institutional custom, in particular in the UCs. A change of transfusion practice favoring SDP will have significant financial consequenses in medical practice.

0394

TRANSFUSION OF PLATELET CONCENTRATES MADE FROM POOLED BUFFY COATS.

R.N.I.Pietersz[1], A.M.Joustra-Dijkhuis[1], M.Ariaansz[1], P.C.Huijgens[2], W.J.A.Dekker[1], H.W.Reesink[1], 1) Red Cross Blood bank Amsterdam; 2) Free University Hospital, Amsterdam, the Netherlands.

Aim: To assess whether the corrected count increments (CCI) after transfusion of platelet concentrates (PC) from pools of 4 buffy coats (PC-4BC) would be comparable to CCI after transfusion of 6 PC made from single buffy coats (PC-6BC).

Method: Pools were prepared by mixing 4 units of 50 ml-BC with 200 ml plasma from 1 of the donors. Following centrifugation for 7 min at 1,250 rpm the platelet-rich-plasma was transferred into a 1,000 ml PL 732 (Baxter) bag and stored at 20 - 24°C for up to 5 days with agitation (PC-4BC). PC from single buffy coats were prepared by centrifugation of a 100 ml buffy coat for 6 min at 380 x g. Immediately prior to transfusion 6 units were pooled (PC-6BC). The PC were transfused to stable trombocytopenic patients, platelet count < 20 x 10^9 /L.

Results:

		PC-4BC	PC-6BC
Number		24	22
Storage	days	4.7 ± 0.45	5 ± 0
Platelets	x 10^9	222 ± 37.8	247 ± 45.5
Leukocytes	x 10^6	25 ± 12.6	32 ± 12.9
CCI 1 h post		16.1 ± 7.7	18.0 ± 6.8
CCI 24 h post		8.6 ± 7.0	10.4 ± 7.4

There was no statistical difference between the data of the PC or the CCI (Student-t test) at any time.

Conclusion: the CCI's were comparable after transfusion of either a PC pool made from 4 BC or a pool of 6 single-BC-PC. The lower number of units per transfusion will contribute to ease the logistic problems caused by the increasing demand for PC.

0395

REFRACTORINESS HLA- AND NON-HLA ALLO-IMMUNIZATION AFTER PRESTORAGE FILTERED PLATELETS AND RED CELLS.

V.M.J. Novotny[1], R. van Doorn[1], M.D. Witvliet[2], F.H.J. Claas[2], A. Brand[1,2].
[1] Red Cross Bloodbank Foundation Leiden, [2] Department of Immunohaematology, University Hospital Leiden, the Netherlands.

The incidence and consequenses of HLA and non-HLA immunization in 194 patients with aplastic thrombocytopenia was evaluated, in relation to transfusion (TR) history and prior pregnancies. Platelet rich plasma and red cells were both filtered before storage leaving respectively < 10^6 and < 5 x 10^6 residual leucocytes.
Patients sera were tested using a lymphocytotoxicity and platelet immunofluorescence assay. Refractoriness was defined as a corrected count increment of < 7.5 at 1 hrs and/or < 2.5 at 20 hrs. HLA antibodies (Ab) developed in 3/112 patients (2.7%) with a negative history, in 21/41 (51%) after non-filtered Tr and in 23/39 (59%) after pregnancy. Non-HLA Ab occurred in 9/194 cases. Refractoriness occurred in 65% of patients with HLA Ab P < 0.0001) and in 44% with non HLA Ab. All patients with a diagnosis expecting multiple platelet TR should be transfused with leucocyte depleted red cells and platelets prepared in a technique that ensures leucocyte depletion to a level of < 5 x 10^6 per transfusate.

0396

THE CLINICAL EFFICACY OF PLATELET TRANSFUSIONS: A Prospective Study.

R H A GREEN[1], J B Palmer[1], A C Parker[2], M J Mackie[3], and W G Murphy[1,4].

[1]South East Scotland BTS, Edinburgh; [2]Depts of Haematology, Royal Infirmary of Edinburgh; [3]Western General Hospital, Edinburgh and [4]University of Edinburgh, UK.

Over a 15 month period all platelet transfusions for prophylaxis or treatment of bleeding in association with chemotherapy-induced or primary marrow failure were analysed for type of platelet preparation, day of storage, platelet dose, filtration and irradiation status; recipients were reviewed pre and post transfusion for risk factors for refractoriness, WHO bleeding grade, platelet count, CCI (at 24 hours), and outcome. Of a total of 1984 transfusions, 283 were excluded from further analysis (no outcome data available or no further transfusions to that patient within the next 8 days). 1701 transfusions in 95 patients were evaluated: 714(42%) were given for haemostasis (bleeding grade >1); 987(58%) for prophylaxis. Haemostasis was achieved in 297/714 (40.2%). Increment in 24 hour post transfusion circulating platelet count (x10^9/L) was 9.97±12(sd) in patients achieving haemostasis, and 7±12.86(sd) in those showing no benefit (NS, t-test unpaired). Prophylaxis was achieved in 793/987 (80.3%): increment in 24 hour platelet count (x10^9/L) in patients achieving prophylaxis was 10±12 and 7±11 in those not benefitting (NS). For both haemostasis and prophylaxis, neither efficacy nor increment depended on platelet age or type, or on the presence of risk factors for refractoriness. This study suggests that the beneficial effect of platelet transfusion is not determined by freshness, method of preparation or increment achieved.

0397

PLATELETS: HLA-MATCHING vs. CROSSMATCHING

P.S. Walker[1], C.S. Evans [2]
1 Irwin Memorial Blood Centers, San Francisco
2 Blood Bank of the ACCMA, Oakland, California

Refractory platelet recipients have traditionally been managed with HLA-matched plateletpheresis products. This study examines the efficacy of a simple, rapid crossmatch technique to select compatible platelets for these recipients from non-HLA-matched donors. In 1993, 80 of 97 recipients were successfully supported with crossmatch-selected platelets. Our data shows that 56 recipients reacted with more than 70% of random donor platelets, and no compatible crossmatches were found for 17 recipients. Of the recipients who had compatible donors, 27% had less than 5 compatible crossmatches; limiting them to single-donor apheresis platelets. 56% of the recipients had 6 or more compatible crossmatches; allowing them to be supported by pooling 6-8 compatible Whole Blood-derived platelets. Although we have a large, active HLA program, the crossmatch also selects platelets that result in successful transfusions, often from available inventory, and permits expansion of our resources for an ethnically-diverse patient population. Without a pool of donors who are typed for platelet-specific antigens, the crossmatch is the only technique to identify donors for recipients with platelet-specific antibodies. In conclusion, we recommend the crossmatch as an adjunct or alternative to HLA-matching to provide compatible platelets for highly-immunized recipients.

0398

PLATELET CROSSMATCHING FOR THE ALLOIMMUNIZED PATIENTS

S. Bejrachandra[1], W. Boonbanggeng[2], D. Chandanayingyong[1]

1 Department of Transfusion Medicine, Faculty of Medicine Siriraj Hospital, Mahidol University, Bangkok, THAILAND.

2 Department of Transfusion Medicine, Bhumipoladulyadej Hospital, Bangkok, THAILAND.

The lymphocytotoxicity test (LCT) and the mixed passive haemagglutination test (MPHA) were used in retrospective platelet crossmatching for detection of compatible random-donor platelets in multiple transfused patients. Thirty-seven episodes of pooled random-donor platelet transfusion were evaluated in thirty patients who were suspected of having refractoriness to platelet transfusion. Effectiveness of the transfusion was assessed by one-hour posttransfusion corrected count increment (CCI). When both tests were used in combination, the concordant results were significantly correlated with the CCI ($p < 0.05$). The outcome of the platelet transfusions was correctly predicted in 88% of the cases. Furthermore, the sensitivity of the combined tests was higher than the sensitivity of LCT or MPHA alone. These results suggest that platelet crossmatching by MPHA should be used when failure of platelet transfusion occurs after using LCT in alloimmunized patients.

0399

Determination of platelet antibodies using Capture-PM, ELISA and MAIPA in relation to transfusioneffect after platelet transfusion

D.Barz, R.Lehmann, D.Staack, O.Anders V.Lakner
University Rostock, Department of transfusionmedicine and Clinic of Internal Medicine, Rostock, Germany

In this study, IgG antibodies to platelets were detected by Capture-PM, ELISA (Thrombomatch) and MAIPA in sera from patients with haematological disease and their role in platelet transfusion refractoriness.

0400

THROMBOMATCH - ELISA FOR DETECTION OF PLATELET ANTIBODIES

V. Lenhard, C. Goy, H. Uthemann
Biotest AG, Dreieich, Germany

In acute thrombocytopenia and refractoriness to platelet substitution due to alloimmunization rapid and reliable tests for donor platelet selection are needed. We describe an assay which recently was developed on the ELISA principle. In precoated 96-well microplates, recipient's plasma/serum (50 µl) is incubated with 5 x 10^6/well donor platelets and washed three times with a specific buffer solution. The binding of anti-donor platelet antibodies is detected by POD-labelled anti-human IgG (100 µl) and subsequent substrate reaction. The optical density is measured at 492 nm. The cut-off-value was defined as 0.150 O.D. Test time is maximum 90 min.

A panel of 10 platelet-specific antisera with specificity for the HPA-1a/1b, HPA-3a/3b, and HPA-5a/5b alloantigens as well as 14 mono- and polyspecific HLA antisera have been tested against 201 platelet preparations in order to evaluate the test system. In the cross-matching technique all donor-specific alloantisera were clearly identified. Even weak reacting HPA-5 antisera or low titer HLA antisera showed unequivocally positive results (O.D. > 0.150). Testing of diluted antisera indicated high sensitivity. In negative samples mean O.D. ranged from 0.022 to 0.079. False negative or positive reactions were not observed.

The Thrombomatch-Elisa described here fulfills the requirements for simple, fast, specific, and reliable pretransfusion platelet cross-matching.

0401

PROGNOSIS OF THERAPEUTIC EFFECT OF PLATELETS TRANSFUSION IN THROMBOCYTOPENIA

T.Dolidze, N.Katanjan, G.Gogichadze, T.Kiknadze. Institute of Haematology and Blood Transfusion, Tbilisi, Republic of Georgia

In general the existance of antiplatelet antibodies (AA) in patients with thrombocytopenia (TP) causes reduction of platelets transfusion therapeutic effect(PTTE). However our clinical data has shown that in some cases the existance and activity of AA is not enough for prognosis of PTTE. We attempted to find more exact prognostic criterion that could enable us to estimate the destruction of platelets exposed to AA. In particular,appart from immunological tests we researched electroconductivity (E) and resistance (R) of donors platelets after their placing into patients serum at 37°, 45 min. At the same time we used the indirect immunofluorescence techniques with allogenic platelets in complex with lymphocytotoxicity and adsorbtion tests for determination and differentiation of allogenic AA from anti-HLA antibodies. Activity of AA was estimated by intensity of fluorescence. We examined 78 patients with TP. In 19 case we did not find correlation between existence or activity of AA and PTTE when only immunological tests were taken into account, while due to investigation of E and R this number was reduced to 8.

0402

FOLLOW UP OF SERUM PROTEINS AFTER IRRADIATED DRIED PLASMA TRANSFUSION IN NUTRITIONAL DISEASES

A.M. Ibrahim,[1] M.F.S. El-Hawary,[1] N.K., Shawarby,[2] R.Sakr. and[2] S.Samuel.

1 National Research Centre,Biochemistry Dept., Dokki, Cairo, Egypt.
2 Childern Hospital , Faculty of Medicine , Cairo University

In relatively advanced countries, as well as in backward areas all over the world, nutritional diseases represent a major economic medical problem. Of these mutritional deseases, which are frequently met with in Egypt are Kwashiorkor, marasmus and nutritional oedema.

In the present work it is felt to study the levels of serum total proteins and their individual fractions in Kwashiorkor, marasmus [at its different grades, I, II and III] and nutritional oedema, as compared to normals, before and at interval periods after transfusion with Courtland normal human irradiated and dried plasma, (at intervals of 15 minutes immediately following plasma transfusion - 72 hours thereafter] with the aim of observing the immediate and late changes in the electropherogram following plasma transfusion.

The material of study comprised 36 Kwashiorkor, 25 marasmic cases and 9 cases of nutritional oedema.

Samples of fasting venous blood were collected and non- heamolysed serum was obtained after centrifugation.

Plasma transfusion [using irradiated dried normal human plasma supplied by courtland laboratories, Pharmaceuticals, Biologicals U.S.A.] was performed.

Regarding to the normal fractions developed on the electropherogram, an additional band appeared in the region between fibriongen and beta-globulin.

Repeating electrophoresis of serum proteins in some cases of these malnutrition diseases as well as a number of normal individuals , 15 minutes after the plasma transfusion, this new band persisted to appear . Re-investigation 72 hours after, revealed its disappearance. These findings indicate that this abnormal band exists in the plasma used in transfusion and its introduction in the body lead to its disappearance in about 72 hours.

It is suggested that this new band present in plasma used for transfusion is most probably due to the process of irradiation manipulated during the process of manufacture. This suggestion receives evidence from studies on the effect of ultraviolet and X- ray irradiation on protein solutions.

0403

TTP and pregnancy. Plasmapheresis therapy during a long period.

Martín A, López R, Cano I, Pinilla J, Rubio M, Castañeda A, Santacreu M, Rios P, Ojeda E, García de Bustos J, Ulibarrena C, Jiménez V, Martín MP, de la Cámara C. y Hdez Navarro F
Servicio de Hematología y Hemoterapia. Hospital "La Paz". Madrid (Spain).

Thrombotic thrombocytopenic purpura (TTP) have been described associated to pregnancy. Plasmapheresis therapy is mandatory but fetal death is even frequent.

We describe the case of a 25-years old woman who was diagnosed of TTP in the 27th week of her pregnancy. It was started treatment with plasmapheresis (1,5 times plasmatic volume exchange every procedure), steroid and antiagregant drugs. The patient clinical status was worsening in spite of an initial good response to this treatment. Fifteen days after diagnosis, the patient had seizures, high blood pressure and gastrointestinal bleeding. Fetal death in uterus happened. After that, the patient was admitted to the Intensive Care Unit, where plasmapheresis treatment was continued until a satisfactory clinical response was obtained. The plasmapheresis number was 38, with infusion of 523 U of fresh frozen plasma.

Plasmapheresis therapy has improved the TTP prognosis. This treatment must be continued until the disease outcome, even during long time periods and in spite of an initial bad response.

0404

CLINICAL EXPERIENCE WITH HUMAN ALBUMIN PRODUCED BY ION EXCHANGE CHROMATOGRAPHY

Olga Todorovska Damevska[1], D. Ivanovski[1], P. Kolevski[1], A. Stojanovic[2], P. Misevska[3]
1. Institute of Blood Transfusion;
2. Clinics of Haematology; 3. Clinics of gastroenterohepatology, Skopje, Macedonia

We studied the effect of chromatographycally produced albumin from human plasma-HPA-(Pharmacia). The product fulfills all Pharmacopeia requirements. During the 12 years period we produced 360 batches of 5 % and 12 % HPA and 300 batches (30.000 bottles) were applied in patients. A study with rigorous clinical monitoring was done on a heterogenous group of 46 patients with hypoproteiniemic syndrome due to gastro-intestinal and hematologic dissorders. Doses were from 1-19 bottles of HPA in a course, altogether 168 bottles. The most preliminary data indicate: a marked rise in serum albumin level with diminuation of clinical signs (loss of oedema, reduction in body weight), rise of diuresis, normalisation of blood pressure, decrease in serum billirubin level and no changes in electrolite concentrations. No case of transmission of HbsAg and HIV was noticed. Negative side-effects (hyperpyretic, alergic) have to be studied and appeared in 7 % of patients. The study indicates a favourable clinical effects of HPA produced by large scale chromatography method (Pharmacia).

0405

A CASE OF ACUTE HEMOLITIC REACTION PRODUCED BY TRASFUSION OF A LARGE AMOUNT OF PLASMA

JingNa Niu and ShuMin Guan
NanFang Hospital, GuangZhou, 510515. P.R.CHINA

A patient with 95% burning area and acute hemolitic reaction after plasma transfusion was reported. The man was of AB blood qroup who had been transfused frozen dry plasma 2600ml and mixed fresh frozen plasma 1200ml within two days. He was found with serious hemoglobinurea: tne urine became dark brown, urobilinogen 4+, urobilin 1+. Free hemoglobulin in blood was 87mg%. Hemoglobin decreased to 58g/L, RBC count was 1.92×10^{12} /mm³ . He suffered from acute hemolyticreaction, but no shock or other allergic reaction was found. The anit-A IgG was found with serological test.

After review of literature and analysis of the case as can be concluded that:

As the subject of AB blood group is supersensative to the uncompatible plasma,it should be strickly to give the isomorphic plasma for the patient of AB group, transfusion of plasma with other group or mixed ones must be avoided. More attention should be paid to the compatility of the transfused plasma group with the acceptors' in clinics.

The capacity of nentralization and dilution of the incompatible antibody is limited to the human body. The hemolytic reaction may occur after a large amount of incompatible plasma transfused, because the antibodies naccumulate and exceed the ability of nentralization and dilution of the body.

In order to prevent the hemolytic reaction the principle of the blood group compatibility should be insisted in the transfusion of plasma.

0406

Transfusion-associated respiratory distress in Taiwan

M. Lin[1], C.C. Chen[1], C.C. Hong[1], W.S. Lin[2], Y.P. Cheng[3]

1 National Health Research Institute Transfusion Medicine Laboratory,Mackay Memorial Hospital, 2 Taichung Blood Donation Center and 3 Taipei Blood Donation Center, Taiwan, ROC

Transfusion-associated respiratory distress occurred more often in the past in Taiwan but recently only very rarely. Also from our studies, it appears very unlikely that the former cases were the result of immune reactions involving either red blood cells, serum proteins (especially IgA), HLA or granulocyte-specific antigens. Detailed clinical and serological studies were performed on 4 cases(one fatal). Recalcified plasma from the donors involved in these cases always gave a positive reaction by the granulocyte microagglutination test and even showed some "apparent" specificity as not all granulocytes reacted. Therefore initially it was thought that granulocyte antibodies was the cause of these transfusion reactions. However,because repeat samples of serum and plasma(nonrecalcified) from some of the donors incriminated in these transfusion reactions gave negative results, it would appear that the recalcification itself was the cause of a false positive reaction in the granulocyte microagglutination test. Because repeat donations from the donors implicated in these cases were transfused to other patients but showed no untoward reactions, non-immune causes, such as improper handling of the blood units could be involved, but further study is also needed to investigate the possibility of the role of cytokine release from leukocytes or other factors in our transfusion-associated respiratory distress cases.

0408

SELECTIVE IgA DEFICIENCY IN CHINESE BLOOD DONORS IN HONG KONG.

S.Cheng, K.H. Mak, J.Chan, S.Leong,
Hong Kong Red Cross Blood Transfusion Service.

Selective IgA Deficiency (SIgAD) is the most commonly recognised immunodeficiency and is characterized by a serum level of below 5 mg/dl[1]. The rate varies from 0.005% (1:18500) [5] to 0.3% (1:328) [4] in different surveys of blood donors. Severe anaphylactic reaction may occur in IgA-deficient patients with anti-IgA on exposure to human IgA. The incidence of SIgAD was determined in 45,798 Chinese voluntary blood donors in Hong Kong by Tanned cells Passive Haemagglutination Inhibition (PHI). Of the blood donors screened, only 5 donors, 0.011%,(1:9169) were found to be IgA deficient (less than 5mg/dl); all negative results were confirmed by nephelometry. No significant difference between the incidence of SIgAD in Chinese male donors, 0.011% (1:9091), and female donors, 0.012% (1:8333) was observed. The incidence in Chinese donors was significantly lower than that in blood donors of European ancestry (P<0.01) and significantly higher than that in Japanese blood donors (P<0.01), (Table [2,3,4,5]). Antibodies to IgA in the IgA-deficient sera were detected by PHI; none of the 5 donors showing less than 5mg/dl of IgA had antibodies to IgA. Difficulty is encountered in the development of an adequate file of IgA-deficient donors in Hong Kong due to the very low incidence of SIgAD. The establishment of a Rare Donor Registry System still remains a matter of urgency.

Table-Summary of survey of Selective IgA deficiency(<5mg/dl) in blood donors

Reference	Country	No. Tested	Incidence	Ratio
(2)	France	15,200	1:2,171	0.05
(3)	Australia	6,191	1:442	0.23
(4)	U.S.A.	6,240	1:328	0.30
(5)	Japan	22,597	1:18,500	0.005
Present Study	Hong Kong Chinese	45,798	1:9,160	0.011

Reference:
1. Ammann,A.J., Medicine 50:223 (1971)
2. Frommel D., Vox Sang. 25:513 (1973)
3. Well,J.V., Aust. N.Z.J. Med. 10:410 (1980)
4. Clark,J.A., Am J. Clin. Path 80:210 (1983)
5. Kanok,T., Vox Sang. 50:81-86 (1986)

0409

LONG-TERM FOLLOW-UP STUDY OF ANTI-IgA ANTIBODIES IN HEALTHY IgA DEFICIENT BLOOD DONORS

S.Koskinen and J.Koistinen
Finnish Red Cross Blood Transfusion Service, Helsinki,Finland

In 1971-80 215 healthy blood donors with deficiency of serum IgA were identified and their anti-IgA antibodies were determined by hemagglutination (HA). After a median follow-up period of 19 years 204 of them were restudied twice in 1990-1992 for serum IgA and anti-IgA antibodies by using an enzyme immunoassay (EIA). The history of IgA exposure was examined. 237 healthy blood donors were studied as controls. The results were as follows:

	total	anti-IgA	no anti-IgA
IgA deficiency (IgA<0.05 mg/L)	159	32	127
Decreased serum IgA (0.05-800 mg/L)	45	0	45
Normal serum IgA	237	0	237

Of the 32 subjects with anti-IgA 20 had the antibody already in 1971-80. 17 of the 32 had a history of pregnancy, gammaglobulin injection or blood transfusion, but only seven had this before the detection of anti-IgA. No anti-IgA could be detected in 49 subjects with IgA deficiency and a history of IgA exposure. On the other hand 13 of the 45 subjects with low but detectable serum IgA had an earlier exposure to IgA, but showed no anti-IgA in their serum.

In conclusion: specific anti-IgA antibodies are found only in subjects with undetectable serum IgA; exposure to IgA can evidently explain anti-IgA formation only in a few cases and on the other hand it leads only occasionally to anti-IgA formation.

0410

AN ENZYME IMMUNOASSAY FOR ROUTINE DETERMINATION OF ANTI-IgA ANTIBODIES OF IgG CLASS

S.Koskinen, M.Hirvonen and H.Tölö
Finnish Red Cross Blood Transfusion Service, Helsinki,Finland.

We have further developed an enzyme immunoassay (EIA) for screening and quantitation of anti-IgA antibodies in serum. This modification uses polyclonal human serum IgA as the coating antigen, commercial affinity purified alkaline phosphatase-conjugated rabbit anti-human IgG and individual sample blanks. Nonspecific reactions are eliminated by blocking vacant protein binding sites by bovine serum albumin. The specificity of the antibody is confirmed by a liquid adsorption test. Pooled normal human serum inhibits the reaction by over 80 %. The same inhibition could also be demonstrated by IgA used for coating but not by serum lacking IgA. A value of 12,000 arbitrary units of anti-IgA per litre (AU/L) was assigned to a patient serum used as standard. This corresponded well with the anti-IgA titres by hemagglutination (HA) observed from the same patient serum in 1970-1989, which made it possible to compare the earlier HA results with those obtained now by EIA.

The predilution requirement was 1/16. The interassay coefficients of variation (CVs) for the controls (35-3770 AU/L) were 9-12 %. The lowest quantifiable concentration was 7 AU/L.

We have used this method for anti-IgA determinations in more than 350 patient samples during four years. It is most suitable for routine use because the process can be easily automated and the plates can be prepared in bulk and stored frozen until use.

0412

THE CONTENT OF FACTOR VIII:C, FIBRINOGEN AND FIBRONECTIN IN CRYOPRECIPITATES PREPARED IN A BLOOD BANK.

F.Tripaldi,A.Esposito.
Blood Bank, Spoleto, Italy.

The quality controls of cryoprecipitates prepared in a blood bank are based on the determination of factor VIII clotting activi ty, secondly on fibrinogen content and ulti- mely the fibronectin amount. The recovery of factor VIII:C has been of the 67.8% with a concentration ratio of 3.5; the recovery of fibrinogen has been of the 36.8% with a con centration ratio of 1.8 and that of plasma- tic fibronectin of the 69.6% with a concen- tration ratio of 3.56 in the cryoprecipita- tes prepared in a blood bank. The authors has discussed even the clinical usage of the cryoprecipitates.

0413

OUR RESULTS IN PRODUCTION OF THE SPECIFIC IMMUNOGLOBULINS

M.Romić, M.Popović, P.Medić, O.Tomović

Blood Transfusion Institute, Beograd, Yugoslavia

Starting row material was plasma of immunisated donors. Using cold ethanol fractionation procedure according to Cohn, Kistler-Nitschmann's modificaton we odtained for production of the specific immuno-globulins.

* Antitetanus immunoglobulin has been produced for fifteen years. During this time 5176 litres was fractionated. Ratio between concetrations of titer antibodies of product and starting plasma is 24,3.

* Anti-D immunoglobulin is in production for the twelve years and in this period 2230 litres of immunisated plasma was fractionated.In this case the ratio of the concentrations was 13,5.

* Human antirabies immunoglobulin has been produced for the perod of the tree years and have fractionated 712 litres of immunisated plasma, with the concentration ratio 13,2.

0414

SHORT-TERM PREDEPOSIT AUTOLOGOUS BLOOD TRANSFUSION

H. Sakamoto, and H. Nakata,
Department of Blood Transfusion Medicine and Immu-nohaematology, University of Occupational and Env-ironmental Health, School of Medicine.

Surgery with autologous blood transfusion is the safest at present except for bloodless surgery. From August 1984 to March 1993, autologous blood has been predeposited in the liquid state for 839 patients in our hospital. They have included 583 cases(70%) of orthopaedic surgery, 117 cases(14%) of cardiovascular surgery, 58 cases(7%) of abdomi-nal surgery, 52 cases of brain surgery and 29 cas-es of other surgery.

Our program of short-term predeposit autologous blood transfusion is costituted of the informed and written consent, medical and laboratoly exami-nation before phlebotomy, iron therapy, 2~3 phleb-otomy, storage about 900ml of blood in the refrig-erator for 10~14 days and pretransfusion testing.

The maximum collectable blood volume(BV) until the concentration of Hb decreases less than 100g/l is estimated by the initial concentration of Hb (preHb) and total blood volume(TBV) of each patient with the following formula : $BV=TBV\times(1-10\div preHb)$

TBV of Japanese adult male and female is calcul-ated with the formula of Ogawa and Fujita.

adult male : $0.168H^3+0.050W+0.444(l)$
adult female : $0.250H^3+0.063W-0.662(l)$
H : Height(m) W : Weight(Kg)

The amount of collected blood each phlebotomy is within 10~12% of TBV and if necessary crystalloid solution is intravenously administered.
The increase of autologous blood transfusion has decreased allogeneic blood transfusion by 36%.

0415

QUALITY CRITERIA AND OPTIMAL STORAGE OF AUTOLOGOUS PLASMA

W. Heller, H.P. Wendel
Dept. of Thoracic- and Cardiovascular Surg., Univ. of Tuebingen, Germany

In each case ten two, three and four years old autologous plasma bags stored at -80°C were thawed and the activity of various factors and inhibitors of the clotting system as well as the concentration of the individual parameters of the complement system investigated. In order to gain an impression of the effects of long storage these proteins were also investigated in 30 samples of briefly stored plasma from the same donor; in the latter case the period of storage was 7 to 14 weeks. The statistical evaluation was carried out using the SPSS software packing. The individual values of the registered activities and concentrations were for the most part within the normal range. Factor VIIIC and the alternative pathway of the complement cascade showed increased activity.

A comparison of the briefly stored autologous FFP with that kept in storage for two, three and four years yielded no significant difference for prekallikrein, factor XII, kallikrein inhibition, kallikrein-like activity, ß-factor XIIa inhibition and C1-inhibitor, the clotting factors VII, VIIIC, IX, the inhibitors antithrombin III, $alpha_1$-proteinase inhibitor ($alpha_1$-antitrypsin), $alpha_2$-macroglobulin and $alpha_2$-antiplasmin, the complement proteins C1q, C4, C3c and C3 activator and for fibronectin. In the case of C1r, C5 and C9 the several weeks old FFP displayed less activity or lower concentrations than in the older samples. Particularly striking are the high KK values during the autologous plasmapheresis. Factor V the two and three years old FFP showed lower values whereby for the briefly stored samples higher activity was to be found. The differences were significant. A microbe contamination could be excluded.

From the present investigation there is nothing to indicate that the transfusion of autologous plasma stored at -80°C for two, three or even four years should not be carried out.

0416

TWO YEARS EXPERIENCE WITH A HOSPITAL-BASED PRE-SURGICAL AUTOLOGOUS BLOOD DONOR PROGRAM.

P.H. Pinkerton, A.S. Coovadia and J. Young, Departments of Laboratory Haematology and Nursing, Sunnybrook Health Science Centre, and Department of Pathology, University of Toronto, Toronto, Ontario, Canada.

Over a 2 year period, 511 patients deposited one or more units of autologous blood in anticipation of surgery. 439 (86%) did not require allogeneic blood; 72 (14%) required no blood at all and 216 (19%) of the units collected were not used.

Procedure (number)	Autologous Units Obtained	Autologous Units Used	Allogeneic Units Used	Allogeneic Units # of Patients
Hip repl.(132)	354	317	46	16
Knee repl.(54)	110	81	15	6
Rad. prost.(73)	190	177	103	22
Hyster.(92) incl. radical	170	138	10	3
Cardiac(56)	106	83	30	12
Other (104)	217	135	54	14
TOTAL (511)	1147	931	258	73

A schedule for six common procedures (2-3 units depending on the procedure), was used, which, if completely collected, would have provided protection from allogeneic transfusion for 84% of patients with 22% wastage. If an additional unit had been collected for each patient, this would have provided protection for 89% of patients with 44% wastage if the same transfusion decisions had been made.

The reduction in haemoglobin between first donation and pre-operative estimate was statistically significant but clinically unimportant (mean ≈2g/L) and only 25 patients failed to complete the donation schedule because of anemia; this calls in question the need for erythropoietin support in autologous pre-surgical blood donor programs.

0417

AN AUTOLOGOUS BLOOD TRANSFUSION PROGRAM IN A REGIONAL BLOOD CENTER.

H.Kiyokawa[1],K.Yamamoto[1],Y.Irita[1],H.Tanamachi[1],N.Ueda[1],T.Kurachi[2], T.Sayama[2], G.Funamoto[2], Y.Maeda[1].
1Fukuoka Red Cross Blood Center, Fukuoka, 2Department of Blood Programme, Japanese Red Cross, Tokyo, Japan.

With recent attention on the risks of transfusion transmitted diseases,the use of autologous blood transfusion has been increasing also in Japan.To prevent posttransfusion hepatitis,a pre-deposit program for cardiovascular and orthopedic surgery in two university hospitals has been implemented in Fukuoka Red Cross Blood Center since October 1983.During 7-year period (from October 1983 through October 1990), 1710 patients (886 cardiovascular, 824 orthopedic) have undergone their operations using cryopreserved autologous blood. For more conventional autologous blood transfusion we introduced liquid storage in SAGM in the end of 1990. We have switched SAGM to MAP (modified SAGM) since January 1992. During 10-year period (from October 1983 through October 1993),7717 autologous units (frozen: 4873 units, liquid: 2844 units) have been shiped to hospitals. After implementing liquid storage,frozen units have been decreasing as expectedly. 1235 of 74305 red cell units (1.7%) in 1992 were shiped for autologous units. As of October 1993, our autologous blood program (predeposit autologous service) is incorporated in 18 hospitals (including 3 large university hospitals) mainly for cardiovascular and orthopedic patients. We are involved in preoperative phlebotomy in hospitals and our blood center, and blood deposit services.

There has been a lack of widespread education concerning autologous blood transfusion in Japan. In 1992 Japanese Society of Blood Transfusion published guidelines for the preoperative autologous blood donation program. As a result, there is now an increasing demand for safer blood and safer transfusion approaches. Japanese Ministry of Health and Welfare required Japanese Red Cross to promote the preoperative autologous blood donation program in March 1993. Following this governmental announcement, Japanese Red Cross published a manual for the preoperative autologous blood donation program in July 1993.Japanese Ministry of Health and Welfare is planning to provide a practical manual for physicians in 1994.

As of March 1993, 46 of 77 Japanese Red Cross Blood Centers were offering preoperative autologous blood deposit services for hospitals. However, activity on it was very low in Red Cross Blood Centers at that time and a few amount of autologous units were deposited for reasons of economy. Governmental supports would be the most important to promote the preoperative autologous blood donation program in regional blood centers further.

0418

EFFECTIVENESS OF AN AUTOLOGOUS BLOOD PREDEPOSIT PROGRAM IN HIP AND KNEE REPLACEMENT

L. Torretta[1], C. Perotti[1], L.Salvaneschi[1], M. Ghidini[2], G. Domenella[2]
1 Servizio di Immunoematologia e Trasfusione 2 Divisione di Ortopedia e Traumatologia, IRCCS Policlinico San Matteo, Pavia, Italy.

Elective orthopaedic surgery is particularly suggested for an autologous preoperative blood donor program because it is generally foreseeable and routinely requires transfusion. We report a retrospective 3 year analysis of the practice with an autologous blood predeposit program in orthopaedic surgical patients undergoing hip and knee replacement. 570 patients (177 males and 393 females) were considered and 248 (group A) of them (44%) (mean age 64.8 y.) were eligible for autologous donation, according to the criteria established by the AABB. The remaining 322 patients (group B) were excluded from predeposit practice because of medical reasons (low hemoglobin or hematocrit level, unstable cardiac disease, recent infection), organizational difficulties and patient's deny of the autologous practice. In table 1 the results are shown for the two groups:

	total patients/ (pd units)	transfused patients	homologous transfused patients	total transfused units	homologous transfused units
A	248 (487)	207 (83%)	28 (11%)	443	57 (12%)
B	322	292 (91%)	292 (91%)	890	890 (100%)

Our experience confirms the effectiveness of the autologous blood predonation in this elective orthopaedic surgery because it permits an important decrease in homologous blood risk exposure (11%) in comparison with a very high percentage of homologous transfusion (91%).

0419

THE PRE-DEPOSIT ORGANIZATION IN A LARGE POLY-SPECIALIZED HOSPITAL.

S.Solinas, M.Screnci, G.C.Ferrazza, A.Roccetti, G.C.Isacchi.
Dipartimento di Biopatologia Umana, Emato logia, Centro Trasfusionale. Universita´ "La Sapienza", Roma, Italy.

Our poly-specialized hospital spreads for a 300,000 sqm area and counts 66 operating theaters (for 1,265 surgical beds).Moreover the Transfusional Service(T.S) is composed of two separate Centers, one inside the hos pital area, while the other is placed outsi de. For these reasons and in order to offer to most (surgical) patients the autotransfu sion opportunity, some diversified proceedi ngs have been adopted, according to various requirements.The outpatients (mostly orthop aedic and gynaecological) pre-collect their blood at the outside Center, while the inpa tients have two possibilities: to undergo the pre-deposit(s) at bedside (bedridden patients) or at intramural Center (all the others).In three big units (urological, vascular and one general surgical) autologo us program is managed by the house physic ians. RESULTS:this kind of organization all owed the T.S. to control such a wide area and the surgeons and anaesthesists to use better the blood especially in some pati ents (orthopaedic, urological and gynaecolo gical) to whom autologous blood has repres ented more than 60% of the transfused blood.

0420

THE PLACE OF AUTOLOGOUS BLOOD TRANSFUSION IN A DEPARTMENT OF GYNECOLOGY : A SURVEY OF1989 TILL 1993

J. Moh-Klaren[1], H. Ben Hadj Amor[1], R. Belhocine[1], G. Andreu[1], P. Girard[2]
1Blood Bank and 2 Department of Anesthesia of the Hôtel-Dieu hospital, Paris, France.

In 1987 we started a Autologous Blood Transfusion (ABT)program with the Department of Gynecology.We checked the evolution of this ABT during the period 1989-1993.

The files of the 602 patients transfused during these years were reviewed.

We noted the diagnoses, the ages, the number and type of blood transfusions, the hemoglobin levels during the critical period and when leaving the hospital.

After a little lost of freshness between 1989 and 1991 (69%, 58% and 46% of blood transfusions covered with autologous blood in 1989, 1990 and 1991) the ABT program took a new start with 70% and 78% of blood transfusions covered in 1992 and 1993.

The reverse is the waste : in 1992 60% of the autologous red cells and 55% of the autologous plasmas were utilized, in 1993 only 55% and 38%. This non-utilization depends on the type of surgery ; for 17 large abdominal operations for cervix and endometrium cancers in 1993 85% and 71% of the collected autologous red cells and plasmas were utilized.

We conclude that a ABT program is proposed to all eligible patients. The patients receiving homologous blood were almost always oncological and a few obstetrical patients.

In future we should better adapt the quantity of ABT donations to the kind of surgery,that is at low or high risk for blood transfusion.

A better utilization postoperatively of the remaining autologous red cells is another goal.

0421

AUTOLOGOUS BLOOD NOT REINFUSED CAN BE TRANSFUSED TO HOMOLOGOUS RECIPIENTS?

C. MAZZEI, G. BARBERIS, G.IMBERCIADORI
G. CAVAGNARO
C. Trasfusionale,Osp.S.Corona,Pietra Ligure

Different opinions are expressed on safety of cross-over to homologous recipients auto -logous blood not reinfused.In our study we evaluated prevalence of infectious disease markers in 21.700 homologous blood units (A) and 3000 autologous blood units (B) from patients scheduled for orthopedic surgery, collected consecutively .Data were riassumed in the following table. For HCVAb were tested only 16.200 homologous blood units and all autologous blood units.

	A	B		A	B
HBsAg+	47	16	HCVAb+	194	40
HBsAb+	2700	386	VDRL+	0	0
HBcAb+			HIVAb+	0	0
HBsAb-	521	7	ALT>45U.I.	731	139

We didn´t found significant difference in infectious disease marker rates between A and B .If the number of units transmitting infection is correlated with the number of test-negative infected units, and the number of test-negative units is correlated with the prevalence of infectious disease markers, we cannot exclude that autologous blood not reinfused,that meet standards of homologous units, is safe for cross-over. However, more data needs and particularly from different areas.

0422

HOMOLOGOUS BLOOD TRANSFUSION BY CELLSAVER IN PUEBLA, MEXICO.

MARIN-LOPEZ A. +* ; HERNANDEZ-DE-LOJO JM*; BRAVO-HERNANDEZ G*; LOPEZ-PARRA S*.
* MEDICINA TRANSFUSIONAL Y HEMATOLOGIA DE PUEBLA.
+ HOSPITAL GENERAL DE PUEBLA

INTRODUCTION.- COMPLICATIONS FOUND WITH HOMOLOGOUS BLOOD TRANSFUSIONS ARE THE RISK OF INFECTIONS, FURTHER STUDIES NEED TO BE DONE OR OTHER ALTERNATIVES FOUND TO PREVENT ITS OCCURANCE. THE AUTOLOGOUS BLOOD TRANSFUSION PROGRAM HAS INCREASED VASTLY.

MATERIALS AND METHODS.- FROM JULY 1991 TO SEPTEMBER 1993, 33 PERI-OPERATIVE CELLSAVER PROCEEDURES HAD TAKEN PLACE USING HAEMONETICS CELLSAVER AND 3 POST-OPERATIVE CASES USING THE SOLCOTRANS METHOD. THE PATIENTS INVOLVED IN THIS STUDY WERE 24 WOMEN AND 9 MEN. THE MEDIAN AGE WAS 48 (RANGE, 7-90).

RESULTS.- ORTHOPAEDICS PROCEDURES: 26, AESTHETIC SURGERY 7. 4 OF THE 33 PATIENTS WERE INCLUDED IN THE PREDEPOSIT PROGRAM. 5 OF THE 33 PATIENTS WERE INCLUDED POSTOPERATELY CELLSAVER PROGRAM. CELLSAVER VOLUMES WERE BETWEEN 250-2500 ml, THE MEDIAN WAS 1375 ml. ONLY 3 OF THE 33 PATIENTS REQUIRED HOMOLOGOUS TRANSFUSION POST-OPERATIVELY. 3 OF THE 33 PATIENTS PRESENTED HIPOTHERMIA POST-OPERATIVELY. 2 OF THE 33 PATIENTS WERE JEHOVAH'S WITNESSES.

DISCUSSION.- 1) AUTOLOGOUS BLOOD TRANSFUSION FOR ANY KNOWN METHOD, TO OBTAIN 100% SAFE BLOOD. 2) REDUCE THE HOMOLOGOUS BLOOD TRANSFUSION TO ONE UNIT. 3) ACCEPTABLE FOR JEHOVAH'S WITNESSES. 4) PERI AND POST-OPERATIVE CELLSAVER SYSTEMS MUST BE INCLUDED IN EMERGENCY OR PROGRAMMED SURGERY. 5) TO COMBINE TWO OR MORE AUTOLOGOUS BLOOD TRANSFUSION SYSTEMS IS MORE EFFECTIVE. 6) PATIENTS OF ANY AGE CAN BE INCLUDED IN THIS PROGRAM, BEFORE A PRELIMINARY VALORATION.

0424

ERITHROPOIETIN AND AUTOLOGOUS BLOOD DONATION IN SURGICAL RHEUMATOID PATIENTS WITH ANEMIA

F. Mercuriali, G. Gualtieri, G. Inghilleri, E. Biffi, A. Vinci, M.T. Colotti, L. Sinigaglia, R. Scalamogna, G. Barosi*.
Orthopedic Institute "G. Pini", University of Milan, Italy -
* Policlinico S.Matteo, Pavia, Italy.

In RA patients (pts) undergoing orthopedic surgery, anemia is the major cause of homologous blood (HB) exposure. To determine whether recombinant human erytropoietin (rHuEPO) could allow preoperative autologous blood (AB) procurement and reduce HB exposure, 11 RA pts candidate to primary total hip replacement, unable to predeposit AB because of baseline hct Hct<34% were treated with 300U/Kg i.v. of rHuEPO (Eprex, Cilag S.p.A., Milano, Italy) in association with iron saccharate (Ferrum Hausman Ag, St Gallen, Switzerland) 100 mg i.v., twice a week for three weeks. The transfusion treatment of this group of pts was compared with that of 12 RA pts with anemia of chronic disease of comparable severity (mean baseline hct 32,4±1.5) treated only with i.v. iron All rHuEPO and control patients underwent the same operation by the same surgeon.
All rHuEPO treated pts but one could predeposit 2 or more AB units (mean 2.6±0.6, range 2-4) while none of the pts in the control group predeposited AB units. Treatment with rHuEPO allowed the production of 295+87mL of RBCs (range 119-395mL). Control group received more HB units (2.6±1.6 vs 0.8±0.8, p=0.009). Moreover 50%of the rHuEPO treated pts vs 23% in control group completely avoided HB transfusion.
It can be concluded that rHuEPO is safe and effective in significantly: 1. increasing Hct before surgery, 2. increasing the yeld of AB donation, 3. reducing the exposure to HB in RA pts unable to fulfil anticipated transfusion needs because of anemia.

0425

RESPONSE OF THE ERYTHRON AND ERYTHROPOIETIN TO AUTOLOGOUS BLOOD DONATIONS. IS ERYTHROPOIETIN SUPPLEMENT NECESSARY?

P. HAN, D. STACY, Dept. of Haematology, Women's & Children's Hospital, North Adelaide, Australia.

Autologous blood donation is commonly used to avoid homologous blood transfusion for blood loss during orthopaedic surgery. 8 adolescents scheduled for correction of scoliosis undertook 3 weekly autologous blood collections. Blood was taken for erythropoietin, Hb, reticulocyte count, percentage hypochromic cells and serum ferritin measurement at each visit and also at the time of admission. The mean Hb fell from 14.5 to 12.7 g/dL at the time of hospital admission. Mean reticulocyte counts at each visit were 2.3, 4.0, and 5.0% respectively. There was no increase in percentage hypochromic cells over this period. Serum Ferritin fell slightly, predonation (37 μg/L), and at admission (23 μg/L). There was a rise in erythropoietin levels, from 12 to 70 pg/ml (mean levels) paralleling the rise in reticulocytes. In adolescents, the endogenous erythropoietin response together with iron supplement appears to maintain a reasonable Hb level even with 3 units of blood donation.

0426

AN EVALUATION OF MINIMUM HEMOGLOBIN(Hb) LEVEL AT WHICH RECOMBINANT HUMAN ERYTHROPOIETIN(rEPO) IS NOT REQUIRED FOR ONCE A WEEK CONSECUTIVE BLOOD COLLECTIONS WITHIN A THREE-WEEK PERIOD.

N.Wakimoto[1)], K.Takahashi, S.Tachibana[2)]
1) Teikyo Univ., 2) Toranomon Hosp., Tokyo, Japan.

Of 584 orthopaedic donor-patients, 279 aged 1 to 79 were analyzed for minimum Hb levels (Hb_0) prior to the first phlebotomy at which three consecutive once a week blood collections are possible without rEPO.
The 279 patients were divided into four age groups; A(78) aged under 20, B(89) 20 to 39, C(65) 40 to 59, and D(47) more than 60, and consecutively donated 8 to 12% of total blood volume up to 400 ml/week twice or more without rEPO, only with Hb level more than 11 g/dl just prior to each phlebotomy. If Hb fell below 11 g/dl, collection was postponed to the next week. Serial Hb levels were analyzed in each group up to the cessation or through the third consecutive phlebotomy. For patients who required only two blood collections, the third Hb level, i.e. one week after the second phlebotomy and just prior to the surgery, was used for evaluation for a third probable blood collection.
In patients with Hb_0 more than 13 g/dl in group A, more than 14 g/dl in group B, and more than 14.5 g/dl in groups C and D, serial Hb changes through the third phlebotomy never fell below 11.0 g/dl.
For three consecutive once a week blood collections, rEPO is not necessary for every donor-patient. However, rEPO may be supplemented for some patients with Hb_0 below 13.0 aged under 20, below 14.0 from 20 to 39, and below 14.5 g/dl more than 40.

0427

A COMPARISON OF EFFICACY OF SUBCUTANEOUS(SC) AND INTRAVENOUS(IV) ADMINISTRATION OF RECOMBINANT HUMAN ERYTHROPOIETIN(rEPO) FOR PREDEPOSIT AUTOLOGOUS BLOOD DONATION(PABD).

N.Wakimoto[1)], K.Takahashi, S.Tachibana[2)]
1) Teikyo Univ., 2) Toranomon Hosp., Tokyo, Japan.

Sixty-six orthopaedic donor-patients, who were between 40 and 75 yrs with 11 to 14 g/dl of Hb level, and who received rEPO from one week prior to the first phlebotomy until one week before surgery, were evaluated to compare the efficacy of SC and IV administration of rEPO.
Of the 66 patients, SC group(32) received rEPO once a week; 200 IU/Kg × 1SC(11), 400 × 1SC(11), and 600 × 1SC(10). IV group(34) was given rEPO once or twice a week; 200 × 1IV(8), 400 × 1IV(10), 200 × 2IV (9), and 300 × 2IV(7). A schedule of two or three once a week blood collections of 400 ml began one week after the initial administration of rEPO.
In comparison of equal dosages of rEPO at equal frequencies, i.e. 200 × 1SC vs 200 × 1IV and 400 × 1SC vs 400 × 1IV, Hb decreases at one week after second phlebotomy compared to the start of the study were not significant in the 200/400 × 1SC, while they were significant in the 200/400 × 1IV. On the other hand, there were no significant differences in Hb changes after phlebotomy between either 400 × 1SC and 200 × 2IV nor 600 × 1SC and 300 × 2IV, respectively.
Our results showed that for PABD, once a week SC administration of rEPO concurrent with phlebotomy is more effective and recommendable than multiple IV injections which require additional hospital visits.

0428

ERYTHOPOIETIN AND AUTOLOGOUS BLOOD DONATION IN CARDIAC SURGERY

B.H. Walpoth[1], P. Spirig[1], B. Galliker[2], A. Rosenmund[2], A. Häberli[2], U. Althaus[1], U. Nydegger[3]
Thoracic and Cardiovascular Surgery[1], Internal Medicine[2] and Transfusion Medicine[3], Inselspital, 3010 Bern, Switzerland

We compared preoperative autologous blood donation (PAD) with and without erythropoietin (r-HuEPO) and iron substitution to reduce the need for homologous blood transfusion. 30 adult elective patients (20 CABG, 5 Valves and 5 ASD) were randomized double blind into the following groups:
I placebo, II r-HuEPO (150 IU/kg), III r-HuEPO (300 IU/kg) given subcutaneously 15 minutes after the 3 isovolemic PAD (3 red packed cells [RPC] + 3 FFP) and preoperatively.

No side effects were noted from PAD, r-HuEPO and iron supplementation. Endogenous r-HuEPO levels were significantly elevated during donation and preoperatively in goups II and III. Red cell requirements were not significantly different due to the fact that 4 patients in the r-HuEPO groups needed reoperations for bleeding. However patients receiving r-HuEPO had a significantly higher hemoglobin concentration preoperatively (13,6 and 13,5 versus 11,8 g/dl; $p < 0,05$) as well as postoperatively (11,2 and 10,6 versus 9,9; $p < 0,05$).

We conclude that isovolemic PAD in weekly intervals is safe and yields 3 units of autologous RPC and FFP for cardiac surgery. In these patients r-HuEPO substitution boosted erythropoiesis such as to allow for a normal hemoglobin concentration preoperatively despite 3 PAD. No significant differences were found among the 2 r-HuEPO doses tested.

0429

ERYTHROPLASMAPHERESIS WITH MCS-3P IN PRE-DEPOSIT BLOOD DONATION

G.Matthes, K.-P.Krause, A.Pruß
Institute for Transfusion Medicine, University Hospital Charité, Humboldt University Berlin, Germany

The consequent application of an autologous blood component programme in hospitals is often limited by missing pre-conditions like equipment, space or staff. This is now easily possible by erythroplasmapheresis with the blood component apheresis system MCS-3P (Haemonetics). With this cell separator one red blood cell concentrate, resuspended in SAG-M solution (RCC-SAGM) and one resp. two units of FFP can be collected in one step.
The donation time for one unit RCC-SAGM with one unit of FFP was 7 min, with two units of plasma 20 min. The quality of the red blood cells (ATP, 2,3-DPG, pII, free Hb, free potassium, glucose, lactose) during the storage up to 42 days was as good as with the traditional blood collection.
First results with the clinical implementation of erythroplasmapheresis are presented. It has been shown that the interdisciplinary establishing of a concept which contains diagnosis groups and corresponding donation quantities offers an essential help at planning and organisation for the implementation phase. The economic aspect is to estimate individually by each institution. Finally should be referred also to further opportunities of this concept such as the application for the rejuvenation of autologous erythrocyte concentrates or the preparation of an autologous fibrin glue from the fresh frozen plasma.

0430

VIRAL MARKERS IN AUTOTRANSFUSION CANDIDATES

F. Durand, B. Danic, A. Beauplet, B. Genetet
C.R.T.S, rue Pierre-Jean Gineste, 35000 Rennes (France)

Autologous transfusion is increasingly used in France. At the Rennes CRTS, differed autologous transfusion uses two techniques : weekly sequential collection and normovolemic hemodilution by apheresis. The products are processed as standard blood products, and all regulatory tests performed. The presence of viral markers may pose problems at two levels :retransfusion of seropositive products, and handling of contaminated products. So far, the Rennes CRTS has not retransfused autotransfusion products when any one of the viral markers was positive. Is this attitude justified? To answer that interrogation, we compared viral marker prevalences between blood donors and candidates for autologous transfusion. The results of screening tests performed in 1992 and 1993 for the 6 regulatory markers were analyzed.
In total, 66,530 donors were screened for HBs antigen, anti-HBc, anti-HCV, anti-HIV, anti-HTLV antibodies and ALAT. Collections totalled 107,935. In parallel, 600 patients followed a protocol of weekly sequential collection (1,503 bags) and 232 followed a protocol of normovolemic hemodilution by apheresis. Prevalence rates (%) were higher in candidates than in donors for all markers except HTLV and HIV (HBs Ag : 0.14/0.03 ; HBc Ab : 2.43/1.29 ;HVC Ab : 1.14/0.05 ; ALAT : 3.01/1.66. Collection from candidates is punctual, making this population less prone to self-exclusion and predominantly at risk of Hepatitis C and B. Greatest care therefore should be observed when interviewing these patients, and in the management of the collection bags when preserved and transfused despite the existence of positive markers. Undoubtedly, excluding these candidates from the autotransfusion protocol would make the transfusion system safer.

0431

CURRENT STATUS OF AUTOLOGOUS BLOOD TRANSFUSIONS IN JAPAN – A REPORT OF A NATIONWIDE SURVEY –

S. Yuasa[1], Y. Ikeda[2], Y. Maeda[3], M. Shimizu[4] and K. Nakai[5]
1. Dept. of Transfusion Medicine, Juntendo Univ.
2.Dept. of Internal Medicine, Keio Univ.
3. Fukuoka Blood Center
4.Dept. of Transfusion Medicine, Tokyo Womens' Medical College
5.Blood Products Research Organization

In 1993, a nationwide survey on the current status of autologous transfusion was done in Japan. Questionnaires were sent to 1,169 institutions with more than 300 beds and were received from 693 institutions (59%).

About half of the hospitals (48.5%) had experienced in autologous transfusion, mostly with a preoperative deposit (67%) and intraoperative salvage (20%). During the 3 months period (Oct. - Dec. 1992), 2,637 patients received autologous transfusions. Twenty-eight per cent of them received homologous transfusions due to unexpected excessive bleeding. The ratio of autologous transfusion in different departments were: 24.1% cardiac, 7.9% orthopedics, 7.8% gynecological, and 5.6% G. I. Interestingly 74% of bone marrow transplantation donors received autologous transfusion.

More than half of the hospitals which had no experience in autologous transfusion hope to do so if the Red Cross Blood Center will collaborate with them.

0432

CEO/CORPORATE CAMPAIGN
CORPORATE-SUPPORTED APHERESIS PROGRAMS

Walter Shipley, Chairman of the Board of a major banking corporation, was the first Chief Executive of a major corporation in the New York area to become an apheresis donor. Shortly after his donation, Mr. Shipley asked his 2,700 multi-donors to join him and become apheresis donors. 250 responded favorably for a 9% response.

Mr. Shipley then held a meeting of approximately 30 of the largest donor groups to encourage them to initiate apheresis programs (included in these groups were another major banking corporation, a major insurance company, a large oil company, and a major government group). Shortly thereafter, these companies initiated their own apheresis programs.

Currently, six of these companies have donated permanent apheresis donor sites throughout the tri-state area and apheresis donations have increased from 4,143 in 1988 to over 40,000 in 1993.

The Vice President and Division Executive, Health Affairs, for a major corporation has recently taken on the position of Apheresis and Bone Marrow Chairperson on the corporate blood donor campaign of our blood center. In addition, this corporation, as well as others, have produced and financed motivational videos on apheresis and bone marrow donations.

0433

IN THE NAME OF GOD

A report on the IBTS Hemapheresis activities(Tehran)

Zohreh Atarchi - M.D

This section has begun its activities since 1977and has taken a cosiderable amount of plasma, during the last seventeen years,in order to produce blood components and hyperimmunoglobulins such as:

AntiRabies Immunoglobulin:	$47x10^6$	IU
blood group reagent:		
Anti A	$78x10^4$	ml
Anti B	$87x10^4$	ml
Anti AB	$46x10^4$	ml
Standard gamaglobulin	$8.5x10^6$	IU
Hepatitis B (HBIG)	600	ml
Normal plasma for fractionation	144500	ml

There are two groups of plasma donors:

- Volunteer plasmapheresis donor 35%
- Paid plasmapheresis donor 65%

At each session (that is every 15 days),500ml of - plasma is taken , during which , the donor is under the control of a doctor , and a series of lab.tests are done such as:

- serum electropheresis.
- HIV AB - HBsAg - RPR - CBC -............

No abnormality has been seen in the donors,due to plasmapheresis.

0434

PRE-PLATELET COUNT IS NOT SUITABLE TO DETERMINE FREQUENCY PROTOCOL FOR PHERESIS DONORS

B. Charvátová[1], J. Charvát[2]
1 Faculty Transfusion Department, Prague, 2 Institute for Clinical and Experimental Medicine, Prague, Czech Republic

AABB standards require a documented platelet count > 150 x 10^9 if the frequency of plateletpheresis is < 56 days.

Platelet counts before and after plateletpheresis were evaluated in 138 donors. Plateletpheresis was repeated in the same patients 14 to 60 days later. A Haemonetics PCS plus was used.

Platelet count decreased from 238 ± 53 to 193 ± 42 x10^9/l. The drop was relatively constant (45 ± 15 x 10^9/l). No influence of plateletpheresis frequency on platelet count before the next plateletpheresis, or the platelet count decrease was observed. No impact of pre-platelet count was noticed on the platelet count decrease either.

We conclude the plateletpheresis frequency (between 14 and 60 days) is not related to post-platelet count. While pre-platelet count is an important parameter, it cannot be used to determine pheresis frequency.

0435

PREPARATION OF SINGLE DONOR PLATELET CONCENTRATES USING AN INTEGRATED LEUCOCYTE FILTER WITH THE CS-3000

L. Steenssens°, J.C. Osselaer °°, E. Goossenaerts °°°, D. De Muylder°, B. Van Camp°
°Blood Transfusion Centre Jette-Belgium, °° Blood Transfusion Centre Mont-Godinne, °°° Baxter Biotec Europe.

A new kit for plateletpheresis, with an on-line leucocyte filter has been evaluated in more than 20 procedures with the CS-3000. The following parameters were used : program n° 1 special ; interface detector offset 8 ; separation chamber TNX-6 ; collection chamber PLT-30 ; whole blood (WB) flow rate 55 ml/min ; ACD-A/WB ratio of 1/9-11 and WB volume treated 5500 ml. After preparation of the concentrates, the platelets were resuspended in autologous plasma and were stored at 20°C with continuous gentle agitation for at least 4 hours before filtration through the integrated device.

Twenty three procedures yielded a mean of 5,21 (± 1,12).10^{11} platelets per concentrate after filtration, which corresponds to a platelet recovery of 87% (± 6%), the initial count being 5,99 (± 1,31).10^{11}. The initial WBC contamination of 6,33.10^6 per concentrate was reduced by filtration to 0,11.10^6, corresponding to the elimination of 96% of the WBC.

This kit is thus a usefull tool for leucocyte reduction, which allows the Bloodtransfusion Center to control the filtration process. Moreover, elimination of the WBC after preparation of the platelet concentrates, prevents the release of cytokines from the WBC and thus prevents transfusion reactions due to these cytokines.

0436

DONOR PLATELET APHERESIS WITH COBE SPECTRA

G Baldini, G Milanti, G Ceccherelli, M De Palma, C Vecchi
Blood Transfusion Service. Policlinico of MODENA-ITALY

To evaluate product quality and donor acceptability, 19 donors underwent platelet (PLT) collection on COBE Spectra performed either by single needle (SN=10) or double needle (DN=9) procedure.
Between the 2 groups there was no difference in donors' age, sex distribution, blood volume and pre-apheresis laboratory data.
RESULTS (Data are reported as mean in the table):

	SN	DN	p
PLT Yield x10e11	3.51	4.83	0.019
WBC Contamination x10e6	29.87	1.59	(0.083)
Blood Processed ml	3571	3753	NS
Average Efficiency %	53	64	0.001
PLT Predonation x10e9/L	211	232	NS
ACD used ml	410	455	NS
Run Time minuts	97	95	NS
Donors with symptoms	0	0	

Ratio between observed and predicted yield was 1.06 for SN and 1.10 for DN. White blood cell (WBC) contamination in PLT Concentrate collected in DN group resulted lower than 1 X 10e6 in 6 out of 9 procedures.
We conclude that COBE Spectra apheresis system appears to couple high average efficiency with extreme purity of final product. No adverse reaction ocurred during procedures, either for SN or DN collections.

0437

QUALITY OF PLATELET CONCENTRATES (PCs) OBTAINED WITH THE HAEMONETICS MCS 3P

R. Moog, N. Müller
Institute for Transfusion Medicine, University Clinics Essen, Germany

The Haemonetics MCS 3p is a discontinuous flow cell separator with the option of low leukocyte solution for single donor platelet concentrates (SDP). The MCS 3P uses a third pump to manage the plasma flow instead of the blood pump. This allows to maintain a constant hematocrit during the filling of the bowl and stabilizes the layer.
We used the software version C with hemocalculator in our institute. Processing a blood volume of 2652 $\pm$ 135 ml, we harvested 2.6 $\pm$ 0.8×10^{11} thrombocytes. Leukocytes contamination of the PCs was 4.7 $\pm$ 5.3×10^{6}.
Measured parameters of product quality were glucose, lactate, lactate dehydrogenase (LDH), morphology score and pH. Glucose level was 398 $\pm$ 37 mg/dl, lactate 1.48 $\pm$ 0.29 and LDH was 102 $\pm$ 15 U/l. Morphology score was 337 $\pm$ 12 and pH was 7.36 $\pm$ 0.26.
We conclude that platelet collection with the SDP results in PC with a leukocyte contamination in the 10^{6} range. The quality of the PCs is fine.

0438

EVALUATION OF MCS CELL SEPARATOR

Ph. Gillet, A. Rapaille, D. Sondag-Thull
Blood Transfusion Centre, Liège, Belgium

Platelets concentrates (PC) were collected from single donor by the MCS cell separator (Haemonetics). One part of bleeding kits (794F) was equipped with a filter Pall PL 50 integrated. Filtration was realised 1 hour after bleeding. We evaluted the separator in term of platelets yield and the efficiency of the filter. All samples were counted by Sysmex 5000. The leukocytes were counted with a Nageotte chamber in Plaxan dilution.

The best results were obtained with a treated blood volume of 3000 ml and a selection of donors with a concentration higher than 210,000 platelets per mm^3. In these conditions, the mean of platelets per PC was 4.21 10^{11} (n=23). The efficiency of filtration was suitable for 13 PC (<10^6 leukocytes per PC) on 14 tested. The recovery of platelets after filtration was 89.6%.

We obtain PC with an appropriate yield of platelets. Filtration one hour after bleeding allowed us to conserve the filtered PC for 5 days as the other PC.

0439

THE EFFECT OF ADJURETIN ON THE YIELD OF CLOTHING FACTORS AND PLATELETS

G.G.Iosava, A.I.Abesadze, S.I.Shelegia, M.Gudjabidze
Institute of Hematology and Blood Transfusion, Tbilisi, Republic of Georgia.

The need in platelet, F VIII and vWF concentrates has increased very much in the recent I0-I5 years. In order to improve their economy some blood banks have combind plateletapheresis and plasmapheresis, thus being able to debit the cost of preparation of several products instead of one. It was found that vasoactive hormons can induce the release of t-PA, PAI, vWF and prostacycline from vessel endothelium in patients. In order to increase the concentration of vWF, FVIII and platelets in blood donors there was made Adjuretin prior to platelet-plasmapheresis (Img/kg intranasal. I0-I5 min prior to donation). The behaviour of t-PA, PAI, vWF and prostacycline as well as platelet amount, their aggregation and life-span were studied in I0 donors. It was found that Adjuretin significantly increased the concentration of vWF, PAI and prostacycline as well as the amount of circulating platelets and their life-span. The release of t-PA and prostacycline was short-lasting (I5-20 min). We conclude that the use of Adjuretin enhances the yield of clothing factors and platelets from the same number of donors.

0440

EVALUATION OF THE HAEMONETICS MCS3p RBCP-PROTOCOL

J.B.M. Guit , R.M.H. Kivit, H.J.C. de Wit
Red Cross Blood Bank Friesland, Leeuwarden,
The Netherlands.

The RBCP-protocol of the Haemonetics MCS-3p is an apheresis procedure in which, from one donor, in a single procedure of about 20 minutes a unit of plasma and a red bloodcellconcentrate (RBC), in 80 ml of SAG-M, can be obtained.

The procedure was performed on 101 fully informed, experienced, non-remunerated plasmapheresis-donors. Procedure time, donordiscomfort and donor-bloodcounts before and after the procedure, weight and hematological parameters of the products were measured. At an intermediate evaluation after 31 procedures (cluster I, 1st and 2nd cycle 175 ml plasma) the hematocrite (Ht) of the RBC appeared to be low (mean 0.51 l/l). The protocol was adjusted to get the maximum Ht, without changing the total volume of the donation (cluster II, 67 procedures, 1st cycle 130 ml, 2nd of 230 ml plasma).

During apheresis and by follow up interview some weeks later no donordiscomfort was reported. The hemoglobine concentration (Hb) decreased 0.5 mmol/l (mean, range 0.2-1.1 mmol/l). Cluster I: Ht of the RBC 0.51 l/l (0.44-0.58), cluster II: Ht 0.55 l/l (0.45-0.61). In cluster I 13% and in cluster II 61% of the RBC's met the Dutch standards (Ht ≥ 0.55 l/l). Other items showed no significant difference between the two clusters. Cluster II, RBC: nett weight 362 g (342-377), leucocytes 7.9 x 10^9/l (3.7-16.8), platelets 91 x 10^9/l (21-408). Mean apheresis time was 21 minutes. One procedure failed due to wrong installation of disposables, 2 due to wrong programming of the MCS3p.

The RBCP-protocol is donorfriendly, easy to perform and yields both RBC and plasma in about 20 minutes. The leucocyte and platelet contamination in the RBC is comparable to a non-buffycoat depleted RBC from whole blood.

0441

REVIEW OF PLASMAPHERESIS WITH THE HAEMONETICS PCS-PLUS

J.B.M. Guit , R.M.H. Kivit, H.J.C. de Wit
Red Cross Blood Bank Friesland, Leeuwarden,
The Netherlands.

To evaluate the donorplasmapheresis proces from appointment up to end of donation, relevant information about donors and donations is recorded.

During 1992 and 1993 eight Haemonetics PCS-plus plasmapheresis units were used, the last three months of 1992 two extra machines were installed. Specifications of the method are: Platelet Poor Plasma (PPP) protocol, blow-molded bowl, sodium-citrate (1:16) or ACD-A (1:12) as anticoagulant, draw speed 70 ml/min. and centrifugespeed of 6000 rpm. The intended donation volume is 650 ml.

In the last 2 years 20,599 appointments were made. Donor show was 18,161 (88.2%). Donation was postponed in 393 cases (2.2%). The most important reasons for postponement were recent inflammation or use of antibiotics (66 ≈ 17%), recent dental treatment (58 ≈ 15%), hypertension (58 ≈ 15%), low hemoglobine concentration (40 ≈ 10%) and herpes labialis (22 ≈ 6%). Of a total of 17,768 performed procedures 17,490 gave the expected result. The most important reasons for stopping a procedure (278 times) were developing hematoma (75 ≈ 27%), high return pressure (51 ≈ 18%), flow-problems (43 ≈ 15%), problems with disposables (34 ≈ 12%), technical failure of the PCS-plus (17 ≈ 6%) and donor slightly unwell during procedure (15 ≈ 5%). No dangerous complications were observed, no donor collapsed. Of all procedures 75% was finished between 45 and 50 minutes.

The Haemonetics PCS-plus appears to be a reliable machine for a safe collection of donorplasma. 98.4% of all procedures results in a acceptable unit of donorplasma.

0442

PLASMAPHERESIS THERAPY IN A PATIENT WITH MYASTHENIA GRAVIS(MG) USING THE HAEMONETICS MCS 3P

J.Ph.H.B. Sybesma[1,2], W.J.J. van Dongen[1], L.I. Hertzberger[2]
1 Bloodbank "South-West Netherlands",Dordrecht,
2 Merwede Hospital, Dordrecht, The Netherlands.

The purpose of this study was to investigate the efficacy of therapeutic plasmapheresis with the new Haemonetics MCS 3p machine in a patient with severe M.G.
A man, 38 years, known with MG during 5 years, was treated with plasmapheresis during a myastenic crisis with respiratory insufficiency for which he needed artificial respiration. His hospitalisation time was 3 weeks, compared with 5 weeks when he was treated elsewere without plasmapheresis.
After 2 months, however, he complained of shortness of breath again and weakness of his muscles. We decided to perform plasmapheresis again. His vital capacity increased and we decided to continue the plamapheresis therapy in a prophylactic way, using the Haemonetics MCS 3p. The MCS 3p was installed with disposable R225 PX, standard protocol (single arm procedure). The default plasma was 2000 ml. As replacement fluid was used albumin solution with a default setting of 100%. Other parameters were: Optics volume:0-20, ACD/Blood ratio 1:12, draw flow rate: 60ml/min, return flow rate: 60 ml/min, centrifuge speed 4800 rpm. The mean time of the procedure was 93 min. The patient was treated 13 x in 12 months. Before plasmapheresis therapy he could not ride a bike nor drive a car. He was not able to dress himself and could only eat mashed or liquid food.
After 6 months treatment he enjoyed a complete normal life again. The improvement was not only clinically, but also demonstrable by measuring vital capacity and acetylcholine receptor antibody levels. (Central Lab of the Bloodtransfusion, AMSTERDAM).

In conclusion: the MCS 3p was succesfully used for therapeutic plasmapheresis in a patient with severe MG.

0443

THE USE OF THERAPEUTIC PLASMA EXCHANGE FOR ACUTE POLYRADICULONEUROPATHY

M.Radović, B.Balint, A.Jovičić
Institute of Transfusiology of MMA
Belgrade, Yugoslavia

The rationale for therapeutic plasma exchange (TPE) in acute polyradiculoneuropathy (APRN) is based on the presence of an immune-mediated process and an circulating immune factor/antibody that causes demyelinization of the patient peripheral nerves.
This study comprises 24 patients, mostly with a neurologic defect of the 4th grade, divided into two groups. One group was treated with immunosuppressive drugs, and TPE, and another group received immunosuppressive drugs only. TPE was performed using blood cell separator (Haemonetics M-30 or IBM 2997), mainly every other day. In average, about 20 L patient's plasma was removed during the whole therapeutic protocol. Treatment efficacy was assessed on the basis of changes of the neurologic deficit grade, and in electrophysiological parameters. It was shown that improvements were better and faster in patients treated by combination of immunosuppressive drugs and TPE, and when TPE was started within the first 7 days of clinical manifestations of disease.
Conclusion: TPE can produce benefit and be effective in the treatment of APRN, but should be applied as early as possible, and in patients with more severe neurologic deficit.

0444

EXTRACORPOREAL DETOXICATION IN HEMOLYTIC ANEMIA THERAPY

A.A.Kerimov, G.F.Gulieva, N.S.Alieva
Institute of Haematology and Blood Transfusion, Baku, Azerbaijan.

We studied the efficiency of some extracorporeal methods in the treatment complex of acquired autoimmune hemolytic anemias (AIHA). In 44 patients having failed to arrest hemolytic crises and to achieve persistent remission, we used plasmapheresis and plasmasorption. 29 of them were patients with idiopathic AIHA and 15 with symptomatic AIHA developed on the background of different hemoblastosis (acute leukemia, chronic lymphoid leukemia, Hodgkin's and non-Hodgkin's lymphomas). During the treatment the humoral and cellular immunity indices and endogenous cortisol levels of patients were defined. Most of the patients who received extracorporeal treatment, demonstrated clinico-hematologic improvement; it was expressed in hemolysis reduction or disappearance, erythrocyte count and hemoglobin increase, reduction of antierythrocyte and antileukocyte antibodies, circulating immune complexes and mid mass molecules. Additional washing of autoerythrocytes of patients before reinfusion appeared to be more effective. Plasmasorption, despite the treated plasma cortisol level reduction under the influence of hemosorbant, reinforced the detoxication efficiency.

0446

FALSELY LOW CALCIUM MEASUREMENTS FOLLOWING PLASMA EXCHANGE IN LIVER FAILURE

J.P. Miller, P.D. Mintz
University of Virginia Blood Bank, Charlottesville, Virginia, U.S.A.

In liver transplantation, plasma exchange (PE) has been employed to correct the coagulopathy of liver failure and in an attempt to arrest humorally mediated rejection. These patients would be expected to have impaired metabolism of citrate (C) and low calcium (Ca). Therefore, we measured serum C as well as total Ca by Ektachem (E) and atomic absorption (AA) before and after PE (n=10) in 3 patients. Prior to PE, Ca measured by either method was similar, however, the post-PE E Ca was significantly lower than the elemental Ca determined by AA (in mg/dL):

	E Ca	AA Ca	P
Pre-PE	8.5	8.7	0.39
Post- PE	10.0	10.6	0.003

There was a correlation between the difference in the Ca measured by the two methods and the serum C concentration (R=0.77, P=0.0001). In the setting of hepatic failure, accumulation of unmetabolized C during PE can cause falsely low total Ca measurements in these critically ill patients because the dye binding method used by E does not measure Ca bound to C.

0447

BIOCOMPATIBILITY IN THE APHERESIS PROCESSES: INTERLEUKIN-6

J. Muñoz, A. Rubió, C. Ferrán, F. Martí*, M. Peiró*, J. García*.
Blood BanK Hospital Bellvitge.Hospitalet.Barcelona. SPAIN.
*Oncologic Research Institut. Barcelona. SPAIN.

The discovery of the interleukin-6 as a T lymphocite activator and differentiation has allowed its use as T lymphocite activity marker. Its confluence with the interleukin-1 for the production of interleukin-2 was demonstrate.

During the apheresis process, we assesed the interl6 levels of twenty-two healty platelets, this was done via six hemodialysis processes and eight aortocoron· bypass processes. Two serum specimens were assesed in each process, one prior and one after. The two samples were taken inmediately befor or after the process.

A noticeable increase of interleukin-6 was observed in those patients underwent an aortocoronary bypass, the hemodialysis processes remained constant as did the apheresis processes.

An increase in the interleukin-6 of patients that underwent bypass surgery was observed, in connection to an increase in the limphocite activity.

0448

RECOMBINANT HUMAN ERYTHROPOIETIN IN TREATMENT OF ANEMIA IN MULTIPLE MYELOMA

G.G.Iosava
Institute of Hematology and Blood Transfusion, Tbilisi, Republic of Georgia.

Anemia freguently occurs in patients with myeloma. It may be due to many factors, but is frequently related to the disease itself with impairment of renal function or to the effect of chemotherapeutic agents. Erythropoietin which is produced in the proximal renal tubules by unrecognised cells, stimulates the erythroid progenitor cells at different levels to develop into mature erythrocytes. We studied the effect of recombinant human erythropoietin (EPRREX) as adjuvant treatment for plasmapheresis and chemotherapy in myeloma patients with severe anemia. Plasmapheresis (4-5 procedures during a fortnight, removing I000-I500 ml of plasma per procedure and concomitant chemotherapy) has been administered in I4 patients. 6 of them received r-EPO at dose 50 U/kg SC 3 times weekly. Hb level of the r-EPO group was compared to Hb level of 8 control patients at days 7-28. R-EPO treated patients showed a significantly higher values of Hb than the control group patients. The results suggest that EPO-deficiency plays a certain role in pathogenesis of anemia in myeloma patients and r-EPO can be useful in the treatment of anemia in these patients.

0449

THE USE OF APHERESIS METHODS FOR THE TREATMENT OF LEUKEMIAS, MULTIPLE MYELOMA AND APLASTIC ANAEMIA.

K. M. Abdulkadirov, A. A. Ganapiev, S. I. Moiseev
Russian Institute of Hematology and Transfusiology, Saint-Petersburg, Russia.

In last 12 years the apheresis methods is used for treatment hematologic diseasis. In 120 patients (pts) with acute and chronic leukemias we used leukaferesis (LF) for removing of the mass of tumor cells. We have established the rise of chemotherapy agents susceptive leukemias cells after the first LF, because the "resting" cells are entering in the active proliferation stage. In that cases we used chemotherapy course in combination with LF for toxic complications prevention. In 45 pts with multiple myeloma and Waldenstrom's macroglobulinemia have used plasmapheresis (PF) as an urgency therapy for treatment hyperviscosity syndrome and toxity complications. In 26 pts with aplastic anemia were effectived the use of PF for the prevention of transfusion reactions and treatment of toxic complications during the course of antilymphocyte globulin. In conclusion, indications for apheresis methods are the level of leukocytes ≥100 $x10^9/l$ and 50% blasts in pts with leukemias, hyperproteinemia ≥100 g/l and hyperviscosity syndrome in pts with multiple myeloma and treatment of transfusion reactions and toxic complications in patients with aplastic anemia.

0450

LYMPHOCYTOPHERESIS IN CHRONIC LYMPHOCYTIC LEUKEMIA (CLL) PATIENTS

T.N.Huseynov
Institute of Haematology and Blood Transfusion, Baku, Azerbaijan.

37 CLL patients in III-IV stages of disease (Rai) received lymphocytopheresis. Disease history lasted several months to 20 years. Indications for the use of lymphocytopheresis were two or three lineage cytopenias (25 patients). The effect of previous cytostatic therapy was not sufficient (12 patients). During each procedure $0.3\text{-}1.32 \times 10^{12}$ cells were removed and in most cases (71.4%) lymphocytes were mobilized from extravasal to circulating pool. It led to the reduction of circulating lymphocyte count, diminishing of lymph nodes, spleen and liver size. In the course of lymphocytopheresis (2-6 procedures) $3.65 \pm 0.28 \times 10^{12}$ cells were removed. The reduction of intoxication symptoms (79.4%), sizes of lymph nodes (89.2%), spleen (88.3%), liver (74.1%) was detected. There was no increase of ^{3}H-thymidine labeled cell count, but we revealed the rise of ^{3}H-uridine labeled cell count and diploid cells with decondensated chromatin according to G1 phase. After every procedure PAS-positive cell count raised. Correlation analysis showed close relation between cytophotometry G1 cells and PAS-positive cell count.

0451

INTRAOPERATIVE BLOOD TRANSFUSION IN PARTIAL LIVER TRANSPLANTATION FROM LIVING RELATIVES

K. Ito[1], H. Yosida[1], K. Yurugi[1], S. Uemoto[2], K. Tanaka[2], Y. Yamaoka[2], K. Ozawa[2]
1Department of Blood Transfusion, 2Second Division, Department of Surgery, Kyoto University Hospital, Kyoto, Japan.

Sixty two patients with intractable liver diseases underwent partial liver transplantation from living relatives and were transfused. Intraoperative blood transfusion to the patients is described. Their diseases were biliary atresia, liver cirrhosis, Wilson disease, Budd-Chiari syndrome, progressive intrahepatic cholestasis, protoporphyrinemia, tyrosinemia, fulminant hepatitis and glycogen storage disease. Most of the patients were less than 15 years old.

Average amounts of blood lost during surgery were 210 ±30 ml / kg of body weight and average amounts of RBC transfused were 0.99 ± 0.13 unit / kg of body weight. One unit is products from 200 ml of whole blood. Leukocyte-poor blood products were irradiated at 15-50 Gy and were transfused. Average amounts of blood transfused to one paitient were 13.6 ± 2.2 units of RBC, 7.3 ± 1.4 units of PC and 2.0 ± 0.8 units of FFP.

Less than FFP reported in liver transplantation from brain-dead donors was transfused.

0452

ASSESSMENT OF BLOOD QUALITY DURING AND AFTER RETRANSFUSION OF AUTOLOGOUS SOLOCTRANS-PLUS BLOOD IN VASCULAR SURGERY

B.H. Walpoth[1], R. Schmid[1], T. Amport[1], H.U. Rothen[2], P. Spaeth[3], U. Althaus[1]

Dept. of Thoracic and Cardiovascular Surgery[1], Anesthesia[2], SRK Central Laboratory[3], University Berne, Switzerland.

Quantitative and qualitative assessment of intraoperative aspiration and reinfusion of autologous blood with the Solcotrans-Plus was carried out in 11 males (52-79 years) undergoing elective resection of abdominal aortic aneurysms. Hematology, blood chemistry, coagulation parameters and complement activation were studied in the patients blood at the following time points: preoperatively, before and after heparinisation, after retransfusion of the first and last Solcotrans, 6 and 20 hours postoperatively. In addition the same laboratory tests were performed in the first and last Solcotrans unit blood.

Results (mean values of 11 patients ± 1 SD): Intraoperatively 2 Solcotrans units were salvaged (total 1'039 ± 565 ml) of which 805 ± 487 ml were retransfused to the patients. As a mean patients required only 1 unit of homologous RBC's (395 ± 781 ml) intraoperatively. Patients intraoperative hemoglobin concentration amounted to 10 g/dl or more. Whereas the hemoglobin level in the Solcotrans attained only 8,2 g/dl. Thrombocyte counts 48 ± 18 x 10^{9}/l) and ionized calcium (0,2 ± 0,4 mmol/l) were significantly depressed when compared to the preoperative patient values (p < 0,05). The protein concentration remained within normal limits in the patients and in the Solcotrans blood. Complement activation (C4a, C5a) showed a significant increase after initiation of surgery but there was no significant difference between the Solco- or patient blood. Whereas plasma free hemoglobin, coagulation and fibrinolytic parameters showed a significant elevation in the Solcotrans blood when compared to the patient's blood (p < 0,05).

In conclusion the Solcotrans-Plus offers a fast, efficient and simple method for salvage and retransfusion of intraoperative autologous blood in vascular surgery.

0453

HAEMOFILTRATION VERSUS AUTOTRANSFUSION EVALUATION OF BLOOD SAVING METHODS IN HEART SURGERY

W. Heller, H.-E. Hoffmeister
Dept. of Thoracic- and Cardiovascular Surg., Univ. of Tuebingen, Germany

Two patient groups (n=40), with an average age of approx. 60 years, who had to undergo an ACVB operation under application of the Cell Saver (CS) or haemofiltration (HF) were investigated up to the 5th. postoperative day regards their need for transfusion, protein substitution, pressure relationships and coagulatory-physiological peculiarities. Blood samples taken at close intervals pre-, intra- and postoperatively ensured the representation of the course of the parameter of fibrinolysis and the contact phase as well as the total protein course. Regards the postoperative need for transfusion, with the application of the Cell Saver 53.8% blood was saved in comparison to the haemofilter group. A total of 27% of the total requirement in group CS was covered with autologous blood, up to 70% of the postoperative requirement could be covered with autologous blood. Intraoperatively group HF was found to need less transfusion. In the total postoperative course the haemoglobin reached a higher value in the CS group; particularly on the 1st. postoperative day, at 13g%, it was clearly higher than the corresponding value, 11.5g%, in group HF.
The mean postoperative drainage loss was higher in the CS group at approx. 100 ml. Regarding the need for transfusion at different initial haemoglobin values, at the end of bypass the Cell Saver is to be preferred to haemofiltration in patients with high preoperative Hb (12.7g%). With the expected lesser intraoperative blood loss and thus low postoperative transfusion volumes this presents the decisive advantage over the Cell Saver group. The postoperative total assessment was identical in both groups although with a different distribution in the protein application. Dependent on the total protein neither of the two methods had a distinct advantage regards the protein substitution or the total protein course. The results of the clotting analyses showed no significant differences between the two groups at any point. The fibrinogen level rose significantly postoperatively in accordance with its function as an acute phase protein.

0454

THE EFFECTS OF 6% HETASTARCH AND DDAVP ON FACTOR VIII:RISTOCETIN COFACTOR ACTIVITY

J. Lazarchick, J.M. Conroy
Medical University of South Carolina, Department of Pathology/Laboratory Medicine & Anesthesiology, Charleston, SC 29425, USA.
The objective of this study was to monitor the effect of sequential hetastarch and DDAVP treatment on factor VIII:ristocetin cofactor activity (Rcof) in 23 patients undergoing surgical procedures. After induction of anesthesia, hetastarch was administered, 20 ml/kg, to maximum of 1500 ml. Patients then randomly received either a 10 ml solution containing 0.3 ug/kg of DDAVP (group I, n=12) or 10 ml of normal saline (group II, n=11). Rcof was measured preoperatively, after hetastarch infusion, and at 30, 60, and 240 mins after study drug infusion. Mean preoperative Rcof was slightly higher for the saline group, 114.5 vs 90.4 U/dl. After the administration of hetastarch, Rcof decreased to 58% (group I) and 55% (group II) of baseline values. After study drug administration, mean Rcof in group I increased to 95% at 30 mins and 107% of baseline at 60 mins. Mean Rcof values remained below baseline in group II at both times, 69% and 57% respectively. There was no statistically significant difference between the two groups before or immediately after hetastarch administration or at 240 mins. No patient had hypercoagulability with DDAVP treatment. DDAVP is a safe treatment for the predictable reduction in Rcof associated with hetastarch use.

0455

SUCCESFULLY TREATING JEHOVAH'S WITNESSES WITHOUT HOMOLOGOUS BLOOD

1. **Introduction:**
   Jehovah's Witnesses and other patients have been treated without homologous blood.
   Avoiding of medical-legal confrontation.
2. **Material & Methods:**
   Hospital Information Services of Jehovah's Witnesses examines c. 3,600 worldwide medical publications on up-to-date alternatives. More than 40,000 physicians in 65 countries are listed as willing to treat without blood.
   More than 60 bloodless medical and surgery centers.
   A thorough review of medical articles:
   Surgical and clinical cases managed without blood.
3. **Strategies Used for Avoiding and Controlling Hemorrhage and Anemia Without Blood Transfusion**
   * Surgical devices and techniques to locate and arrest internal bleeding
   * Techniques and devices to control external bleeding and shock
   * Operative and anesthetic techniques to limit blood loss during surgery
   * Blood-oxygen monitoring devices and techniques that limit blood sampling
   * Volume Expanders
   * Hemostatic agents for bleeding/clotting problems
   * Therapeutic agents and techniques for managing anemia

0456

ANTI-HCV PROFICIENCY TESTING. H. F. Polesky and M. Hanson. Memorial Blood Centers of Minnesota, Minneapolis, MN., USA.

Since 1990 the College of American Pathologists/ American Association of Blood Banks Viral Markers proficiency testing program has included samples to be evaluated for antibody to hepatitis C virus (anti-HCV). Approximately 500 participants receive 5 samples quarterly in each of two surveys; W1/DC which includes tests performed on blood donors and W2 which is designed to monitor diagnostic testing. Expected sample reactivity is determined by pretesting with multiple methods. Prior to 1992 a first generation recombinant immunoblot assay (RIBA-1, Chiron) was used for pretesting. The 1992-93 panels were pretested with RIBA-2.

From July 1990 through 1991 >90% of participants correctly identified 25/26 EIA reactive (R) samples. Responses on non-reactives (NR) were less consistent with >90% agreement on only 16/24 samples. Four NR samples were reported as R by >90% of labs using an Abbott assay while > 95% of Ortho users reported these samples as NR. One sample reported as NR by >95% of Abbott users was reported as R by >95% of labs using Ortho. Two samples were reported as NR by 50-80% of both Abbott and Ortho users. Results on samples included in the 1992-93 surveys were more consistent with > 90% agreement reported on 23/25 NR and 33/35 R samples. Two weakly reactive samples were detected by 60-80% of both Abbott and Ortho users.

These data suggest that the specificity of EIA screening tests has improved with the introduction of 2nd generation assays in 1992.

0457

EVALUATION OF THE ANTI-HCV ELISA: ABBOTT 2 AND ABBOTT 3. J. R.Villanueva, J .M .M. de Segovia , M. Ferreiro. Hospital Provincial Pontevedra. Spain

Second generation HCV ELISA (Abbott) AND RIBA 3 (Ortho) were compared with ELISA 3 (Abbott).

AIM and METHODS : 124 samples were tested for Anti-HCV ELISA 2, RIBA 3 and Anti-HCV ELISA 3.

A: Samples ELISA 2 were nonreactive with AB/CO 0,5-1.
B: Samples ELISA 2 were reactive with AB/CO 1-1,5.
C: Samples ELISA 2 were reactive and RIBA 3 nonreactive.
D: Samples RIBA 3 were indeterminate.

RESULTS:

	RIBA 3	ELISA 2 Ab/Co	ELISA 3 Ab/Co
Panel A **n=60**	N.R. 42 IND. 13 R. 5	0,5-0,9 0,5-0,9 0,5-0,9	0,1-0,9 (38) 1-1,3 (4) 0,2-0,9 (9) 1,6-2,3 (4) 0,6 (1) 2-2,5 (4)
Panel B **n=23**	N.R. 7 IND. 5 R. 11	1-1,4 1-1,4 1,2-1,5	0,16 - 1,4 1,4 - 3,7 1,6 - 4,9
Panel C **n=18**	N.R. 18 IND. 0 R. 0	1-2 (13) 2-3 (3) 3-4 (2)	0,5-1 (7) 1-2 (6) 2-3 (2) 4-5 (3)
Panel D **n=23**	N.R. 0 IND. 23 R. 0	0,5-1 (11) 1-2 (6) 2-3 (6)	0,5-1 (8) 1-2 (4) 2-3 (3) 3-5 (8)

CONCLUSION: The new HCV ELISA 3 Abbott is more sensitive and more specific than HCV ELISA 2 Abbott.

0458

COMPARISONS BETWEEN SECOND AND THIRD GENERATION SCREENING AND SUPPLEMENTAL TEST FOR THE DETECTION OF ANTI-HCV IN BLOOD DONORS AND THALASSAEMIC PATIENTS.
C. Politis, Cl. Tsiolkas and Cl. Richardson.
Hellenic Red Cross Blood Center, Athens.

In this study we compared the results between: 1) EIA-2 HCV and EIA-3 HCV Abbott and 2) Chiron RIBA-2 and RIBA-3 HCV Test System. Immunoblot Assays in the investigation of a) 21 blood donor samples positive with EIA-2 and RIBA-2 and b) 11 samples from multitransfused thalassaemic patients EIA-2 positive and RIBA-2 indeterminate. The results of the comparison between the Elisas are shown in table.

Blood donors

	O.D	EIA-2 <1	1-3	>3	TOT
E	<1	0	0	0	0
A	1-3	0	1	0	1
3	>3	0	3	17	20
	TOT	0	4	17	21

Patients

	O.D	EIA-2 <1	1-3	>3	TOT
E	<1	0	0	0	0
A	1-3	0	1	0	1
3	>3	0	7	3	10
	TOT	0	8	3	11

The overall aggrement between the RIBAs is 54% (6 specimens were found positive with RIBA-3, while the rest 5 remain indeterminate.

Conclusion: Third generation assays are more sensitive for testing and confirming anti-HCV reactivity.

0459

Comparative evaluation commercially available second generation test kits for hepatitis C virusdiagnosis. Preliminary results.

P.P.Michielsen[1], A.M.Ramon[1,2],P.A.Berg[3],L.Muylle[4],D.De Groof[5], P.A.Pelckmans[1].
[1]Division of Gastroenterology University Hospital of Antwerp,Belgium; [2]International Institute of Immunopathology,Inc. Cologne, FRG, [3]Department of Internal Medecine, University Tübingen, FRG[4], Belgian Red Cross, Bloodbank Antwerp (Belgium), [5]Belgian Medical Cooperation, Niamey (Niger)

Second generation assays have improved the accuracy of detection of Hepatitis C virus (HCV) infection (Hepatology 1992; 16:300).
In order to compare the diagnostic value of different commercially available testkits, a prospective study is being performed.
Apparently healthy voluntary blood donors from Antwerp and Cologne (n=550, group 1), and from Niger (n=100, group 2) and patients with liver diseases [NANB hepatitis (n=22, group 3), primary biliary cirrhosis (n=100, group 4), autoimmune hepatitis (n=100 group 5)] are studied by second generation EIA tests (Abbott, Organon-UBI, Innotest, Ortho) and blotting tests (Inno-LIA, Ortho RIBA II). In some samples, HCV-RNA testing is performed by reverse transcriptase PCR using primers from the 5'UTR.
In group 1, 4 samples scored (+) in at least one test. In group 2, 22 scored (+) in 1 or more EIA tests; in 14/22 the blottings were negative, in 8/22 Ortho RIBA was indeterminate. In group 3, all samples scored (+) in all tests, confirmed by PCR. In group 4, 5 samples scored (+) in 1 or more EIA tests, only 1 also in the blottings. In group 5, 10 samples were (+) in 1 or more EIA and blotting tests, confirmed by PCR, 20 scored (+) in Ortho EIA, not confirmed in blottings and PCR.
It can be concluded that second generation HCV tests detect HCV antibodies in all patients with NANB hepatitis, but also in a high proportion of patients with autoimmune hepatitis and blood donors from Niger. These data have to be further evaluated by means of a "gold standard" for which to date only HCV-RNA detection by PCR is available.

0460

Supplemental Single Marker EIA's for HCV Testing

Bonnie Moore and James Scheffel. Hepatitis Diagnostic Products Research and Development. Abbott Laboratories, Abbott Park, IL 60064.

A series of EIA's containing single domain (e.g. Core, NS3, NS4, NS5 only) HCV targets have been developed as alternative tests for confirmation of HCV antibody status. A given HCV domain is represented by 2-3 distinct EIA's containing the same HCV antigen expressed in different recombinant hosts, or a combination of recombinant target and a corresponding synthetic peptide. Reactivity of a specimen with multiple recombinant/synthetic antigens from a single HCV domain constitutes serologic confirmation of the presence of antibody to that domain. These assays have been used as an aid in clarification of screening assay positive, Matrix HCV indeterminant or nonreactive specimens. Since only a single antigen target is represented (as opposed to multiple targets) these assays are more sensitive than the currently licensed screening tests. From seroconversion panel, dilution panel and concordance testing these assays are equivalent to or slightly more sensitive than Matrix HCV. When testing populations negative by the screening test additional serologically confirmed reactives on the order of ~2-3% are detected. Essentially all of these incremental reactives are negative for HCV RNA. The predominant reactivity is for Core or NS5 only, but NS3 and NS4 only reactives are also seen. Rarely a double marker incremental reactive is seen. Do these low-level single marker reactives represent prior HCV infection, or a result of exposure to a cross-reactive stimulus? In order to assess the risk of disease transmission of these samples, several follow-up and transmission studies are underway.

0461

Discordancy of New Generation HCV Screening Assays with Current Generation Tests.

James Scheffel, Kevin Callear, and Bonnie Moore. Hepatitis Diagnostic Products Research and Development, Abbott Laboratories, Abbott Park, IL 60064.

Two new generation EIA's for HCV screening containing NS5 targets were evaluated vs. a panel of current generation repeat reactive plasma donor samples. The Abbott third generation assay (3.0) was tested on a group of 200 Abbott second generation (2.0) repeat reactive plasma donor samples representing approximately 40,000 donations. There were 8 2.0 reactives negative by the third generation test. Matrix HCV supplemental testing of these revealed that all 8 were indeterminant (7 NS3 and 1 Core only reactives). None of these samples were positive for HCV RNA, and all were negative on two additional supplemental EIA's for E2 and for the epitope between aa1911-1940. The Ortho third generation assay (3.0) was evaluated on a group of 600 Ortho 2.0 repeat reactives representing approximately 144,000 donations. There were 60 Ortho 2.0 repeat reactives testing negative with the new generation Ortho test. Matrix HCV supplemental test results on these discordants were as follows: there were 3 Matrix confirmed reactives (1 Core/NS3; 1 Core/NS5, and 1 Core/NS4), 24 Matrix indeterminants and 33 Matrix nonreactives. Among the Ortho 2.0/3.0 discordants were two RNA positives and 3 sporadic reactives by PCR. One of the PCR positives was also E2 positive. Another of the Ortho 2.0/3.0 discordants (NS3 only) was reactive for the 1911-1940 epitope.These data indicate that the addition of an NS5 target to existing HCV EIA targets, while adding incremental NS5 antibody detectability, may also produce discordancies with current (2.0) generation assays.

0462

A NEW SCREENING ASSAY FOR THE DETECTION OF ANTI HCV ANTIBODIES : " MONOLISA ANTI HCV NEW ANTIGENS" TEST

F. Aubrit[1], F. Lunel[2], P. Gruson[1], C. Lesieur[1], E. Ripoche[1], J. P. Bourgeois[1], J. F. Delagneau[1]
[1]SANOFI DIAGNOSTICS PASTEUR, Marnes la Coquette , [2]Hépatologie, CHU Pitié-Salpétrière, Paris, FRANCE

Introduction
In order to improve the detection of anti HCV antibodies in serum or plasma of patients during or after infection with the hepatitis C virus, we have developed a new test which includes several modifications compared to the first SDP test "MONOLISA ANTI HCV" .

Materials and Methods
The major improvement concerns the solid phase ; HCV immunodominant antigens are coated on the solid phase as two capsid synthetic peptides, a previous recombinant NS3 protein which now encompasses additional upstream epitopes, and a recombinant coded by the NS4 region.

Results
Improved sensitivity of the MONOLISA ANTI HCV NEW ANTIGENS was demonstrated by testing seven seroconverter samples previously detected by the first kit version. Seroconversion, in two patient samples, was detected earlier with the new reagents : one sample was reactive with the NS3 antigen and the other with the capsid antigens. The specificity assessed by testing 2,000 fresh samples from volunteer blood donors was greater than 99.7%. No cross reactions were obtained with sera from patients infected with HIV(10),HTLV(10),CMV(10),and HBV(10).

Conclusion
This MONOLISA ANTI HCV NEW ANTIGENS test with a totally modified solid phase provides better sensitivity and specificity for detecting HCV antibodies in serum and plasma.

0463

EVALUATION OF ANTI-HEPATITIS C VIRUS SCREENING USING 2ND GENERATION PASSIVE HEMAGGLUTINATION ASSAY IN DONOR BLOOD

S.Sato[1], S.Kishimoto[1], H.Ihara[1], T.Kato[1], H.Ikeda[1], S.Sekiguchil[1], Iinuma[2], S.Tokita[2], Y.Komagoe[2]
1 Hokkaido Red Cross Blood Center, 2 Dainabot Co., Ltd., JAPAN

Currently, anti-HCV screening of Japanese blood donor is carried out by 2nd passive hemagglutination (PHA) assay with 3 recombinant polypeptides (Dainabot). The purpose of this study is to evaluate the sensitivity and specificity of anti-HCV PHA assay in donor screening. PHA positive samples were tested for the presence of HCV-RNA by RT-PCR. Of 122 samples with the highest PHA titer ($\geqq 2^{12}$), 117 (95.9%) were PCR positive and 7 of 170 (4.1%) weakly-positive samples (2^5~2^{11}) also contained HCV-RNA. In contrast, 792 seronegative samples were negative for HCV-RNA. These results indicate that PHA can detect PCR-positive specimens and PHA strongly-positive result closely associate viraemia. Panel sera were used for comparative study on the sensitivity with PHA and EIA-2 (Abbott). In core dominant panels, EIA showed slightly better sensitivity than PHA. In c33 dominant panels, PHA exhibited obviously higher sensitivity than EIA. Eight PCR-positive panels were examined by MATRIX (Abbott), RIBA3.0 (Ortho) and single- peptide-coated PHA. Anti-core reactivity of the 8 samples could be detected by any of the three assays. As to anti-c33 reactivity, only 2 of 8 were positive by MATRIX, whereas all samples were positive by RIBA3.0 and c33-coated PHA. Fifty-two samples with PHA(+)/EIA(-) were also tested by the three assays. These samples were PCR negative. Anti-c33 reactivity was detected in 7, 17 or 50 samples, while anti-core reactivity was detected in 14, 12, or 2 of the 52 samples by MATRIX, RIBA3.0 or core-coated PHA, respectively. These results indicate that c33 is mainly responsible for PHA reactivity. In our prospective study of anti-HCV screening with PHA, no definite case of post-transfusion hepatitis C has found. We conclude that PHA is sensitive and specific enough for donor screening of HCV infection.

0464

HCV ANTIBODIES IN POST-TRANSFUSION NANB-HEPATITIS : DETECTION AND ANALYSIS BY THIRD GENERATION ANTI-HCV ASSAYS

S.Kikuchi[1], R.Masamune[1], Y.Kunii[1], N.Endo[2]
1 Sendai National Hospital, 2 Miyagi Red Cross Blood Center, Sendai, Japan

Objective: The purpose of this study is to assess third generation anti-HCV assays in comparison to second generation assays on the time of appearance of anti-HCV in post-transfusion NANB-hepatitis patients and to analyze seroconversion patterns by strip immunoblot assays.

Methods: Serial bleeds from 28 patients who developed post-transfusion NANB-hepatitis were retrospectively tested by the HCV 2.0 and 3.0 ELISAs (Ortho), and RIBA HCV 2.0 and 3.0 immunoblot assays (Chiron).

Results: Of the 28 patients, 16 seroconverted, while 12 did not seroconvert in either ELISA 2.0 or 3.0. Although passive antibody acquired by transfusion was detected in 10/16 cases, apparent anti-HCV seroconversion was detected and substantiated by concomitant detection of antibody profile and intensity by RIBA 2.0 and 3.0 in 13 cases. In 9/13 cases, ELISA 2.0 and 3.0 detected seroconversion at the same bleed.
In 4 cases, HCV 3.0 assays detected seroconversion 50.8 days(ranged from 34 to 71 days)earlier than HCV 2.0 assays. Initial seroconversion was contributed by antibody against c33c in 4 cases.

Conclusion: Ortho HCV 3.0 assays demonstrated increased sensitivity for the detection of anti-HCV seroconversion and antibody against c33c contributed to increasing sensitivity.

0465

DONOR ANTI-HCV TESTING: COMPARISON OF 2ND AND 3RD GENERATION ELISA AND RIBA

A Heethuis, B de Vries, RL McShine, PC Das, CTh Smit Sibinga.
RC Blood Bank Groningen-Drenthe, Groningen, NL

Since the introduction of the 3rd generation Ortho anti-HCV kits for ELISA screening and RIBA confirmation, 32,163 donations were routinely screened in ELISA and 52 Repeatable Reactives (RR) were tested in RIBA. The results of the 3rd generation tests are compared to 2nd generation tests (n=55,197).

RESULTS:	2nd gen. ELISA/RIBA	3rd gen. ELISA/RIBA
Donations (n)	55,197	32,163
RR (ELISA)	128 (0.23%)	52 (0.16%)
RIBA		
Neg	49 (38%)	31 (60%)
Indet. Reactive	75 (59%)	18 (35%)
Pos	4 (3%)	3 (6%)

CONCLUSION: The use of synthetic peptides in the 3rd generation ELISA and RIBA assay shows a significant improvement:

- Percentage of RR in anti-HCV screening decreases from 0.23% to 0.16%.
- Percentage of RIBA 3rd generation Indet. Reactives decreased significantly, an important factor for re-entry policy.

0466

ORTHO HCV 3.0 ELISA - A HIGHLY SENSITIVE TEST FOR THE DETECTION OF HEAPTITIS C VIRUS

H.I. Joller-Jemelka[1], A.N. Wicki[2]
1Section of Clinical Immunology, University Hospital Zürich, Switzerland,2ANAWA Laboratories Inc. Wangen, Switzerland.

To detect a hepatitis C virusinfection, highly specific and sensitive test methods are necessary. ELISA assays detect antibodies against HCV. The PCR method detects viremia. Epidemiologically it is of prime importance to find all patients with past or ongoing hepatitis C, but for the monitoring of the patients it is important to know the present status.

Material and Methods: 283 sera ORTHO HCV 2.0 ELISA negative, retested by ORTHO HCV 3.0 ELISA and at the same time by HCV-RNA (PCR) were tested.

Results:

ORTHO HCV 2.0 negative	ORTHO HCV 3.0 ELISA negative (definition ORTHO*)					ORTHO HCV 3.0 ELISA (positive or indeterminate)		
Patients	OD Patients 0.020-0.200**		OD Patients 0.200-0.500**		HCV-RNA (PCR)	OD Patients 0.500-3.0		HCV-RNA (PCR)
	n	x̄ OD	n	x̄ OD	positive	n	x̄ OD	positive
i.v. drug user (n=69)	62	0.092	5	0.378	3	2	1.422	1
hepatopathy(excl. HBV,AIH) (n=30)	21	0.074	6	0.407	5	3	3.627	3
dialysis,TPL (n=46)	36	0.124	8	0.399	6	2	2.879	1
gravidae (n=129)	127	0.083	1	0.369	0	1	2.453	0
needlesticks (n=9)	6	0.064	2	0.341	0	1	1.932	0
total (n=283)	252(89%)		22(8%)		14(64%)	9(3%)		5(56%)

* cutoff = (OD negative controls + 0.600)
** less than cutoff range

Conclusion:

The ORTHO 3.0 ELISA is a highly sensitive and specific diagnostical method for the detection of hepatitis C virus infection. For clinical purposes, it would be desirable to change the cutoff definition for ORTHO HCV 3.0. To assess viremia, only the PCR will give a valid answer.

0467

EVALUATION OF THREE ANTI-HCV ELISAs: ORTHO 2.0, Ortho 2.5 AND ORTHO 3.0.

H. Vrielink[1], C.L. van der Poel[1],H.W. Reesink[1], H. Zaaijer[2], P.N. Lelie[2], H.T.M. Cuypers[2]. 1)Red Cross Blood Bank Amsterdam, 2)Central Lab Blood Transfusion Service Amsterdam, The Netherlands.

Aim: Three commercially available HCV ELISAs (Ortho 2.0, Ortho 2.5 and Ortho 3.0) were evaluated with panels consisting of cDNA-PCR and RIBA-2 confirmed serum samples.

Methods: Panel A consisted of serum samples (n=530) from blood donors who were reactive in anti-HCV ELISAs from various manufacturers. RIBA-2 and PCR were performed on all samples. Panel B consisted of serum samples (n=185) from clinical non-A, non-B hepatitis patients. RIBA-2 and PCR were performed on all samples.

Results:

Panel	PCR	RIBA-2			Ortho 2.0		Ortho 2.5		Ortho 3.0	
		+ve	ind	-ve	+ve	-ve	+ve	-ve	+ve	-ve
A	+	81	2	0	83	0	83	0	83	0
(n=530)	-	22	254	171	251	196	201	246	165	278
B	+	109	13	0	122	0	122	0	122	0
(n=185)	-	18	11	34	29	34	23	40	23	40

ELISA +ve = repeatedly reactive

Conclusions: The new Ortho 3.0 was at least as sensitive as the previous 2.0 and 2.5 versions. No PCR +ve samples were missed in any test. In ELISA reactive (PCR -ve) blood donors, Ortho 3.0 was significantly more specific than Ortho 2.5 and 2.0 ELISA ($p<0.02$ and $p<0.001$ respectively).

0468

EVALUATION OF TWO 3RD GENERATION ANTI-HCV ELISAs: MUREX-VK47 AND ORTHO 3.0.

H. Vrielink[1], C.L. van der Poel[1], H.W Reesink[1], H.L Zaaijer[2], P.N. Lelie[2], H.T.M. Cuypers[2]. 1) Red Cross Blood Bank Amsterdam, 2) Central Lab Blood Transfusion Service Amsterdam, The Netherlands.

Aim: Two commercially available 3rd generation anti-HCV ELISAs (Murex and Ortho) were evaluated in various serum panels. Both ELISAs apply Core, NS3, NS4, and NS5 antigens of the HCV genome.

Methods: Panel A consisted of serum samples (n=401) from blood donors who were repeatedly reactive in 1st and/or 2nd generation anti-HCV ELISAs from various manufacturers and who were also indeterminate or positive in RIBA-2 (Ortho). cDNA-PCR was performed on all samples.
Panel B consisted of serum samples (n=1,054) from first time blood donors not tested in any screening test before. RIBA-3 and cDNA-PCR were performed on all ELISA repeatedly reactive samples.

Results:

Panel	PCR	n	Murex +ve[1]	Murex -ve	Ortho +ve[1]	Ortho -ve
	+ve	86	86	0	86	0
A (n=401)	-ve	315	53	262	159	156
B (n=1,054)			8[2]	1046	2[3]	1052

[1] ELISA +ve = repeatedly reactive. [2] 1 sample reacted +ve in RIBA-3 and cDNA-PCR, and 7/8 samples were RIBA-3 -ve and PCR -ve.
[3] 1 sample reacted +ve in RIBA-3 and cDNA-PCR, and 1 sample was NS5 only reactive in RIBA-3 and was cDNA-PCR -ve.

Conclusions: In both ELISAs no cDNA-PCR positive samples were missed. The specificity of the Murex-VK47 versus Ortho 3.0, as calculated in the blood donor panel was 99.3% and 99.9% respectively (not significant, Chi-Square).

0469

HEPATITIS C VIRUS. INDETERMINATE SEROLOGICAL SAMPLES.
E.I.A. THIRD GENERATION AND IMMUNOBLOT ASSAY (RIBA 3.0-SIA).

Lucinda Queiros, Alzira Tender, Manuela Mateus, Marilia Morais.
REGIONAL BLOOD CENTER OF PORTO
PORTO - PORTUGAL

A group of 35 sera of volunteer blood donnors, positive in E.I.A. second generation (Abbott and Ortho) and RIBA-2 Indeterminate, was further evaluated by E.I.A. third generation (Ortho) and by Immunoblot assay RIBA-SIA.

RIBA-2	EIA 3th neg.	EIA 3th pos.	RIBA-SIA neg.	RIBA-SIA react.	RIBA-SIA ind.
C100-3 n=11(31.4%)	11	0	8	0	3
C22-3 n=18(51.5%)	5	13	8	4	6
C33-c n=6(17.1%)	5	1	1	5	0
Total	21 60%	14 40%	17 48.6%	9 25.7%	9 25.7%

The table shows 60% of the samples was negative in E.I.A. 3th, all of the samples positive for protein C100-3 has shown negative by this test. 74.3% of the indeterminate samples could be solved with RIBA 3.0 - SIA.
In this evaluation we have verified some discrepancies in the results, so we think that it is important to be carefull and prudent in the evaluation of the results of all the samples HCV indeterminate.

0470

ANTI-HCV CONFIRMATION TESTING: COMPARISON OF INDETERMINATE RESULTS OF 2ND AND 3RD GENERATION RIBA

A Heethuis, RL McShine, PC Das, CTh Smit Sibinga. RC Blood Bank Groningen-Drenthe, Groningen, NL

A. RIBA 3rd gen. results of new samples (n=28) tesed negative in the 3rd gen. anti-HCV ELISA and previously known with Repeat Reactive (RR) results in ELISA 2nd gen. and Indeterminate Results (IR) in RIBA 2nd gen. were compared.

RESULTS	Previous sample 2nd gen. assays		New sample 3rd gen assays		
ELISA RR	28		NEG	28	
RIBA IR	28		NEG	26	
C100		18	IR	2	
C33		1	C33		2
C22		8			
SOD + C100		1			

B. The IR RIBA patterns in 2nd and 3rd gen. were compared after tested RR resp. in 2nd and 3rd gen. ELISA's.

RESULTS	2nd gen RIBA		3rd gen RIBA		
Donations	n = 55,197			n = 32,163	
RIBA IR	75	0.136 %		18	0.056 %
5-1-1	0		NS5	13	0.040 %
C100	36	0.065 %	C100p	0	
C33	7	0.012 %	C33c	3	0.009 %
C22	31	0.056 %	C22p	0	
SOD+	1	0.002 %	SOD+	2	0.006 %

CONCLUSION: There is a significant decrease of C22 and C100 IR antibody patterns after testing in 3rd gen. ELISA and RIBA.

0471

FOLLOW UP OF HCV ANTIBODY MARKERS IN BLOOD DONORS BY SUPPLEMENTAL ASSAY

P.C. Das, A. Heethuis, J. Simileer, R.L. McShine, C.Th. Smit Sibinga.
Red Cross Blood Bank Groningen-Drenthe, Groningen, The Netherlands

With 2 supplemental assays (RIBA, Ortho & Innolia, Innogenetics) we have re-tested 73 repeat reactive (RR) sera derived from 25,000 blood donor screenings, by 2 supplemental assays. 66 donors were followed up to 15 months.
RESULTS: 42/73 sera were reactive by RIBA: 39 indeterminate reactions (ID) and 3 positives; Innolia: 11 reactives, (6 ID + 5 positives). 3 of the 5 Innolia positives were also positive in RIBA. Male was predominant in the 66 RR donors (M 48, F 18), of which 30 were ID on initial RIBA (M 21, F 9). Follow up 5-15 months later: 25 remained ID (M 16 and F 9) and 1 was positive (M), maintaining a higher male percentage. There was a shifting of band patterns between initial and recent RIBAs: 5-1-1, C-100 and C33 antibodies were inconsistant while C22 bands are generally repeatable during follow up.
CONCLUSION: The recent RIBAs seem to identify early seroconversion. A second supplementary test may help to reduce the false positive and ID reactions. Sera with only C-100, 5-1-1 bands are likely to be false reactives. The presence of higher incidence to HCV antibody markers in male remains to be clarified.

0472

DOES DUAL POSITIVITY IN TWO ANTI-HCV ELISA'S DEFINE TRUE ANTI-HCV REACTIVITY?

Williamson LM[1], Reeves I[1], Petrik J[1], Contreras M[2], Aloysious S[2], Barbara J[2], Harrison J[3], Kitchen A[3], Allain J-P[1].
[1]Division of Transfusion Medicine, University of Cambridge, [2]North London and [3]Brentwood Transfusion Centres, UK.

Objective: To establish whether the result of an alternative anti-HCV ELISA can predict the true reactivity of anti-HCV reactive blood donations.
Study design: Samples from blood donors giving positive results in a single anti-HCV ELISA were retested by a generically different ELISA as follows:-

No samples screened	First assay(S1)	Second assay(S2)
25,000	Murex VK 45/46	Ortho 2.0
31,700	Abbott 2.0	Murex VK 45/46
19,000	Ortho 2.0	UBI

Samples positive in any assay were tested by RIBA 2/3 and by PCR for HCV RNA, using primers to the conserved non-coding region.
Results: 223 samples (0.29%) were repeatably reactive in S1 assays, of which 37 (0.05%) were reactive in both S1 and S2. Of the 37, 28 were RIBA positive, 8 indeterminate, and 1 negative. Of the 186 samples which were reactive in S1 but not S2, none was RIBA positive, 53 were indeterminate, and 133 were negative. Most `indeterminates` reacted as single c22 or c100 bands in RIBA 2. RIBA 3 and PCR examination is ongoing.

0473

THE VALUE OF HCV-RNA DETECTION BY PCR FOR CONFIRMATION OF HCV-INFECTION. N. Lelie, T. Cuypers, H. Zaaijer, H. Reesink. Central Lab. Blood Transfusion Service, Amsterdam The Netherlands.

Objective: To determine the proportions of HCV-RNA positives among patients and donors with and without anti-HCV antibodies.

Methods: we determined the proportions of HCV-RNA positives according to their anti-HCV status in RIBA among the following populations: A) anti-HCV ELISA positive blooddonors, B) anti-HCV negative blooddonors with high ALT-values above 100 U/l, C) non-A,non-B hepatitis patients and D) hemophilia patients who had been treated with HCV unsafe clotting products in the past.

Results: Proportion HCV-RNA positive in relation to RIBA-result.

	negative	indeterminate	positive
A	0/426	11/754 (1.5%)	180/234 (77%)
B	0/86		
C	2/178 *	30/67 (45%)	372/428 (87%)
D	0/43	4/11 (36%)	178/214 (83%)

* One transplant and one AIDS-patient became anti-HCV negative. Futhermore in a lookback procedure we discovered a highly viremic HCV window donation that was implicated in a case of post-transfusion hepatitis C. 89% of HCV-RNA positive hemophilia patients and 48% of blooddonors had elevated ALT-values, whereas among HCV-RNA negative subjects with apparently resolved infection the proportions with elevated ALT-levels were not higher than those found in anti-HCV negative individuals.

Conclusion: In spite of earlier reported results (among others Sugatani et al; Lancet 1992:1:1018; M. Alter et al New Engl. J. Med. 1992:327: 1899) we did not observe HCV-RNA positive patients who were (persistently) anti-HCV negative. Our data indicate that the sensitivity of the 2nd and 3rd generation ELISAs is close to 100%. About one fifth of blooddonors and hemophilia patients manage to clear HCV-infection as indicated by negative HCV-RNA results and normal ALT-values. Application of HCV-RNA-PCR for confirmation of HCV-infection is necessary for careful counseling of blooddonors

0474

COMPARISON OF 5 NEW HCV IMMUNOBLOT ASSAYS.

H.Zaaijer,H.Vrielink,H.Cuypers,H.Reesink,P.v.Exel-Oehlers,P.Lelie.
Central Lab Blood Transfusion Service, Amsterdam, Netherlands.

Objective: Evaluation of 5 anti-HCV immunoblot assays.

Method: We determined sensitivity and specificity of the Riba-3 assay (Chiron); Liatek-III (Organon-Teknika); HCV Western blot (Murex); Matrix (Abbott) and HCV Blot-2 assay (Diagnostic Biotechnology) on 5 panels of samples:
panel A: Riba-2 indeterminate; HCV-RNA pos; n=31 donors/patients.
panel B: Riba-2 indeterminate; HCV-RNA neg; n=39 donors.
panel C: Riba-2 positive; HCV-RNA pos; n=48 donors and patients.
panel D: Abbott 2nd gen and Ortho 3rd gen EIA neg; n=31 donors.
panel E: 4 post-transfusion hepatitis C seroconversions (n=4x8).
For detection of HCV antibodies, all assays employ HCV core, NS3 and NS4 antigens. In addition Riba-3, Liatek-III and Murex include an NS5 antigen; Liatek-III additionally contains an E2/NS1 antigen.

Results:		Chiron Riba-2	Chiron Riba-3	Organon Liatek-III	Murex W.blot	Abbott Matrix	D.Biotec. Blot-2
A	sens:	0%	90%	94%	61%	55%	39%
B	specif:	0%	67%	77%	49%	15%	33%
C	sens:	100%	100%	100%	100%	96%	98%
D	specif:	n.a.	100%	97%	100%	100%	97%
E	sens:	n.a.	50%	47%	44%	44%	44%

In 6 samples in panel A, anti-NS5 reactivity was essential for a positive test result in 1 or 2 assays, but other assays found these samples to be positive without contribution of NS5. E2/NS1 reactivity was not essential for positive test results.

Conclusion: Liatek-III. Riba-3 and the Murex-blot assay resolved the majority of Riba-2 indeterminate samples (panel A and B). HCV antibody detection was not refined by additional 'new' HCV antigens (NS5, E2/NS1), but by improved classical HCV antigens (core, NS3, NS4). Replacement of the commonly used Riba-2 assay will resolve a high number of Riba-2 indeterminate test results.

0475

COMPARISON OF TWO 3D GENERATION ANTI-HCV RIBA VERSIONS IN RIBA-2 INDETERMINATE DONORS.

C.L. van der Poel[1], H. Vrielink[1], H.W. Reesink[1], H.L. Zaaijer[2], H.T.M. Cuypers[2], P.N. Lelie[2], S. Quan[3], A. Polito[3]. 1) Red Cross Blood Bank Amsterdam, 2) Central Lab RC Blood Transfusion Service Amsterdam, The Netherlands, 3) Chiron Corp, Emeryville CA, USA.

Objective: To compare 2 versions of 3d generation anti-HCV recombinant immunoblot (RIBA-3.0 and RIBA 3.5, Chiron) in RIBA-2 indeterminate blood donors.

Methods: RIBA-3.0 and -3.5 employ C22, C100 peptide and C33c, NS5 recombinant antigens, RIBA 3.5 employs modified C33c antigen. RIBA-2 indeterminate blood donors (n=103) were tested with RIBA-3.0 and -3.5 and cDNA-PCR (5'-UTR). All blood donors were interviewed with standardised protocols for risk factors.

Results:

RIBA-2 indet PCR -ve donors		RIBA-3.5 results		
RIBA-3.0	n	-ve	ind	+ve
-ve	66	61	5	0
ind	29	12	17	0
+ve	6	0	1	5
total	101	73	23	5

Of 2 RIBA-2 ind / PCR +ve donors, 1 was +ve, the other indeterminate in both 3d gen RIBA's.

Conclusion: RIBA-2 indeterminate / PCR negative donors were resolved as negative by RIBA-3.0 and -3.5 in respectively 66% and 73 % of the cases.

0476

DETECTION OF ANTI-HCV SEROCONVERSION WITH 3d GENERATION ASSAYS.

C.L. van der Poel[1], H. Vrielink[1], H.W. Reesink[1], H.T.M. Cuypers[2], P.N. Lelie[2], S. Quan[3], A. Polito[3]. 1) Red Cross Blood Bank Amsterdam, 2) Central Lab RC Blood Transfusion Service Amsterdam, The Netherlands, 3) Chiron Corp, Emeryville CA, USA.

Objective/Methods: Third generation HCV ELISA (ELISA-3, Ortho) and RIBA (RIBA-3.0, Chiron) were compared with ELISA-2 and RIBA-2 during seroconversion of 9 HCV infected (PCR +ve) recipients of blood. Serum samples, obtained before, and at regular intervals after transfusion were tested. To exclude passive antibody, sera were also tested in dilutions.

Results:

	Anti-HCV seroconversion in weeks after transfusion			
Recipient	ELISA (+ve)		RIBA (+ve)	
	2	3	2	3
R1	11	11	17	9
R2	8	8	13	13
R3	12	12	26	14
R4	20	20	-	25
R5	12	12	17	17
R6	23	12	26	26
R7	9	9	9	9
R8	12	12	-	-
R9	20	11	20	20

Conclusions: ELISA-3 and RIBA-3.0 are more sensitive than ELISA-2 and RIBA-2 in early HCV infection.

0477

COMPARATION OF THE METHODS : RIBA HCV 3 AND MATRIX HCV.

J. R .Villanueva[1], J. M .M. de Segovia[1], M. Ferreiro[1] A. Aguilera[2] . [1] Hospital Provincial Pontevedra. [2]Hospital Xeral de Galicia. Spain.

Two confirmatory methods RIBA HCV 3 and MATRIX HCV were compared with serum panels.

AIM and METHODS : 63 samples were tested for Anti-HCV ELISA 2 (Abbott) , RIBA 3 (Ortho) before, MATRIX HCV assay was performed.

A: Samples were reactive in HCV ELISA and RIBA 3 nonreactive (NON SPECIFIC).

B: Samples were nonreactive in HCV ELISA with AB/CO 0,5-1 (NON REACTIVE).

C: Samples were reactive in HCV ELISA and RIBA 3 (REACTIVE).

RESULTS:

	HCV ELISA AB/CO	RIBA 3	MATRIX HCV NR	IND	R
NON SPECIFIC n=16	>1	N.R. : 16	8	8	0
		IND. : 0	0	0	0
		R. : 0	0	0	0
NONREACTIVE n=18	0,5-1	N.R. : 0	0	0	0
		IND. : 11	2	8	1
		R. : 7	1	3	3
REACTIVE n=18	>1	N.R.: 0	0	0	0
		IND. : 13	3	7	3
		R. : 16	0	3	13

n=12	1	2	1	1	2	4	1
RIBA 3	IND.	IND.	R.	R.	N.R.	N.R.	IND.
MATRIX	R.	N.R.	IND.	N.R.	N.R.	IND.	IND.
P.C.R.	-	-	-	-	-	-	-
HCV IgM	-	-	-	-	-	-	-

CONCLUSION: The method RIBA 3 is more specific and more sensitive than MATRIX HCV.

0478

PATTERN OF ANTIBODIES REACTION AGAINST HEPATITIS C VIRUS IMMUNOBLOT ANTIGENS AMONG BRAZILIAN BLOOD DONORS

Parise, E.[1]; Wendel, S.[1,2]; Biagini, S.[1] and Batemarchi, M.V.[2]
1- Hospital Sirio-Libanês - Blood Bank - São Paulo, Brazil
2- Centro de Imunologia e Imunogenética - São Paulo, Brazil

From a total of 10.300 blood donors, 138 (1,34%) had their blood repeatedly reactive for 2nd generation Anti-HCV tests. Frozen samples from these donors were further tested by immunoblot for HCV (Inno-Lia, Innogenetics, Belgium) and 39 (28,3%) of them were considered as negative, 22 (15,9%) as indeterminated and 77 (55,8%) as positive. The positive samples were divided into two groups according to the ALT level, with the cut-off value >75IU/L (1,5 times greater than upper normal value). These samples were also tested against Anti-HBc. The percentual of positive reactions against each immunoblot antigens are shown in the table below.

PATTERN		n	NS4	NS5	C1	C2	C3	C4
			BAND					
	Indeterminated	22	18%	36%	45%	23%	4%	0%
	Positive + ALT >75UI/L	32	81%*	81%	84%	97%	84%	81%
	Positive + ALT <75UI/L	45	53%	67%	73%	93%	71%	69%

(*) = p <0,01, comparing both positive groups

No donor from the indeterminated group was also positive for Anti-HBc or elevated ALT. On the other hand, Anti-HBc was found in 18 (23,4%) HCV positive donors, with 34% (n= 11) in those with elevated ALT and 15,5% (n= 7) in the normal ALT group (p= 0,06). Among those donors Anti-HBc(+) / HCV(+) 94% showed reactivity against NS5 band, with only 66% in the Anti-HBc negative samples (p <0,01). In addition, Anti-HBc seems to be more prevalent in these donors than in historical controls (mean prevalence= 10,2%)[1].

We conclude that in donors HCV(+), Anti-NS4 seems to be more prevalent in those with ALT >75UI/L and that Anti-NS5 is linked with Anti-HBc(+)/HCV(+) donors, whereas Anti-C4 (core) is not found in the indeterminated group.

REFERENCE

1- Wendel, S. et al. - Rev Paul Med 109: 77-83, 1991

0479

SCREENING OF BLOOD DONORS FOR ANTI-HCV WITH AN ASSAY INCLUDING NS5 ANTIGEN

M. Senn, J.J. Burckhardt
ZLB Central Laboratory, Blood Transfusion Service SRC, Berne, Switzerland

The Central Laboratory employed in 1993 the Murex anti-HCV test, which includes a recombinant protein from the NS5 region. This offered the unique opportunity to find NS5-reactive donor samples in a previously NS5 unscreened population. We selected 100 subsequently screening repeat reactive (RR) donor samples, tested them with the Wellcozyme HCV Westernblot (WB) and determined HCV-RNA by nested PCR.

ALAT normal	elevat.	WB indet.	positive	PCR negative	positive
87		71		68	3
			16	2	14
	13	1		1	0
			12	2	10
50	1	51 NS5 only		51	0

87 anti-HCV RR donors presented with a normal ALAT value (male ≤ 70, female ≤ 50 U/L). Among all 100 RR was a significant correlation between a positive WB and positive PCR (X^2=68). In 24 of the 28 WB positive samples was HCV-RNA detectable. All 51 "NS5 only" samples were PCR negative. Thus, donor screening without NS5 antigens missed few, if any, potentially infectious units in our blood supply.

0480

IMPROVEMENT IN DETECTION OF HEPATITIS C VIRUS ANTIBODIES BY NEW SUPPLEMENTAL ASSAYS.

M.Macrì,[1], R.Colucci[1], E.Perna[2] and S.Formisano[2].
[1] Transfusion Service - Foligno , Italy
[2]Immunohematology-Medical School University "Federico II" Naples

Objective: The purpose of this study was to evaluate the performance of the new assays for the supplemental investigation of anti-HCV antibodies in blood donors sera.

Methods: We selected 35 anti-HCV antibody ELISA reactive samples based on reactivity to Recombinant Immuno Blot Assay (RIBA 2.0). The samples were then assayed with the new RIBA 3.0 SIA (Ortho), MATRIX (Abbott), and DECISCAN (S.Pasteur), according to the recommended protocols. The samples selected were single antibody band present (n.23), two band present (n.8) and all band present (n.4) on RIBA 2.0 .

Results: RIBA 3.0 results showed a significant improvement in sensitivity as 56% of samples indeterminate by RIBA 2.0 became reactive and 17% no-reactive by the new test. The 34% of samples indeterminate by RIBA 2.0 became reactive and 8% no-reactive by MATRIX; the 69% of samples indeterminate by RIBA 2.0 became reactive and the 17% no-reactive by DECISCAN (see Table).

Table. RIBA 2.0 Indeterminate Samples (n=23)

	Reactive	No-reactive	Indeterminate
RIBA 3.0	13 (56%)	4 (17%)	6 (27%)
MATRIX	8 (34%)	2 (8%)	13 (56%)
DECISCAN	16(69%)	4 (17%)	3 (14%)

The 74% of single C-22 band present indeterminate samples became reactive by the new tests; the samples wich were no-reactive on new tests had weak reactions on 5-1-1 and C-100 on RIBA 2.0.

Conclusion: The new supplemental assays are more sensitive and more specific tests than their predecessors. The data suggest that the additional information provided by new supplemental assays may be useful for counseling donors at low risk for HCV exposure and who have tested as repeatedly reactive in an anti-HCV screening test.

0481

COMPARISON BETWEEN SECOND AND THIRD GENERATION ANTI-HCV EIA ASSAYS APPLIED TO BLOOD DONORS.

U.Margraff, Chr.François-Gérard, B.Donéa, D.Sondag-Thull
Immuno-Hématologie et CTS de Liège, Belgium.

OBJECTIVE: To evaluate a third generation enzyme immunoassay (EIA3) for Hepatitis C virus (HCV) antibodies in parallel with the previously available second generation test (EIA2) in blood donors (BD).
SERIES: Serum samples from 5040 volunteer BD, collected between 20/09/93 and 13/10/93 at the Blood Transfusion Centre of Liège.
METHODS: Fresh serum samples were simultaneously screened with both EIA2 and EIA3 HCV assays (ABBOTT GmbH, Germany). Complementary testing of repeatedly reactive samples (Test Ratio > 0.80) was realized by using Matrix HCV 2.0 immunodot assay (ABBOTT).
RESULTS:

Screening		Rate		MATRIX HCV 2.0		
EIA3	EIA2	N	%	Neg	SAR *	R**
+	+	6	0.12	1	1	4
+	-	21	0.42	9	12	0
-	+	0	0			
-	-	5013	99.46	nt	nt	nt

** SAR = Single antigen reactivity* *** R = Reactive*

CONCLUSION: When considering SAR as a specific HCV antibody reactivity, the EIA3 specificity is 99.80% and the seroprevalence (SP) of HCV antibodies in Belgian BD is 0.33%. Whereas when considering R as the only True Positive, the EIA3 test specificity is 99.54% and the SP, 0.10%. In 1991, the SP in Belgian BD with 1st gen EIA was 0.55%. In 1993, the SP with 3 rd gen EIA was found to be between 0.10 and 0.33%.

0482

CONFIRMATION OF HEPATITIS C VIRUS ANTIBODY IN BLOOD DONORS. COMPARISON OF TWO IMMUNOBLOT ASSAYS.

C. Politis, Cl. Tsiolkas and Cl. Richardson.
Hellenic Red Cross Blood Transfusion Center Athens Greece.

Immunoblot assays are universably used for confirmation of screening assays for antibodies against HCV (anti-HCV). However, the interpretation of indeterminate results remain as a problem. In this study we evaluated two immunoblot assays, the Chiron RIBA HCV Test System Strip Immunoblot Assays 2.0 (RIBA-2) and the Abbott MATRIX HCV. We tested 21 blood donor samples repeatetly reactive with Abbott HCV EIA-2. The results of the study are showed in table 1.

		MATRIX POS	MATRIX NEG	MATRIX IND	TOTAL
	POS	17	0	0	17
	NEG	0	1	0	1
RIBA-2	IND	1	0	2	3
	TOTAL	18	1	2	21

The distribution of the HCV antibody patterns was with RIBA-2 71%, 76%, 81%, and 95% for the antigens C22-3, C33-c, 5-1-1 and C100-3 respectively and with MATRIX 90%, 86%, 86% and 81% for the core, NS-3, NS-4 (yeast) and NS-4 (E. Coli) respectively.
Conclusion: The overall aggrement of RIBA-2 and MATRIX is 95%. One sample was confirmed to be positive with MATRIX but remained indeterminate with RIBA-2. It is postulated that both assays are rebiable supplemental tests for confirming anti-HCV reactivity in blood donors.

0483

INDETERMINATE HEPATITIS C IN BLOOD DONORS

M. da Silva Cardoso, K. Koerner, K. Siemoneit, S. Epple, B. Kubanek
German Red Cross Blood Bank Ulm and Department of Transfusion Medicine, University of Ulm, FRG

In an attempt to establish the prevalence of HCV-RNA positive in the recombinant immunoblot assay RIBA-2 indeterminate donations, we submitted all 124 RIBA indeterminates out of 292 ELISA-2 (Ortho) positive samples (42,5%) to HCV RT/PCR. These positive samples were obtained after screening 52,124 donors for HCV-antibodies. The PCR protocol is based on the use of two sets of nested primers: one set for the 3' non-coding and one for the core region. From the 124 indeterminate samples, 58 (46.8%) showed reactivity to c-100-3, 57 (46%) to c-22, 7 (5.6%) to c33c and finally 2 (1.6%) to 5-1-1. HCV-RNA could be found in 15.5% of the c-100-3 positive subgroup and in 14% of the c-22 positive subgroup. Due to the extremely low number of samples positive to c33c or 5-1-1 we could not establish the prevalence of HCV-RNA positive in these subgroups.
Our result suggests that reactivity in RIBA II to either c-100-3 or the c-22 alone have the same predictable value for HCV infection in blood donors. This contrasts with data from high risk populations, where c-22 seems to be a better marker than c-100-3.

0484

MULTICENTRIC QUALITY CONTROL OF HEPATITIS C VIRUS RNA POLYMERASE CHAIN REACTION (PCR)

J.J.Lefrère* for the French Study Group for the Standardization of Hepatitis C virus PCR
***INTS, hôpital St-Antoine, Paris, France.**

Nine French laboratories initiated multicentric quality control study to assess and to improve the specificity and sensitivity of their procedures of PCR for detection of HCV RNA. The study was performed in three rounds, based on coded panels consisting of positive controls (anti-HCV +) and of negative controls (anti-HCV -). For the first panel, each laboratory followed its own PCR procedure : 100% sensitivity was observed in 2 laboratories, 100% specificity in 7 laboratories. For the second panel, all laboratories were required to use both their personal procedure and a consensus procedure established from that of the laboratories which provided the best results on the first panel. This common procedure was a nested PCR performed with primer pairs in 5' non coding region. Results were analysed by electrophoresis on 2% agarose gel containing BET. With personal procedure, 100% sensitivity was observed in 5 laboratories and 100% specificity in all. With common procedure, 100% sensitivity was observed in all but one, and 100% specificity in all. False results were more often observed with personal primers than with primers of common procedure.The third panel included 3 positive samples with 4 successive dilutions. For 2 samples, 8/8 laboratories had positive signals until the 1/100 dilution and discrepant results beyond this dilution; for the third sample, the signals were more discrepant. Conclusions : The results show that the variability of both sensitivity and specificity was strongly reduced in the second round for which all laboratories used the same PCR procedure. The results also indicate that optimization and standardization of PCR may help laboratories to improve their procedure.

0485

CONFIRMATORY TESTS IN RIBA-2 INDETERMINATED BLOOD DONORS SAMPLES

Jorge Pereira; Isabel Neves; Fátima Nascimento
Centro Regional de Sangue de Lisboa. IPS
Lisboa, Portugal

In Portugal we discard all blood units with anti-HCV positive by EIA, not taking in consideration the results of the confirmatory tests.

The blood donors with confirmatory tests positives are informed about the results, they are not admitted for further donations and they are instructed to consult an hepatic diseases doctor.

In what concerns the blood donors with indeterminated results in confirmatory tests, we have been studing 41 blood samples of donors RIBA-2 indeterminated using four differents confirmatory tests: RIBA-3 (Ortho), Matrix (Abbott), Western Blot (Murex), Liatek (Organon).

When these different tests are employed 41.5 to 48.8% of the samples are positives, 12.2 to 29.3% are negatives and 26.8 to 41.5% remain indeterminated.

RIBA-3 and Liatek have showed us 70% of positivity in indeterminated samples with anti-C22 and all of them show only 0 to 10% of positivity with anti-C100.

We conclued that in spite of the high percentage of positivity (41.5 -48%) only ten samples (24.4%) are positives simultaneously with the four tests.

RIBA-3 gives a great percentage of positive results when the samples are anti-C22 or C33 and 90% become negative when the samples are anti-C100, in second RIBA generation

0486

PREVALENCE OF ANTI-HTLV-I/II IN THE BLOOD DONOR POPULATION OF MARTINIQUE

R. CESAIRE, O. BERA, B. KEROB-BAUCHET, H. MAIER, K. OULD AMAR, CDTS Fort-de-France (Martinique.FWI)

OBJECTIVE

To determine the prevalence of anti-HTLV-I/II in the blood donor population of Martinique, an endemic area for HTLV infection.

METHODS

7500 blood donors were included in the study. The antibodies anti-HTLV-I/II were screened by ELISA technique (PLATELIA HTLV-I NEW - Sanofi Diagnostics Pasteur). The confirmation was performed by Western Blot :Cambridge Biotech or Diagnostic Biotechnology.

RESULTS

Out of the total testing, the initial and repeat ELISA positive rates were respectively 1.47% and 1.35%. A confirmed 0.53% positive rate and a 59% indeterminate Western Blot rate were seen.

Moreover, the seroprevalence increased with the age of donors, especially after 50 years (1.7%). In addition, we noted that the frequency of positive serologies for the new donors was 0.64 %.

CONCLUSION

Five years after the systematic screening of anti-HTLV-I/II antibodies in the French West Indies (january 1st 1989), the prevalence of anti-HTLV-I/II antibodies in Martinique blood donors remain high, in particular for older blood donors.

The levels of HTLV-I/II seroprevalence are inferior to the ones observed with anterior studies (2% in 1987) including the new donors.

This can be explained by the modification of confirmation criteria (French SNTS retrovirus group), the improvement of the specificity of the techniques and the reinforcement of predonation selection.

0487

"SCREENING FOR ANTI-HUMAN T-LYMPHOTROPIC VIRUS ANTIBODY IN BLOOD DONORS POPULATION OF SPOLETO"

F.Tripaldi, A.Esposito, A.M.Di Virgilio, M.R.Briguori, A.Fulvi, F.De Motoli.
Blood Bank, Spoleto, Italy.

OBJECTIVE: to evaluate the prevalence of antibodies of anti-Human T-lymphotropic virus I/II in periodic blood donors population of Spoleto.

MATERIAL AND METHODS: from the 1st of August 1992 to the 30st November 1993 in 2635 period blood donors of Spoleto (639 females and 1996 males, average years 40 +/- 2 for males and 38,5 +/- for females) the prevalence of antibodies to HTLV I/II virus was studied Antibodies to HTLV I/II were screened by Elisa HTLV I/II(Alfabiotech S.p.A.).

RESULTS: 13 (0,49%) periodic blood donors, 12 males and 1 female, were repeatedly positives to screening for HTLV I/II Ab; of 13 anti-HTLV I/II positive reactions, 4 (3 males and 1 female) was positives (of 3 males, 2 for HTLV I and 1 for HTLV II, and 1 female for HTLV II), 6 indefinite and 3 negative to Western blot assay. The real prevalence of HTLV I/II Ab in periodic blood donors was 0,15% (4/2635).

CONCLUSIONS: the presence of HTLV I and HTLV II infection within periodic donors population, evidentiated by these data, suggest the search of a economical, ethic and scientific solution whether introduce or not this test as screening for blood donors population.

0488

IDENTIFICATION AND MAPPING OF NEUTRALING EPITOPES OF HUMAN T-CELL LYMPHOTROPIC VIRUS TYPE-I BY USING HUMAN ANTIBODIES

Y.W.Inoue, H. Shiraki, H. Sato and Y. Maeda
Fukuoka Red Cross Blood Center, Fukuoka, Japan

We identified and mapped the region responsible for neutralization in the human T-cell lymphotropic virus type-I (HTLV-I) structural proteins.

We obtained 18 kinds of site-specific antibody (2 in the p19 gag, 10 in the gp46 env and 6 in the gp21 env proteins) from seropositive human plasma by means of an affinity chromatography coupled with the synthetic peptides corresponding to the antigenic regions of the HTLV-I structural proteins. These antibodies were highly specific in the ELISA using synthetic peptides as an antigen. We examined the neutralizing activity of site-specific antibodies for its inhibitory efect against syncytium formation induced by co-cultivation of 8C cells with KT_{252}, T-cell line established from ATL patient.

The inhibitory activity of each antibody was determined by the IgG concentration having 50% inhibition in the syncytium formation assay with serially diluted antibodies. Two antibodies recognized the sequence amino acids 89 to 115 and 175 to 199 of the gp46 protein have potent inhibitory activity in syncytium formation assay.

The antibodies derived from the p19 gag protein, gp21 env protein and the sero-negative plasma used as the control showed no significant activity.

These observations suggest that the middle region corresponding to amino acids 89 to 199 of the gp46 env protein participates in the cell-to-cell infection with HTLV-I.

0489

PREVALENCE OF ANTI-HCV AND ANTI-HTLV-I/II ANTIBODIES IN CURAÇAO.

H. Vrielink[1], M. Woerdeman[1], C.L. van der Poel[1], H.W. Reesink[1], C. Winkel[2], PN Lelie[3], 1)Red Cross Blood Bank Amsterdam, 2)Blood Bank St. Elisabeth Hospital, Curaçao, 3)Central Lab Blood Transfusion Service, Amsterdam, The Netherlands.

Aim: To assess the prevalence of anti-HCV and anti-HTLV-I/II antibodies in blood donors in Curaçao.

Methods: All donations (n=7,614) (March 1991 to November 1992) were screened with HCV ELISA (Ortho Diagnostics) and with HTLV-I/II ELISA (Murex Diagnostics). ELISA positive samples were confirmed by RIBA-2 (Ortho) for anti-HCV antibodies and by Western Blot (Diagnostic Biotechnology) for anti-HTLV-I/II antibodies.

Results: 45/7,614 (0.6%) were anti-HCV and 98/7,614 (1.3%) were anti-HTLV-I/II ELISA positive.

ELISA +ve		Immunoblot confirmation			
		+ve		ind	
		n	(%)	n	(%)
HCV	(n=45)	6	(13)	22	(49)
HTLV-I/II	(n=98)	84	(86)*	14	(14)

*]72/84 (86%) were anti-HTLV type I, 0/84 was type II and 12/84 (14%) were double reactive for HTLV-I and HTLV-II.

Conclusions: The prevalence of confirmed anti-HCV and anti-HTLV-I/II antibodies in blood donors in Curaçao was 0.1% and 1.1% respectively. No blood donors with exclusively anti-HTLV-II antibodies were found.

0490

PREVALENCE OF ANTI-HTLVI IN BLOOD DONORS OF BASQUE COUNTRY.

M.A.Pérez[1], M.A.Vesga[1], M.Monasterio[2], J.M.Cárdenas[2], A.Renovales[3], M.A.Basaldua[3].
1.Centro Vasco de Transfusión. 2.Banco de Sangre de Guipúzcoa. 3.Banco de Sangre de Alava. Spain.

During last year we have studied 7776 blood donors of several regions of Basque Country to know the prevalence of antibodies to HTLVI virus.
The samples were screened for HTLV antibodies with ABBOTT HTLV-I EIA (Abbott Laboratories) (n= 6524) and BIOELISA HIV-1+2 + HTLV-I+II EIA (n= 1252).
ELISA repeteadly reactive samples were confirmed by Western Blot (Diagnostic Biotechnology) and radioimmunoprecipitation assay (RIPA).
Of 7776 blood donors, 8 (0.10%) were reactives repeteadly to ELISA screening. Of these 8, 7 were indeterminate to Western Blot assay (5 to p24, 2 to p19) and all of them were negative to RIPA.

In conclusion, in our blood donor population we have no found any positive result. Provided we have found some HTLV positive results in our intravenous drug abuser population it is necessary to continue studying the epidemiology of HTLV I-II in our blood donor population.

0491

HTLV I/II SEROPREVALENCE IN BLOOD DONORS OF PIEDMONT (NORTH ITALY) AND IN SUBJECTS AT RISK

D. Testa(1), G.M. Peano(2)
(1)Servizio di Immunoematologia e Trasfusionale di Savigliano (CN) e di (2) Cuneo, Italy.

The purpose of the study was to value the presence of HTLV I/II virus in a sample of blood donors of our geographic area and in a group of subjects at risk. We evaluated 4821 blood donors belonging to our Transfusional Services; 175 HCV positive and 83 HIV positive subjects; 37 polytransfused patients.We used as screening test Abbott HTLV-I Eia and Retro-Tek HTLV-I Elisa Medical Systems. Reactive sera with a kit were tested with the other one and those repeatedly reactive were studied with a confirmatory test (WB,Ripa,Matrix). Among blood donors 15 (0,3%) were positive to screening test (7 only with one of two tests,8 with both); at confirmatory test 6 were negative,9 indeterminate (single reactivities to p19,p24 p53 antigens). Among HCV positive subjects nobody was positive to the screening test. Conversely 2 HIV positive subjects and 1 polytransfused was positive with high "ratio" values: all they were confirmed positive, but for HTLV-II. Our data are reassuring with regard to HTLV-I circulation among our blood donors and among subjects at risk, even if is difficult to understand the meaning of indeterminate results. More inusual is the positivity for HTLV-II in the polytransfused patient.

0492

HTLV1/2-Ab IN PATIENTS AT HIGH RISK FOR TRANSFUSION TRANSMITTED INFECTIONS

C.MAZZEI,M.A.VERATTI*,G.CAVAGNARO
G.BARBERIS,F.NOTARIS, G.IMBERCIADORI
C.Trasfusionale Osp. S.Corona Pietra Ligure
*C. Trasfusionale Osp. A.Pugliese-Catanzaro

While blood and blood products are tested for HBsAg, VDRL, HCVAb, HIV1/2-Ab in Italy, screening for HTLV1/2-Ab is not suggested. In this study we evaluated prevalence of HTLV1/2-Ab in a group of polytransfused patients , from different area of Italy (North and South Italy).Sera from 182 patients (100 with Thalassemia, 42 with hemofilia,40 affected by other hematological diseases) were screened in EIA for HTLV1-Ab (Abbott),HTLV2-Ab(Olimpus),and reactivities expressed as C.I. (Cut-off Index):

C. I.	HTLV1-Ab	HTLV2-Ab
0.000 - 0.300	112	114
0.301 - 0.600	62	56
0.601 - 0.900	8	12
> 0.901	–	–

We didn't find significant reactivities for HTLV1-2-Ab in , our patients.Data confirm that viruses don't circulate also in donors whose blood was utilized for their transfusional needs.On the other hand , we cannot exclude that removal of leucocytes by filtering blood protected patients [illegible] transmission of viruses.

0493

ANTI-HTLV1/2 ANTIBODIES IN VARIOUS SUBIECTS GROUPS.

S. Barbante, A. Rughetti.
Blood Bank and Trasfusion Service,
General Hospital, Rieti, Italy.

It had been demonstrated that blood-trasfusion and its components is an efficacious means of HTLV-1/2 infection trasmission. In fact antibodies had been demonstrated in subjects that had been taken blood and/or its components by blood-donors anti HTLV-1/2 positives. Sera of 39 at risk subjects, 42 politransfused patients, 61 in haemodialysis patients and samples of 2204 blood-donors were tested for the presence of antibodies to HTLV-1/2 with Elisa method. The sera repeteadly positive was confirmed by two Western Blot (W.B.) method. Any politransfused patients and any in haemodialysis patients were repeteadly reactive. One at risk subject resulted indeterminate by W.B.(only band p24).Of the 11 chance blood-donors repeteadly reactive, 3 of them resulted indeterminate and I showed positive to band p24 and rgp21 by W. B.. Of the 16 sera repeteadly reactive periodic donors, 8 of them were indeterminate and 1 was reactive to band p19 and rgp21. The second kit W.B. gived discordant results as no one samples had specific band rgp46-1/2. Is confirmed the high number of indeterminates with reactivity for the band rgp21.

0494

PREVALENCE OF HTLV 1/2 ANTIBODY REACTION IN BAVARIAN BLOOD DONORS

W. Weise*, C. Fleischer+, C. Kücherer+, P. Michel*, G Pauli+

* Blood Transfusion Service, BRC, Munich, FRG
+ AIDS-Center, Berlin, FRG

Beside of HIV 1/2 the human lymphotropic virus type 1 and 2 (HTLV 1/2) are additional retroviruses known to be transmissible by blood transfusion. While routine screening for HTLV 1/2 antibodies is recommanded in USA, France and Netherlands in Germany this test is done volontary. In a preliminary study 1989/90 the Blood Transfusion Service of Bavarian Red Cross analysed 0.07 % repeated reactive HTLV samples against HTLV by ELISA. 0.02 % of these samples have shown positive results in Westernblot and/or RIPA, while 0.05 % were indeterminated. In a following investigation in 1991 till 1993 we tested about 600 000 blood donors. Out of them 2741 were repeated reactive in ELISA (0.004 %). More than 500 sera have been tested in Westernblot. All of them were reactive for unless internal protein (343 = 61.8 % with p19; 63 = 13.2 % with p24) or more rare with recombinant envelope protein rgp 21 (3 = 0.54 %). These samples have been classified as indeterminated. The reported prevalence of HTLV 1/2 in our blood donor population represents the epidemiological situation in Bavaria and gives the opportunity to interpret the various indeterminated reactions.

0495

ANTI-HIV PREVALENCE AND EPIDEMIOLOGIC DATA IN FRENCH BLOOD DONORS

P. MAISONNEUVE, AM COUROUCE and the Retrovirus Study Group of the French Society of Blood Transfusion - FRANCE

Blood Transfusion Centers involved in the Retrovirus Study Group are collecting an average of 1 million blood donations a year. Their data concerning anti-HIV positive donations are :

Year	Number		Prevalence per 1.000 blood donations			Anti -HBc
	HIV1	HIV2	Total	First-time	Regular	%
1987	356	5	0.319	1.45	0.097	60
1988	176	0	0.165	0.92	0.052	50
1989	124	2	0.118	0.56	0.053	41
1990	105	3	0.104	0.43	0.044	35
1991	105	1	0.090	0.38	0.040	36
1992	64	1	0.059	0.25	0.028	29
1993 (6months)	31	0	0.058	0.23	0.030	29

Sex ratio was close to 5 until 1989, 3.5 in 1990-1991 and 5.5 in 1992 ; age was below 30 in more than 45% ; homo and bisexual men still represent the major transmission group.

Conclusion : HIV prevalence was six-fold lower in 1993 than in 1987. HIV2-infected subjects represent 1.4% of the total anti-HIV positive blood donations. No change in the sex ratio and risk group was observed in the recent years.

0496

SEROPREVALENCE OF HIV1 ANTIBODIES IN BLOOD DONORS

G.Isacchi, V.Filoni, T.Bighiani, A.Roccetti, L.Piro.
Department Human Biopathology, Transfusion Center University "La Sapienza" of Rome.

We evaluate the prevalence of HIV1 in blood from established (ED) or occasional donors (OD), tested by ELISA technique and confirmed to be positive by W.B. analysis, over the period January 1,1991 - March 31,1993. 62700 blood units from 50681 subjects we screened ; 22960 of them were OD, whereas the remaining 27721 were ED. 1,24 control/year were performed for each donor. Only 74 blood samples (out of 62700) were positive at the time of the second ELISA test, which corresponds to 0,12%. When 54 donor sera were re-examinated according to our protocol, only 47 resulted ELISA positive to HIV1. The W.B. provided us with 28 negative results (17 ED and 11 OD), 8 positive results (6 ED and 2 OD) and 11 undefined results (8 ED and 3 OD). The percentage of positive results is 0,013% if we consider the blood units (8 out of 62700) and 0,016% about the blood donors (8 out of 50681). The positive results account for by 0,02% and 0,009% in ED and OD, respectively. As for the W.B. undefined results, their percentage appears to be similar to that observed for the positive results: 0,017% total, 0,028% for the ED and 0,013% for the OD. These data confirm the necessity of a routinely control and follow-up of blood donors.

0497

ANNUAL INCIDENCE OF HIV SEROPOSITIVITY IN A COHORT OF IVDUs FOLLOWED 7 YEARS

S.Ciaffoni[1], F.Schiesari[1], F. Lugoboni[2], P.Mezzelani[3].
1 Blood Transfusion Service, Bussolengo (Verona)
2 Center for Drug Addicts, Bussolengo (Verona)
3Institute of Clinica Medica, University of Verona ITALY

Objective. To evalue annual incidence of HIV seroconversions in a cohort of Intravenous Drug Users (IVDUs) followed 7 years.
Methods.We studied (in ELISA and Western-Blot) 84 IVDUs that were all seronegative in 1985 and we followed up to 1993. All IVDUs enrolled in this study were voluntary.In 1985 the HIV seropositivity in Verona area was very low (12%).
Results.The results are shown in table

years	85	86	87	88	89	90	91	92	93
n.IVDUs	84	75	65	57	52	48	43	32	21
% in follow up		89.3	78.3	69.5	65	60.8	56.6	42.7	29.2
n.seroconversions	0	0	0	0	1	2	0	0	0
n.IVDUs died	0	1	1	2	0	1	1	3	0

It's important to note that the IVDUs died or seroconverted are not in the sequent number of seroconversion or in % of follow up. Pearl's index (seroconversions/100 years of observation) is 0.77.
Conclusions. We have found two very important results in our study : the low incidence of seroconversion and the high percent of IVDUs who were been in follow up during theese years. Both theese conlusions show that the compliance to our follow up in IVDUs has been very high.

0498

LACK OF HIV SEROCONVERSIONS AMONG INJECTING DRUG USERS PARTICIPATING IN A HEPATITIS B VACCINATION STUDY

S. Ciaffoni[1], G.L. Bovo[1], F. Schiesari[1], N. Pauletto[1], F. Lugoboni[2], P. Mezzelani[3].
1 Blood Transfusion Service, Bussolengo (Verona)
2 Center for Drug Addicts, Bussolengo (Verona)
3Institute of Clinica Medica, University of Verona ITALY

Objective. To assess HIV seroconversions among injecting drug users in a hepatitis B vaccination program.
Methods. An HBV vaccination program was offered to 185 HBV and HIV negative injecting drug users attending the Center for Drug Addicts n. 26 of the Veneto Region of Italy. Among them 162 accepted and 31 declined. Both groups were followed over time and tested for at least twice for HIV with a mean of 5,3 tests over 4252 person-months for the vaccination group and a mean of 3,5 tests in 887 person-months for the non-vaccination group.
HIV seroprevalence is approximately 10% among injecting drug users in the district.
Results. 93% of the HBV vaccination group successfully completed the vaccinations. None of the vaccination group seroconverted for HIV during follow up compared to 4 of the non-vaccination group (5.4/100 persons-years at risk) ($p<.02$ by exact binomial test). Seven HBV seroconversions occurred in non-vaccination group.
Conclusions. There are excellent adherence to the vaccination protocol and the vaccination program, along with frequent HIV testing and counseling, appears to have lowered HIV risk behavior. This suggest that ethical testing of HIV vaccines should be possible with high risk subjects.

0499

IS INCORRECT USE OF CONDOM A MAJOR RISK OF HIV INFECTION?

T. Nuchprayoon[1], C. Nuchprayoon[2], T. Chuni-akjaraki[1]; 1. Dept. of Prev. and Soc. Med. Faculty of Med., Chulalongkorn Univ.
2. Nat. Blood Centre, Thai Red Cross Society (RCS), Bangkok, Thailand

Due to the policy of the National Blood Centres, Thai RCS to screen all donors blood for HIV-ab and HIV-ag, an unmatched case-control study was carried out during Jan. 1992 - May 1993 to study sex behavior and incorrect use of condom among male donors. 298 male pos. HIV-ab donors who ever used condom during sexual intercourse were cases, while 625 neg. anti-HIV were randomly chosen as controls. The history on sex behavior and technique of using condom was collected by questionaires. The study revealed that the ones who had sex contact other than wife had 5.9 x the risk of HIV infection to those who had sex contact only with his wife. In singles who were homo-sexuals, bisexuals and heterosexuals had 8.34, 6.93 and 4.72 x respectively the risk of HIV infection compared to singles who did not have sexual contact. The frequency of contact with prostitutes ever once per month gave the risk of HIV infection 7.8 x of those who had sex only with his wife. The incorrect use of condom showed significantly higher risk for HIV infection.

0500

EFFECTS ON VIROLOGICAL PARAMETERS OF PASSIVE IMMUNOTHERAPY BASED ON INFUSIONS OF PLASMAS RICH IN ANTI-p24 ANTIBODIES IN AIDS PATIENTS

Joubert L(1), Chevret S(2), Vittecoq D(3), Lefrere JJ(1) and the Passive Immunotherapy Collaborative Study Group
(1)Hôpital St-Antoine (2)Hôp.St-Louis (3)Hôp.Paul Brousse

Objectives: To study the biological effects of passive immunotherapy in AIDS on usual virological parameters.
Patients and methods: 82 CDC IV patients were included in a double blind phase II trial and randomized between 2 groups: infusions of plasma rich in anti-p24 antibody (HIV+P) or standard seronegative plasma (HIV-P). Each patient received infusion every 14 days over a one-year period and every 28 days beyond. p24 antigen (ag) titer was quantified through monoclonal assay (Abbott) before and after immune complex dissociation (ICD); the specificity of the low + result (<30 pg/mL) was confirmed by a neutralization assay. Anti-p24 antibody (ab) titer was determined (Abbott)
Results: Among the 46 patients positive for p24 ag before inclusion, p24 ag was found negative in 100 % of treated patients in a median delay of 77 days, vs in 24 % of controls in a median delay not reached at 1091 days ($p=0.0001$,log-rank). The reapparance of a positive p24 ag was less frequent in treated patients (19%) than in controls (50 %); among the 54 patients positive for ICD-p24, p24 ag was found negative in 52 % of treated patients in a median delay of 310 days vs 17 % of controls (median not reached) ($p=0.006$, log-rank). Anti-p24 titers were negative or weak in most controls while treated patients had a titer variable according to both the ab titer of HIV+P and the ag p24 of recipients.
Conclusion: the negative p24 ag without ICD observed in all treated patients reflects a complexation with ab; the results observed with ICD-ag assay suggest that this decrease of ag in treated group could also be due to a slower release of ag.

0501

"TRANSIENT" ANTI-HIV-1 SEROPOSITIVITY

Transfusion Safety Study Group[1] represented by M.J.Nowicki[2], T.F. Unger[3]
1Participating institutions, 2Univ. Southern California, Los Angeles, 3Miragen, Irvine, CA, USA.

Background: Short-lived anti-HIV-1 and/or HIV-1 PCR positivity has been reported, but may be due to handling errors (*JAMA* 1993;269:2876).
Aim: To evaluate cases of "transient" seropositivity.
Methods: In follow-up of 2,905 subjects, 7 otherwise anti-HIV-1 (-) persons had an unexplained, repeatably (+) serum on a single visit. For 6, we had plasma and frozen cells separated in a different laboratory; these were tested for anti-HIV-1, pro-viral DNA, protein isotyping, and antibody fingerprinting (Miragen).
Results: Pertinent results and our evaluations are:

ID	EIA serum S/CO	EIA plasma	Pro-viral DNA	Iso-type	Mira-gen	Eval.
A1	1.7	(-)	(-)	Same	Same	Cont.
A2	7.7	(-)	(-)	?	Diff.	Label
A3	2.5	(-)	(-)	Same	Same	Cont.
A4	1.7	(-)	(-)	Same	Same	Cont.
B5	2.5	(-)	(-)	Same	Same	Cont.
A6	2.0	(-)	(-)	Same	Same	Cont.

Same = same as person's other sera; ? = previously (-) mother of (+) son; Cont. = low-level contamination.

Among 6 clinical centers, 5/6 subjects were at center A and occurred in the 1st 18 months of the study.
Discussion: The fingerprinting method is useful for mislabelled sera, but low-level cross-contamination may give weak anti-HIV-1 reactivity without being detectable by the tests used. (NHLBI Contracts No. NO1-HB-4-7003 and 9-7074.)

0502

HUMAN IMMUNODEFICIENCY VIRUS TYPE 1 (HIV-1) INFECTED ASYMPTOMATIC BLOOD DONORS: EPIDEMIOLOGIC CHARACTERISTICS AND CLINICAL EVOLUTION.

A.Altès,E.Muñiz-Díaz ,P.Madoz,R.Martino R,LL.Puig.
Hemotherapy service. Hospital de Sant Pau. Barcelona (SPAIN).

OBJECTIVES: *To ascertain the epidemiologic characteristics and the clinical evolution of asymptomatic HIV-1 infected blood donors during the last eight years.*
MATERIAL AND METHODS: *From 1986 to 1993, all seropositive blood donors for HIV-1 were interviewed about their epidemiologic data. Afterwards, clinical status (according to Centers for Diseases Control criteria) and evolution were evaluated.*
RESULTS: *HIV-1 seropositivity was confirmed for 57 (43 men and 14 women, median age 31 years) out of 67532 blood donors (0.84 per thousand). At the beginning, all were classified as stage II. The route of HIV exposure was: Heterosexual activity 30 (53%), Homosexual 10 (18%), Intravenous drug use 11 (19%), and unknown 6 (10%). Heterosexual donors were unaware of their risk behavior at donation. Sixteen patients were followed for up to 2 years. Four (25%) progressed to stage IV (3/7 homosexuals and 1/1 drug user). None of the 7 heterosexual donors progressed from the initial stage. 4/7 homosexual patients reached a CD4-cell count lower than $0.2X10^9/L$, and the 7 heterosexual never reached this count. 29% of these patients had a previous history of venereal disease, and 24% had a positive HBsAg test.*
CONCLUSIONS:*Heterosexual activity with different partners has become the most frequent route of HIV exposure in our blood donors. Protocols of self exclusion should discourage donation by these people. The progression to the illness has been clearly more frequent in the group with homosexual activity. It seems that a previous history of venereal disease or positivity for HBsAg test are good indirect markers to detect an important part of these donors.*

0503

LOOK BACK STUDY OF THE GERMAN RED CROSS BLOOD BANKS

D. Glück, B. Kubanek et al.
Dept. Transfusion Medicine, University of Ulm and German Red Cross Blood Bank Ulm for all Red Cross Blook Banks in the FRG.

The HIV study group of German Red Cross Blood Banks tried to identify retrospectively HIV-infections in transfusion recipients who received blood from donors who tested HIV-positive at a subsequent donation. These look back data were traced back as completely as possible to answer the following questions: 1) How many transfusion recipients were infected before HIV-testing was routinely applied in 1985; 2) To estimate the risk of HIV-infection from donors infected but not yet HIV-antibody positive.
The study comprises look back data from more than 200 Western blot positive donors found among the 20 million blood donations given to the German Red Cross Blood Banks since 1985. We found 9 HIV-ab-positive recipients of blood components which had been tested negative thus confirming the estimation of the HIV-risk of tested blood products in the FRG is smaller than 1 : 1 million.
The look back data identified 25 HIV-antibody-positive recipients of blood before testing was introduced, 11 in 1985, 10 in 1984 and 4 in 1982 and 1983. No infection was found before 1982. From the data of this look back study can be concluded that the total number of HIV-infections by blood products of the Red Cross Blood Banks before 1985 will be less than 150 and less than 20 thereafter.

Supported by grants from BMFT.

0504

RESULTS OF THE SWISS NATIONAL TRANSFUSION ASSOCIATED HIV- INFECTION LOOK BACK STUDY

M. Frey-Wettstein (l), H. Bosshard (2)
l Zurich Blood Transfusion Service SRC, Zurich / 2 Swiss Federal Office of Public Health, Bern, Switzerland

In l993 the Swiss Red Cross Blood Transfusion Service and the Swiss Public Health Authorities have carried out a donor related Look Back with the ame to uncover additional TA HIV-Infections in living patients and their partners. All Swiss Blood Donation Facilities had to register blood units donated between l982 and l985 by persons found Anti-HIV positive after introduction of HIV-Screening. The ID-numbers of these blood units were transmitted to the transfusing institutions which were asked to locate the receivers of the according blood transfusions. Living receivers had to be contacted, informed about the implications of the Look Back Study and after consent tested for Anti-HIV. In HIV positive blood receivers search was done for secondary HIV-infections in the patients family or partners.
396 blood units were registred as possible sources for TA HIV-infection. In 59 cases the delivery documents were destroyed or missing and the transfusing institution could not be determined. An other 22 units never left the Blood Donation Centers. In 73 of 315 units with known destination the receivers could not be determined due to non-response of treating hospital or destroyed, missing or incomplete documentation. Additional l7 units never were transfused. Of the 224 documented receivers (one patient received two possibly HIV-positive blood units), 50 were HIV positive, with 47 of these having been reported as HIV infected before this Look Back Study was initiated. Not more than 3 additional cases were discovered as beeing Anti-HIV positive, of these 1 in a deceased patient (diagnosed retrospectively on autopsy material) and 2 in living receivers. In 131 receivers, HIV-status remained undocumented, mainly because of a high mortality after transfusion (104 receivers dead at time of the study).Of the 8 cases of secondary TA-HIV-Infection, all had been known before initiation of this study.
In summary, in 264 (67%) of 396 suspected products the fate of the blood units could be determined. 3 additional cases of TA-HIV Infections were detected by this nationwide Look Back Study.

0505

THE ITALIAN LOOK-BACK PROGRAM FOR TRANSFUSION-ASSOCIATED (T-A) AIDS.

R. Arcieri[1]; N. Schinaia[1], C. Valdarchi[1], A. Ghirardini[1], M.C. Berra[1], G.A. Sciorelli[2], and the ICBTG. [1]AIDS Unit, Lab. of Epidemiology and Biostatistics., Istituto Superiore di Sanità, Rome; [2]Immunohemat. Departm., Civil Hospital, Monza, Italy.

Objective: To investigate in depth the circumstances of HIV infection for those patients with AIDS that are considered T-A.
Methods: Patients with AIDS are reported to the National AIDS Registry (NAIDSR) by physicians at clinical settings throughout the country. Persons whose sole risk factor is having received blood transfusions after 1978 according to the physician's report, for whom no other risk factor or behavior for HIV infection can be determined are considered as T-A cases. Only are cases included that are known to have received blood in Italy.
Results: As of September 30, 1992, out of 14,783 cases of AIDS reported in Italy at the National AIDS Operational Centre, 199 were T-A. Of these, only 127 (63.8%) were eligible for investigation, as 32 (16.1%) were transfused abroad, for 28 (14.1%) the place of transfusion is unknown and for 14 (7.0%) the year of transfusion is unknown. 15 (11.8%) T-A cases were re-attributed to other risk factors after the investigations. Out of 119 on going investigations 186 donors were identified: 150 (80.6%) were repeat and 31 (16.7%) were first-time donors; 146/186 (78.5%) had been tested for HIV; 7 (4.8%) were HIV-positive and 2 developed AIDS. During the same investigations, 20 blood recipients were also identified; of these, 7 were tested for HIV: all were HIV-positive and 5 developed AIDS.
Conclusions: Active surveillance of T-A AIDS enables better ascertainment of the mode of acquiring HIV infection, and it allows to identify subjects, that may have been exposed to HIV infection.

0506

EVALUATION OF OLYMPUS-PK TPHA 1000 FOR BLOOD DONORS SYPHILIS SEROLOGY

C. Cherby[1], B. Bertin[2], M. Poitevin[3]
1.Regional Blood Bank, Clermont-Ferrand, France. 2.Army Blood Bank, Clamart, France. 3.Institut Alfred Fournier, Paris, France.

Purpose : OLYMPUS-PK TPHA 1000, is a treponemal test for the serologic detection of syphilis, based upon the passive agglutination of chicken erythrocytes sensitived with T. pallidum antigens and antibodies found in the patient's serum, directly used on the blood grouping automates OLYMPUS PK7100 and PK7200.
Methods : Two French Blood Banks, one with the PK7100, the other with the PK7200, have studied the reagent, in order to determine its specificity and its sensitivity. The specificity is measured with 2000 plasma samples from blood donors in each evaluation site. The sensitivity is measured with a specific panel from Alfred Fournier Institute ; This panel is composed with 80 TPHA negative serums, 1 spontaneous agglutination serum, 119 TPHA positive serums with different titles ranging from 1/80 to 1/40960.
Results : Specificity : 2 plasmas gave a false positive reaction (spontaneous agglutination). Sensitivity : Real good results are obtained with all the 200 samples of the panel.
Conclusion : With this study, it's possible to choose the better thresholds to read automatically the reactions, in order to have a good specificity (99,95%) and a good sensitivity (100%).

0507

FURTHER EVIDENCES SHOWING THE ABSENCE OF SEROLOGICAL SURROGATE MARKERS FOR *Trypanosoma cruzi* INFECTED BLOOD DONORS

Wendel, S. and Biagini, S.
Hospital Sírio-Libanês Blood Bank, São Paulo, Brazil

Previous data have shown that no surrogate markers could be linked with current serological tests used in blood donation screening[1]. We extended our results in order to confirm or not these data.

From Jan. 88 to Dec. 93, 26,365 blood donors (male= 21,053 - 79.85%, female= 5,312 - 20.15%), resulting in 29,801 blood donations were tested for HIV, Syphilis, HBsAg, ALT, Abnormal hemoglobin (AbHb) and *T. cruzi* antibodies - (TcAb - by IFI, HAI and/or ELISA). Other markers were introduced in a later period such as: Anti-HBc (n= 19,455), -HTLV-I/II (n= 16,334) and -HCV (n= 14,802).

A total of 380 donors (1.44%) were found to have TcAb, either isolated (n= 317 - 83.42%) or associated with other serological marker (n= 63 - 16.58%). We have only found an association between syphilis tests and TcAb in the female group (p= 0.005), but only 4/72 cases were observed with both markers; no linkage could be proved neither in the male donors (8/386), nor in the whole group (12/458) regarding syphilis and TcAb (p= 0.466 and 0.053 respectively). No other linkage could be shown concerning: serological markers (-HCV, HBsAg, -HBc, HIV, -HTLV-I/II, ALT or AbHb), age (male= 35.77 ± 10.54 yrs, female= 38.95 ± 10.64 yrs p= 0.071), gender (male= 315 - 82.89%, female= 65 - 17.11% , p= NS). In addition, when age is divided into 6 (six) different groups (≥ 26, 27-35, 36-44, 45-53, 54-62 and ≥ 63 years), no association could be found.

We conclude that, despite a slight association between syphilis in females and TcAb, no other serological markers than those specific for TcAb will ensure an addition protection to detect *T. cruzi* infected blood donors in our population.

REFERENCE

1- Wendel, S. and Biagini, S. - Transfusion 33: 9S (Abstract S156), 1993

0508

BACTERIAL GROWTH IN POOLED PLATELET CONCENTRATES (PC) WITH AND WITHOUT LEUKODEPLETION (LD).

S.Wagner[1], E.Snyder[2], L.Friedman[1], A.Katz[1], G.Moroff[1]
1American Red Cross, Rockville, MD, 2Yale Univ. School of Medicine, New Haven CT, USA.

In the U.S., PC must be transfused within 4 hours of pooling. Extending the post-pooling storage period would provide logistical flexibility. However, reports of sepsis from PC transfusions led us to examine whether the total bacterial levels (TBL) during storage of deliberatedly inoculated (DI) PC pools would be significantly different than in an unpooled but contaminated PC. A single PC was DI on day 0 with one of 3 bacterial species (0.4-5.0 colony forming units/mL). On day 1, the DI PC was divided into 3 equal parts and either pooled with 5 half-volume PC, similarly pooled and leukodepleted (Asahi PL10-A LD filter), or kept as a control. Sterile connections were used during pooling, and modified PL732 (Baxter) containers provided storage with the correct surface to volume ratio. Results (n≥9 per bacterial species) indicated that by day 2-5 of storage, many LD pools had substantially more TBL than did the paired single PC. For *S. epidermidis*, a number of LD pools had higher TBL by day 5. For *S. aureus*, there was rapid growth in either pooled or unpooled PCs by day 2; by day 3, ≈6-fold higher levels were present in LD pools compared to single PC. For *E. coli*, LD pools had ≈9-fold higher TBL by day 2 than did controls. Growth in the LD and non-LD pools was not significantly different. Thus, there is potential for increased TBL during storage of pools prepared with a DI PC.

0509

POST-TRANSFUSION SURVIVAL OF PRIMATE PLATELETS AFTER PHOTOCHEMICAL DECONTAMINATION (PCD) : A TWO COLOR ASSAY.

L.Corash and W. Liu, University of California, San Francisco, CA, USA.

Pathogenic bacteria seeded into human platelet concentrates (PC) can be inactivated by 8-methoxypsoralen (8-MOP) PCD (**Blood 82: 205a, 1993**). Because *in vitro* platelet function tests inconsistently predict *in vivo* post-transfusion platelet recovery (R) and mean life-span (MLS), we developed a method to measure R and MLS in a primate transfusion model after bactericidal 8-MOP PCD. Rhesus monkey (*M. mulatta*) PC (N = 6) prepared from CPD-A_1 whole blood (WB), were treated (8-MOP = 25 µg/ml, 320-380 nm UVA = 5 J/cm^2), labeled with a green fluorescent probe (PKH-2), stored for 18 hr at 22 °C with shaking, and transfused into autologous donors (N = 7). Similar studies using control PC were carried out. Blood volume (BV) was independently measured using a red fluorescent probe (PKH-26). WB samples obtained 0.5, 3, 6, 20, 30, 44, 54, 68, 78, and 92 hr post-transfusion were assayed by fluorescent cytometry to determine BV, R, and MLS. Average BV = 43 ± 8.0 (SD) ml/kg (N = 6). Average R for (N = 6) controls = 75.5 ± 12.7%(SD). Control MLS = 118.8 hr derived from a pooled, linear fitted survival curve (r = 0.88). Average R for PCD treated PC = 69.8 ± 12.8% (SD) with a pooled MLS of 104.1 hr (r = 0.92). Bactericidal PCD conditions did not significantly impair *in vivo* post-transfusion R and MLS of sub-human primate platelet concentrates.

0510

BACTERIAL LEVELS (BL) IN COMPONENTS PREPARED FROM DELIBERATELY INOCULATED (DI) WHOLE BLOOD (WB) HELD FOR 8 AND 24 HOURS AT ROOM TEMPERATURE (RT).

S. Wagner, G. Moroff, A. Katz and L. Friedman. American Red Cross, Rockville, MD, USA.

Increasing the WB RT hold from 8 to 24 hours would facilitate blood component preparation. The potential for bacterial growth during such an extended holding period needs to be evaluated to ensure product safety. We studied the growth of DI bacteria during the extended WB RT hold and after component preparation. Two-unit pools of ABO/Rh identical WB were DI on day 0 with one of 8 bacterial species (primarily 1-2 colony forming units/mL). DI pools were then divided at once into 2 identical units and stored at 20-24°C. Adsol red cells ($RBC_{8 \text{ or } 24}$), platelet concentrates ($PC_{8 \text{ or } 24}$), and fresh frozen plasma ($FFP_{8 \text{ or } 24}$) were prepared after 8 or 24 hours. RBC_{24} samples were taken before and after leukodepletion (LD) (Pall, BPF4); no LD was performed on RBC_8. Bacterial growth was monitored during 42 day storage of RBC, 5 day storage of PC and after thawing FFP. With 4 of 8 organisms (n≥6), there were significantly higher bacterial levels in WB_{24} compared to WB_8. The same strains were also present at higher levels in unfiltered RBC_{24} than in RBC_8. However, LD significantly reduced the levels for 3 of these 4 strains, with RBC_{24} levels similar or lower than those of RBC_8. Generally, BL of thawed FFP_{24} and PC_{24} were comparable to FFP_8 and PC_8. Thus, BL appear to be similar in components prepared from 8 and 24 hour-held DI WB, provided that RBC_{24} are LD.

0511

EXPERIMENTAL STUDY OF HUMAN POLYMERIZED HEMOGLOBIN (PPHb)

E.Selivanov[1], I.Bystrova[1], N.Kochetygov[1], K.Gerbut[1], Molokovskaya[1], I.Kuznetsova[1], L.Gudkin[2], R.Mishaeva[2]
Russian Research Institute of Hematology and Transfusiology-1, Institute of High-Molecular Compouds of the Russian Academy of Sciences2,St.Petersburg, Russia

Human hemoglobin free of stroma was pyridoxylated and polymerized. Its medico-biological and physico-chemical parameters were studied. PPHb has a P_{50} 28 torr,Bohr-effect 0.4, M_W 120 kD, /MetHb/ 3%, time of half-release 12-18 hr. It is established that PPHb solutions of 0.2-1.0 gr/dl concentration are not toxic, nor teratogenic or mutagenic and do not affect the immune and coagulation systems. In experiments with hemorrhagic shock, PPHb reconstituted the systemic circulation, carryed and unloaded the oxygen. PPHb can be stored in the lyophilized form for 2 years without losing its functional properties. PPHb dose of 3-4 gr/kg of animal body has an effect on the immune, nervous, coagulation and other systems. Further studies are necessary to improve the safety of PPHb solution to be used in clinic.

0512

FIBRINOPEPTIDE A GENERATION IN THE GUINEA PIG AS AN IN VIVO MODEL FOR MEASURING COAGULATION EFFECTS OF HEMOGLOBIN SOLUTIONS.

P.T.Biessels, G.M. Rigter, J. Agterberg, F. Meijer-Huizinga., K. Mertens and J.C. Bakker; Central Laboratory of the Netherlands Red Cross Blood Transfusion Service, Amsterdam, the Netherlands.

Hemoglobin (Hb) solutions are known to produce coagulation problems, probably due to membrane contaminants, in particular, by negatively charged phospholipids, that play a role in the coagulation cascade. Therefore, an animal model was developed to study activation of coagulation in vivo in a non-stasis model. A polyclonal antiserum against human fibrinopeptide A (FPA) was used to detect FPA generation in the plasma of a guinea pig. FPA is generated when fibrin is formed from fibrinogen and is a very sensitive marker for activation of coagulation.

This model was used to study the effects of Hb solutions in vivo. One-third of the blood volume of a guinea pig was replaced with a Hb solution, and blood samples were taken and assayed for FPA. Fifteen min after the end of the exchange transfusion basal values were reached (1.2± 0.4 ng FPA/ml plasma). To create a stressed animal model FXa was injected in a dose (9 µg/kg) that did not resulted in FPA generation unless phospholipids were present.

After an exchange transfusion with albumin (control), polyHb, purified SFHb or SFHb contaminated with stroma, we found a small increase in FPA levels during the total duration of the experiment (60 min). When FXa was injected there was a small increase in FPA with SFHb (5.2±0.7 ng FPA/ml plasma) and a clear increase with contaminated SFHb, depending on the amount of stroma added. Albumin and polyHb together with FXa caused no increase in FPA levels.

Conclusion: Only in a stressed model, i.e. after injection of a small amount of FXa, we found activation of coagulation with both contaminated and purified SFHb solutions (PL content about 2.5 nmol/ml). No increase in FPA levels was found after an exchange transfusion with polyHb (PL content <1 nmol/ml)

0513

EVALUATION OF IMMUNOGENICITY OF MODIFIED HUMAN HEMOGLOBIN SOLUTIONS

W.K. Bleeker, E.M. Zappeij, P.J. den Boer, J.A. Agterberg, G. Rigter, J.C. Bakker
Central Laboratory of the Netherlands Red Cross Blood Transfusion Service

We are currently developing a blood substitute based on human hemoglobin that is modified by intra- and intermolecular crosslinking with glutaraldehyde. In the present study we investigated the possibility that neoantigens are introduced by the modification.

To investigate the potential immunogenicity of the polymerized hemoglobin (polyHb) we analyzed antibody responses of rabbits after intramuscular adminstration with Freunds complete adjuvant. In view of the species differences we also tested polymerized rabbit hemoglobin. Thereafter, we also studied the antibody response after weekly intravenous infusion of relatively large doses of polyHb (100 mg/kg), to evaluate whether an immune response is likely to occur when modified hemoglobin is used as blood substitute.

The occurrence of an antibody response was tested for using an enzyme immunoassay (ELISA). To find out whether antibodies were directed against neo-epitopes on human polyHb we used competitive ELISA in which native hemoglobin competes with modified hemoglobin that is immobilized on the solid phase. The results showed that polymerized hemoglobin carries neo-epitopes that may activate the immune system in special conditions, but are unlikely to do so when polyHb is used as blood substitute.

0514

Human Hemoglobin-based Blood Substitutes

Diana H. Pliura, Ph.D.

Hemosol Inc. 115 Skyway Ave, Etobicoke, Ontario, Canada M9W 4Z4

The clinical use of human hemoglobin-derived blood substitutes has the potential to be jeopardized by factors other than those inherent to the product. It is essential to show that both the hemoglobin and its modified product are free of contaminants. This is particularly important when attributing pharmacologic effects observed in preclinical and clinical trials to the product or to impurities. Unequivocal demonstration of freedom from infectious agents is mandatory. The product requires detailed characterization such that sites of protein modification are understood and controlled. Proof of safety and freedom from serious side effects, beyond the levels for existing products, are necessary preliminaries to undertake new clinical studies. *In vivo* effects of Hemolink™ on hemodynamic parameters, renal function, immune response and microcirculatory function have been determined. The distribution and rate of product clearance have been characterized. Finally, since red blood cells have established a cost target, blood substitute pricing will have to be competitive. To achieve this, an efficient manufacturing process providing high product yields at relatively low costs is required. Hemosol's product meets all of these criteria.

0515

DIASPIRIN CROSSLINKED HEMOGLOBIN (DCLHb™): EFFICAY IN THE TREATMENT OF HYPOVOLEMIC HEMORRHAGIC SHOCK

K.E. Burhop[1], J. McKenzie[2], E. Dunlap[1], and D. Malcolm[2]. Uniformed Services Univ.[2], and Baxter Healthcare Corp.[1]. Blood Substitutes Program, Round Lake, IL., 60073. U.S.A.

DCLHb is a highly purified, alpha, alpha-crosslinked human hemoglobin solution that is currently under investigation in human clinical trials. The purpose of the current studies was to examine the potential efficacy of DCLHb in a variety of animal models of hemorrhagic shock. In swine (n=6/gp) subjected to hemorrhage of 30 mL/kg over 20 minutes, resuscitation with 0.5 mL/kg DCLHb increased MAP from 45±1 mmHg to 102±8mmHg within 5 min and was as effective as 90 mL/kg of lactated Ringer's (LR) solution. Other studies in swine and rats will be presented.

Conclusion: preclinical studies in a variety of animal models demonstrate that DCLHb at low doses restores mean arterial blood pressure, increases blood flow to a variety of critical organs when administered to hypovolemic animals, and positively affects a number of physiologic indices of perfusion.

0516

LARGE SCALE PRODUCTION OF A NEW CONTROL SERUM FROM PLASMA FRACTIONATION WASTE PRODUCTS

N. Shafaghi-Nejad & I. Majd Teimuri
Iranian Blood Transfusion Service,
138, Nejatollahi Avenue, Tehran, Iran.

A new control material can be prepared inexpensively using plasma fractionation waste products. This can be produced on a very large scale and with as many constituents as required, the only additives being enzymes extracted from human and non-human sources. One major problem with routine or commercial lyophilyzed sera has so far been their turbidity (especially after reconstituting the lyophilyzed material) which can lead to inaccurate data, where blanks can not be used and in the case of autoanalyzers which can get clogged up.

Our control material which is a mixture of various waste products (i.e. final waste product of alcohol-water containing all the electrolytes from which alcohol is evaporated, fraction III containing the lipids as well as fractions V &/or VI which is failed due to, for example, bacterial or fungal growth and is pre-filtered before use) plus crude enzymes (Alanine Aminotransferase, Aspartate Aminotransferase, Creatine Kinase, Lactate Dehydrogenase, Alkaline Phosphatase, Acid-Phosphatase & Amylase) retains its clarity even after reconstitution following lyophilyzation and carries a relatively lower risk of HBs antigen transmission than commercially prepared controlled sera on account of its being previously treated and controlled.

0517

Purification of Factor VIII and von Willebrand Factor from Human Plasma by Anion Exchange Chromatography

Dj. Josic, H. Schwinn, M. Stadler,
Octapharma Produktionsges.m.b.H., Oberlaaer Str. 235, A-1100 Wien, Austria
A. Strancar: BIA d.o.o., Adamiceva 4, SLO-61000 Ljubljana, Slovenia

Factor VIII (anti-hemophilia A factor) is isolated from human plasma. Purification is carried out by a combination of precipitation and chromatographic procedures. The precipitate after cryo-precipitation is dissolved in the buffer, and bulk proteins such as prothrombin factors, factor I and factor V are removed by adding of $Al(OH)_3$ and subsequent cooling down to 16°C. This aluminum hydroxide precipitation also removes several additional proteins from the clotting cascade. Although only traces of such proteins, e.g., factor Xa, are found in the cryoprecipitate, they may activate factor VIII (FVIII) during subsequent steps of the isolation process, thereby reducing both yield and stability of the product.
The first step in virus inactivation is achieved through the effect of a non-ionic detergent such as Triton X 100 or Tween 80, and a solvent, e.g., Tri-n-butyl-phosphate (TnBP). By a subsequent anion exchange chromatography step, a highly enriched product is isolated, consisting of a complex formed by factor VIII and von Willebrand factor (F VIII-vWF). This treatment also reduces the virus-inactivating reagents to quantitites in the low ppm range.
The second step in virus inactivation is aimed specifically at the non-enveloped viruses and consists of pasteurization at temperatures greater than 60°C for 10 hours. In order to preserve the activity of the clotting FVIII during heating, sugars, amino acids and bivalent cations are added as stabilizers. They are subsequently removed by ion exchange chromatography, along with possibly denaturing proteins. In this step, additional vWF is removed. Through the addition of stabilizers, between 80% and 90% of the initial activity of FVIII is preserved during the modified pasteurisation. The twofold virus inactivation, by solvent/detergent treatment and subsequent pasteurisation, allows the destruction of both lipid enveloped and non-enveloped viruses. During this procedure FVIII is stabilized through the high content of vWF. The complex consisting of FVIII and vWF can be dissociated by adding calcium ions. Subsequently both glycoproteins from this complex are separated from one another by further anion-exchange chromatography.

0518

PURIFICATION OF ALPHA$_1$-PROTEINASE INHIBITOR (α_1-PI) FROM WASTE FRACTIONS OF THE COHN PROCESS.

I.R. MacGregor, J. Campbell, O. Drummond.
National Science Laboratory, Scottish National Blood Transfusion Service, 2 Forrest Road, Edinburgh, EH1 2QN, United Kingdom.

α_1-PI (also known as α_1-antitrypsin) is the major plasma inhibitor of neutrophil elastase. Severe deficiencies are associated with emphysema and the efficacy of replacement therapy is now being assessed in clinical trials in the USA and Europe. We have evaluated the α_1-PI content and properties in waste fractions of the SNBTS continuous-small-volume cold ethanol fractionation process to establish if they could be a useful source for purification. We have also investigated published methods of purification to ascertain their suitability for such material.

Fraction IV-1 paste was best suited as source material based on solubility and stability measurements. However this fraction only contained about 6% of the total α_1-PI available in plasma. Optimisation of solubilisation and precipitation steps combined with acid-elution after DEAE-Sepharose FF chromatography yielded α_1-PI of 80-90% purity. Pasteurisation at 60°C for 18hr with stabilisers resulted in only minimal loss of activity (<10%) and no generation of aggregates. Further investigations are necessary to improve overall recovery. For example, by altering the conditions for producing IV-1 paste, it may be possible to increase the yield of α_1-PI.

0519

STERILIZING 100°C (BOILING) TERMINAL DRY HEAT TREATMENT OF FACTOR VIII CONCENTRATES ADDITIONAL STUDIES

[1]J. Lew, D.S. Pinkney, [2]A. Rubinstein, [1]Hematology Laboratory, Department of Clinical Pathology, MS-32; Childrens Hospital Los Angeles, Los Angeles, CA; [2]Smith Research Building, Childrens Hospital of Los Angeles

Because solvent-detergent will not inactivate nonlipid enveloped viruses such as Hepatitis A and parvovirus, 100°C terminal dry heat has been added by at least one major manufacturer (Aima Derivati) and is undergoing evaluation by other companies. 100°C terminal dry heat for 7-1/2 minutes has been reported to inactivate over five (5) logs of a nonlipid enveloped virus (poliovirus) (Franco, E., et al., World Fed. of Hemophilia, 1992 [Abstract #181]). An important and necessary advantage of terminal high temperature dry heat is that it will assure sterility if there has been in process contamination.

Liquid heating (60°C/10 hours in solution) because of high concentrations of stabilizers has also been reported to transmit Hepatitis C (Lancet, 1993). We have thus immersed in boiling water (100°C), a Factor VIII concentrate (Humate) - P Lot #719011) for 15 minutes and showed approximately 16.5% loss of VIII:C. Reaction with a high titred inhibitor (19.5 BU) showed no significant change from unheated control. High temperature terminal dry heat should be added to all Factor VIII concentrates to: (1) assure sterility if there has been in process contamination and (2) inactivate nonlipid enveloped viruses.

0520

An improved chromatography method for production of IgG from Human Plasma.

I. Andersson, L-O Lindquist, J. Berglöf
Pharmacia BioProcess Technology AB,
S-75182 Uppsala, Sweden

Chromatography is today a well established technique for the purification of IgG from human plasma. The Pharmacia method based on a mixed bed of Arginine-Sepharose 4B and DEAE-Sepharose Fast Flow has now been improved by use of Q-Sepharose Fast Flow alone, which eliminates the draw-backs of the mixed bed such as packing, mixing of two media together and process control of a mixed bed. With Q-Sepharose the flow rate properties are improved and the cost for the media is at least 2X less.

This poster describes the whole procedure for purification of IgG from plasma using ion exchange chromatography on DEAE Sepharose Fast Flow, Q-Sepharose Fast Flow and CM-Sepharose Fast Flow including virus inactivation with the solvent detergent method. Methods for removal of virus inactivation chemicals are perhaps also applicable to recombinant proteins produced in mammalian cell lines.

The obtained IgG preparation is more than 99% pure and contains less than 1% of aggregates other than monomeric IgG. Typical recovery from normal plasma is 5.0-5.5 g/l.

0521

PURIFICATION AND BIOLOGICAL ACTIVITY OF A RECOMBINANT HUMAN ERYTHROPOIETIN PRODUCED BY LYMPHOBLASTOID CELLS

P. Lambin[1], A. Ben Ghanem[1], J.J. Winchenne[1], C. Lopez[1], S. Chrétien[1], P. Rouger[1], J.P. Cartron[2].
[1]Institut National de Transfusion Sanguine Paris France
[2]INSERM U 76 Paris France.

A recombinant human erythropoietin (rH-EPO) was obtained from the culture supernatants of human B-lymphoblastoid cells transfected by the human EPO gene. rH-EPO was purified by a two-step method based on immunoaffinity and ion exchange chromatography. The first step was achieved with an anti-EPO monoclonal antibody (Mab). This Mab, immobilized on Sepharose 4B, allowed a 410-fold purification of the protein. The second step consisted of ion exchange chromatography on DEAE Sephacel. The combination of these two steps results in a highly purified rH-EPO with a global yield of about 50 %; the specific activity of the protein was 176,000 IU/A_{280}. The NMR spectrum was characteristic for a well structured, single-conformation protein. The purified protein was analyzed by SDS-PAGE and Western blot. With both procedures, the molecular mass of the isolated protein was identical for urinary human EPO and rH-EPO produced in an other mammalian cell. The biological activity of purified rH-EPO was measured in vivo, by the incorporation of ^{59}Fe into red blood cells (RBC) of polycythemic mice and in vitro by the proliferative response of an EPO-dependent cell line. The purified protein expressed in lymphoblastoid cells of human origin had the same biological activity as that of urinary EPO and rH-EPO produced in other mammalian cells.

0522

CLONING AND EXPRESSION OF A HUMAN MONOCLONAL ANTI-RHESUS (D) ANTIBODY.

T Paterson, S.S. Armstrong[1], I. Downing[2], S.J. Thorpe[3], S. Moore & M.C. McCann Carter, National Science Laboratory, Scottish National Blood Transfusion Service, 2 Forrest Road, Edinburgh, EH1 2QN Scotland. [1]Aberdeen and NE Scotland BTS; [2]Glasgow and W Scotland BTS; [3]NIBSC Potters Bar.

The availability of human monoclonal antibodies to Rhesus antigen D offers the possibility of alternative therapy for the prevention of Haemolytic Disease of the Newborn. We report here the cloning and expression of the cDNAs coding for the IgG expressed by a heterohybrid cell-line (ESD-1) secreting anti-D. We present data comparing the parent heterohybrid and transfected NS-0 cell lines in terms of antibody production. Additionally, we present information on the serological and biochemical characteristics of both native and recombinant antibody and on their ability to mediate in vitro biological function in assays of monocyte and lymphocyte mediated red cell destruction.

0523

CONVERSION OF VARIOUS GROUP A RED CELLS BY DEACETYLATION TO REACTORS WITH MONOCLONAL ANTI-ACQUIRED B REAGENTS

Y.Okubo, T.Seno, M.Tanaka, H.Yamano, T.Nakade, H.Yamaguchi
Osaka Red Cross Blood Center, Osaka, Japan

Using monoclonal anti-acquired B we tested artificial acquired Bs converted from group A_1, A_1B, A_2, A_3, cisA_2B_3 and Amos red cells treated with a deacetylase prepared by the ammonium sulfate fractionation method from the liquid medium in which *Clostridium tertium* has grown.

Samples of the monoclonal anti-acquired B that we used here were OSK21 produced by the routine hybridization method using the spleen cells of the mouse immunized with the red cells of a group A_1 patient with acquired B, and E231 antibody sent kindly by Dr.Janvier, Paris, France. We used agglutination tests and thin layer chromatograph (TLC)-immunostaining method for detection of acquired B.

The red cells from an acquired B group A_1 patient with ileus were agglutinated strongly with both reagents. But both reagents agglutinated neither intact group A_1, A_1B, A_2, A_3, cisA_2B_3, B, O red cells nor Tn, Th, Tk, T polyagglutinability red cells.

All the A_1, A_1B, A_2, A_3, cisA_2B_3 and Amos red cells treated with the deacetylase reacted with both OSK21 and E231 reagents and after being acetylated with acetic acid these red cells no longer did. By TLC-immunostaining using glycolipids prepared form red cells of group A_1 acquired B patient and each of the artificial acquired B red cells converted from A_1, A_1B, A_2, A_3, cisA_2B_3 and Amos, we detected two or three bands in the same locations.

0524

IN VIVO SURVIVAL OF At(a$^+$) RED CELLS IN AN At(a-) RECIPIENT WITH ANTI-At^a. J.D.Sweeney, S.Holme, L.A.McCall, D.Huett,*J.Storry, *M.E.Reid. American Red Cross, Mid-Atlantic Region, Norfolk, VA; *New York Blood Center, New York, NY

The August (At^a) negative phenotype is exceedingly rare and, to date, less than fifteen subjects have been described, all of whom are of African origin. The finding of a positive direct antiglobulin test on cord blood has been the most common event leading to the detection of propositi. No infant had evidence of hemolytic disease of the newborn (HDN), raising questions regarding the clinical significance of this antibody.

A 35-year-old female delivered a healthy neonate. Cord blood showed a positive direct antiglobulin test. Maternal serum contained an anti-E and a second antibody, identified as anti-At^a. Eluate from the cord blood contained anti-At^a only. Subsequently, family studies revealed two of seven siblings who were At^a(a-), neither of whom had detectable anti-At^a. Due to concerns regarding blood availability in an emergency setting, 2 mLs of ^{51}Cr-labeled allogeneic At^a(a$^+$), but otherwise phenotypically matched, red cells were infused. Survival results are reported below as (time after infusion/ %survival): 5 min/100%; 15 min/98%; 30 min/96%; 45 min/96%; 1 hr/95%; 2 hr/88%; 3 hr/76%; 1 day/18%; 2 day/6%; 3 day/4%; 4 day/2%. The survival pattern is exponential. Early survival, however, at 1 hour is 95% and predicts that At^a(a$^+$) red cells could be transfused in an emergency setting. The late survival (Day 1-Day 4) would predict that a hemolytic reaction, of later onset, could be a possible, subsequent event. Anti-At^a is a clinically significant antibody in this case, despite the absence of reported HDN in infants of At^a(a-) women with At^a.

0525

A NEW MONOCLONAL ANTI-LW (BS 87)

H.-H. Sonneborn[1], M. Ernst[1], D. Voak[2]
1Biotest AG, Research Dept., Dreieich, FRG
2Division of Transf. Medicine, Cambridge, UK

By immunizing mice with human red blood cells a new monoclonal anti-LW (BS 87) was raised. The reactivity and specificity of this new mab was evaluated in comparison to the well known mabs BS 46 and BS 56. All three antibodies are of the IgG1 type. BS 87 showed stronger reactions with D-positive red blood cells compared to D-negative cells as is known for other anti-LW's. Using saline tests BS 87 was more reactive, but less effective in AHG technique.
All three antibodies were positive with HT (LW a-b+) using the 2 stage papain technique, whereas BS 87 failed to react with these cells using AHG.
All three antibodies showed negative reactions with well documented LW (a-b-) cells, demonstrating the anti-LW specificity. This was also proven by treating cells with dithiothreitol (DTT) or pronase, which are known for destroying the LW antigen. None of the antibodies reacted with cells treated in this way.
The minor differences in reactivity and differences in the thermal optimum of these antibodies indicate, that they might recognize different "epitopes".
Reactivity with partial- and weak-D cells is currently under investigation.

0526

RED CELL CHIMAERISM IN TWINS AND TRIPLETS

B.A. van Dijk[1], D.I. Boomsma[2], A.J.M. de Man[1]
[1] St Radboud University Hospital, Nijmegen, [2] Free University, Amsterdam, The Netherlands

Mixed erythrocyte chimaerism (MEC) is common in cattle twins, but very rare in man. It can only be demonstrated in non-monozygotic multiples. Until now some 40 human twins are described with MEC. Usually it is found in routine blood grouping. Only gross mixtures (50/50, 30/70 or 10/90% at most) of two blood groups are detectable with the technicians eye; smaller percentages are not recognised. We wondered if MEC is really so rare in man, and investigated the blood of 352 dizygotic twins and 22 di/trizygotic triplets using a very sensitive fluorescence assay (sensitivity 0.01%). This technique is routinely used in our hospital for the monitoring of bone marrow transplant patients, in whom an artificial MEC of gradual degree is created (Vox Sang 1988;55:37-41). The 374 multiples were investigated using blood group differences in one of the following systems: ABO, CcDEe, MNSs, P1, Kk, Kp^aKp^b, Fy^aFy^b, Jk^aJk^b, Lu^aLu^b.
Fifteen cases (4.0%; 9 twins, 6 triplets) of MEC with values ranging 0.1-11% were found, usually in one of the children. Another 17 cases (4.6%; 12 twins, 5 triplets) with marginal values (0.01-0.04%) were seen. Repeat testing after 18 months showed fluctuating results: decrease or abolishment of MEC, as well as some new cases or increase of former values. This fluctuation in time in one individual is a known feature of MEC.

0527

PATERNITY EXCLUSION WHERE THE BIOLOGICAL MOTHER AND ALLEGED FATHER WERE DECEASED.

MA Spivey, PV Genco, A Cannon. Medical University of South Carolina, Charleston, SC, USA.

In a paternity study involving a question of monetary inheritance, only the child (C) of the trio was living. Since the alleged paternal grandmother (AGM) and four siblings of the alleged deceased father (AF) were available for testing, information obtained from their blood types could possibly link C to AF with a high degree of probability or lead to exclusion of paternity. The validity of the conclusions had to rest on the assumption that the deceased alleged paternal grandfather (AGF) was the father of AF as well as his four siblings. After the red cell and HLA phenotypes of AGM and four siblings were determined, we were able to ascertain the obligatory genes (OG) of AGF and most of the genes that AF could have inherited (some genes may have been passed to AF that were not inherited by any of his four siblings). There were no exclusions in 7 red cell systems. There was a valid second order exclusion involving HLA. Four haplotypes were demonstrated in AF's siblings: A2,B27; A3,B56; A3,B35; A3,B7 (or AX, B7). AF would have inherited two haplotypes and transmitted one to a child. C's HLA phenotype was A1, A25, B14, B18. Therefore, he possessed none of the four identified haplotypes.

0528

ANTI-FY^a, FY3, FY5 IN 15 BLACK FY(a-b-) PATIENTS. A NATIONAL TRANSFUSION PROBLEM.

P.Y. Le Pennec, M.T. Klein, M. Le Besnerais, P. Rouger.
Centre National de Référence pour les Groupes Sanguins (CNRGS), 53, bd. Diderot, 75012 PARIS, FRANCE.

The Fy(a-b-) phenotype which is rare among Caucasians, is common in the black population, its frequency ranging from 60 to 100 %. It was commonly accepted that anti-Fy^a, -Fy^b, -Fy3 and -Fy5 were very rare in transfused Fy(a-b-) black patients. Recent studies have suggested that the presence of such antibodies is not as rare as previously believed. We have found 8 anti-Fy^a and 8 anti-Fy3 or Fy5 (sometimes associated with anti-Fy^a) in the sera of 15 Fy(a-b-3-) black subjects. The common features of these findings are : the patients presented a sickle cell disease ; the antibodies were found during the investigation of a hemolytic reaction ; these antibodies appeared on a short period of time associated with immune or naturally occuring alloantibodies (from 1 to 8 in 13 cases) and autoantibodies. These findings, the low number of black blood donors, the number of infectious diseases excluding these donors from blood donation, make a real national health problem.

0529

GERBICH NEGATIVE PHENOTYPE (YUS TYPE) IN TWO UNRELATED JEWISH ETHIOPIAN WOMEN.

E. Sigler[1], C. Levene[2], E.J. Vorst[1], G. Lugassy[3], J. Poole [4], J.L. Daniels[5].
1 Blood Bank and Hematology Institute, Kaplan Hospital, Rehovot, 2 Reference Laboratory for Immunohematology and Blood Groups, Ministry of Health, Jerusalem, 3 Hematology Institute and Blood Bank, Barzilay Medical Center, Ashkelon, 4 International Blood Group Reference Laboratory, Bristol, 5 M.R.C. Blood Group Unit, London.

The Gerbich blood group antigens (Ge) were discovered in 1960 and are found on the majority of human red blood cells (RBC) (>99%), except those from some ethnic groups within the Melanesian population. There are four main types of Ge negative RBC's, the Gerbich type (Ge:-2,-3), the Yus type (Ge:-2,3), the Leach type (also Ge:-2,-3) and a type (Ge:-1,2,3) that so far has been found only in Melanesians. We describe 2 unrelated women of Ethiopian Jewish origin, with the Gerbich negative Yus phenotype and anti Ge(Yus) in there serum, that were discovered during pregnancy. The serological results were confirmed by examination of the RBC's membranes by immunoblotting. A monocyte monolayer assay (MMA) of the serum did not indicate that there was any clinical significance to this antibody at the time of testing. The RBC's of the mother of one propositus and from 34 other Ethiopian Jews from the same region were found to have normal Gerbich antigens. This is the first report of the Ge-Yus type phenotype in the Ethiopian Jewish population.

0530

GENETIC LINKAGE DATA FOR CO RELATIVE TO CHROMOSOME 7p LOCI EGFR, D7S132, D7S135, D7S370, ASSP11 AND D7S149.

T. Zelinski, L. White, S. Philipps and G. Coghlan
Rh Laboratory, Depts. of Pediatrics and Human Genetics, University of Manitoba, Winnipeg, Canada.

In 1990, the Colton blood group locus (CO) was assigned to the short arm of chromosome 7 through family linkage studies (1). Despite the assignment, the precise location of CO was not known, nor had the genetic relationships between CO and other 7p markers been established. In an attempt to resolve these issues, we examined a series of families segregating for CO and six other 7p markers.

The DNA markers selected for this study were purchased from the American Type Culture Collection Repository of the NIH. All reveal restriction fragment length polymorphisms using standard recombinant DNA methodologies. The MARK III computer program was used for linkage analysis.

Our results indicate that CO is linked to all 6 markers. The poor regional localization of all but two of these markers (EGFR and D7S132) does not allow us to assign CO to a specific 7p band. However based on our genetic data, the Colton blood group locus should reside within 7p15-7pter and the best fit for order and distance is as follows :
7p12 - EGFR - 20cM - D7S132 - 9cM - CO/D7S135 - 6cM - D7S370 - 3cM - ASSP11 - 8cM - D7S149 - 7pter.

(1) Zelinski et al., (1990) Genomics 6, 623-625.

Work supported by the Medical Research Council of Canada and The Children's Hospital Research Fdn.

0531

Tn EXPRESSION CAN ARISE THROUGH DIFFERNT GLYCOSYLTRANSFERASE DEFECTS

A.P. Corfield[1] and M-J King[2]
1. Department of Medicine, Bristol Royal Infirmary
2. IBGRL, Bristol, UK

Tn erythrocytes carry mainly α-N-acetylgalactosamine in O-glycosidic linkage to serine or threonine residues (Tn antigen) on Glycophorin oligosaccharides due to a deficiency in the β(1-3) galactosyltransferase. Tn antigen has also been described as a general carcinoma marker in man and monoclonal anti-Tn antibodies raised against Tn erythrocytes and tumour tissues have the same specificity. We compared the glycosylation defects in colorectal cancer by determination of the glycosyltransferase activities in mucosal tissue from control and cancer patients using asialo-ovine submaxillary - and antifreeze glycoproteins as sugar acceptors. The results show a reduction in β(1-3) N-acetylglucosaminyltransferase activity to N-acetylgalactosamine with no significant loss of β (1-3) galactosyltransferase activity in cancer patients. Therefore, the Tn antigen in Tn erythrocytes and in colorectal cancer result from different glycosyltransferase defects in separate biosynthetic pathways for haematopoietic and epithelial tissues.

0532

UNUSUAL EXPRESSION OF Wr^b IN A Wr(a-) INDIVIDUAL

J Poole[1], J Banks[1], C Levene[2], N Hemming[1]
1. IBGRL, Bristol, UK
2. Reference Lab, Jerusalem, Israel

The serum of a previously transfused male patient (EH) contained an alloantibody to a high incidence antigen lacking on M^kM^k and En(a-) cells. Wr(a+b-) cells reacted more weakly than control Wr(a-b+) cells. The determinant was sensitive to papain, reduced by ficin and resistant to trypsin, α-chymotrypsin & AET. EH cells were positive with seven human polyclonal anti-En^a but were weakly reactive with some sera. Monoclonal antibodies to Glycophorin A (GPA), GPA/GPB and Band 3 reacted normally in serological tests and by immunoblotting. Sialic acid content and polyacrylamide gel electrophoresis patterns were normal. A novel pattern of reactions was obtained with anti-Wr^b: negative with three human polyclonal and four monoclonal (BRIC's 201, 204, 89 and BRAC 13); weak with one monoclonal (BRIC 93) and normal strength positive with six monoclonal (BRIC's 14, 199, 202 and BRAC's 19, 27 and R7). EH cells were Wr(a-) but several antisera revealed a low incidence antigen not previously recognised.

Expression of the Wr^b antigen involves interaction between Band 3 and GPA. It is therefore likely from the results obtained in this study that EH has a structural change within either Band 3 or GPA. DNA sequencing of both are currently in progress.

0533

AN UNUSUAL PROTEASE RESISTANT M ANTIGEN DETECTED IN JAPANESE

M.Uchikawa[1], H.Tsuneyama[1], T.Juji[1], M.Kikuchi[2].
1Central Blood Centre, Tokyo, 2Miyagi Blood Centre, Miyagi, Japan.

Red cells from Japanese blood donors with a frequency of 0.07% gave a previously undescribed pattern of reaction with anti-M antibodies. The M antigen of red cells was trypsin, chymotrypsin, papain, ficin, bromelain resistant. The protease treated red cells did react with human, rabbit and murine monoclonal anti-M. The red cells did not express Vw, Hut, Mur, Hil, Anek, Mut, St^a, Dantsu, SAT, M^g, Mit, Os^a, and did not appear to have any obvious reduction in sialic acid levels using *Glycine soja*. Immunoblotting experiments with antibodies to M and an epitope common to GPA and GPB revealed an abnormal band of apparent Mr.20,000 , as compared to Mr.25,000 of GPB , and aggregates of the components. No abnormal bands were present on blots with various antibodies to N terminal and cytoplasmic C terminal of GPA, and s determinant of GPB. The result of PAS staining showed they had normal amount of GPA and reduced amount of GPB. Study on 6 protease resistant M red cells with S-s+, using anti-s in the fluoresent flow cytometry, showed that they bound, on average, a little over half the amount of anti-s bound by normal S-s+. Two unrelated propositi were S+s-. Their family showed that *S* was not inherited to other members with protease resistant M antigen. These result strongly suggested that the unusual M produced GPA, but did not GPB.

0534

A NOVEL AMINO ACID SEGUENCE RESULT IN THE EXPRESSION OF THE MNS RELATED PRIVATE ANTIGEN, SAT.

M.Uchikawa[1], H.Tsuneyama[1], L.Wang[1], K.Tokunaga[1], T.Juji[1], K.Tadokoro[1]. T.Enomoto[2].
1Central Blood Centre, Tokyo, 2Ina Blood Centre, Saitama, Japan.

Red cells of Japanese donors, M.H. and M.A., did react with antibodies to SAT(MNS36), a low frequency antigen of the MNS blood group system. M.H. and M.A. cells were M+^{w}N+S-s+U+, M-N+S-s+U+ respectively, and were positive with *Glycine soja*. SAT antigen is associated with two different types, GPA-GPB hybrid and apparently normal GPA and GPB, by immunoblots. SDS polyacrylamide gel electrophoresis followed by immunoblotting with various monoclonal antibodies to GPA and GPB showed M.H. had abnormal band, of apparent Mr.38,000, were identified on blots by antibodies to the M and other outer portion of GPA but not with antibodies to the cytoplasmic portion of GPA and N. The result suggested M.H. cells had a hybrid GPA-GPB carring N terminus of M-specific GPA. M.A. had no abnormal band, and the family study showed SAT antigen of M.A. was related with N antigen. cDNA were synthesized from total RNA of reticulocytes obtained from M.A. and M.H. and analysed by the polymerase chain reaction. Sequencing of the amplified products of M.A. showed 9 bases addition (CTC CTG TAG) between exon 4 and exon 5 of GPA. Thus M.A. possesses 134 amino acid residues in the mature form, result in the generation of the novel sequence. M.H. had a hybrid gene composed of exon 1 to exon 4 of GPA linked to exon 4 of GPB. These results suggested that M.A. and M.H. shared the same amino acid sequence S-E-P-A-P-V, which were responsible for the expression of SAT antigen.

0535

FURTHER STUDIES ON THE GENOTYPIC HETEROGENEITY AMONG LEWIS-NEGATIVE INDIVIDUAL.

A. Elmgren, L. Rydberg, G. Larson.
Department of Clinical Chemistry and Transfusion Medicine, Sahlgrenska Hospital, Göteborg, Sweden.

Recently four $\alpha(1,3)$ fucosyltransferases (FT-III, FT-IV, FT-V, FT-VI) were cloned and sequenced and their enzymatic activities determined (1). The FT-III was very similar in its activity to the human blood group fucosyltransferase isolated from human milk. In order to outline the genetic basis for Lewis-negative individuals we have used the PCR-technique to analyze the coding sequence of FT-III in the genome of 40 individuals. The published nucleotide sequence of FT-III, FT-V and FT-VI were used to design oligonucleotide primers specific for the respective transferases. The resulting DNA amplificates were characterized by restriction enzyme cleavage and by DNA sequencing. We found a specific base mutation in the coding sequence of FT-III at nucleotide position 314 (C to T). This could be found on both alleles in 5 of 18 Lewis negative (le) individuals but in none of 22 Lewispositive (Le) individuals (2). Other mutations have recently been described (3; 4 and R.Oriol pers. com.). We have now found another mutation at position 202 (T to C). This could be found on both alleles in 5 out of the 18 le- but in none of the 22 Le-individuals. The mutation was found on both alleles in 4 of the 5 individuals who were mutated on both alleles for the previous one.

1. Van den Eijnden DH et al. Cur Opin Struct Biol 1993;3;711.
2. Elmgren A et al. BBRC 1993;196;515.
3. Nishihara S et al. BBRC 1993;196;624.
4. Koda Y et al. Blood 1993;9;2915.

0536

NO EVIDENCE FOR AN ASSOCIATION BETWEEN NON-SECRETOR STATUS AND COELIAC DISEASE.

L.M. Sollid[1], J. Ek[2], B.G. Solheim[3]
1Inst. of Transplant. Immunol., 2Dept. of Paed., 3Blood Centre, Rikshospitalet, Oslo, Norway.

Coeliac disease (CD) is probably a polygenic disease with HLA as one genetic factor. The other genetic factors are unknown. Recently it was reported that among Northern-Irish CD patients there was an overrepresentation of non-secretors and it was suggested that a gene linked with the secretor locus on chromosome 19 is a susceptibility gene (Dickey & al. Gut:34, S23, 1993). The present study was undertaken to reproduce these findings. Secretor status was inferred from determination of red cell Lewis (Le) antigen phenotype in CD patients and controls using monoclonal antibodies. The unrelated CD patients were diagnosed according to the ESPGAN criteria of 1970. They were all in remission on a gluten-free diet.

Results:

	CD pts.		Ctrls.	
	N	%	N	%
Le(a+b-)	7	15	40	20
Le(a-b+)	34	72	142	71
Le(a-b-)	6	13	18	9

It follows that the prevalence of non-secretors was 17% in the CD patients and 22% in the controls. In contrast to the Northern-Irish study we find no evidence for an association between a non-secretor status and CD. Lewis blood type antigens are produced by the secretory epithelium in the gastrointestinal tract. Staining of biopsies with lectins has previously shown that the oligosaccharide antigens of jejunal epithelial cells are altered in untreated CD patients. The discrepancy between the two studies may thus possibly relate to the disease status (i.e. treated/untreated) of the patients tested.

0537

ABH SECRETOR STATUS, AS JUDGED BY THE LEWIS PHENOTYPES, IN NORWEGIAN SURVIVORS FROM MENINGOCOCCAL DISEASE

L. Kornstad, A.-L. Heistø, T.E. Michaelsen, G. Bjune
National Institute of Public Health, Oslo, Norway.

A study of various immunological parameters was performed in 1992 on persons who had suffered from invasive meningococcal disease in the period 1988-91. Since it has been claimed that non-secretion of ABH substance is a predisposing factor for such infection, it was decided to include Lewis grouping in the study.

Blood samples were collected from 98 survivors from meningococcal disease. They were tested in parallel with samples from 200 Oslo blood donors. All samples were tested against two different anti-Le^a and two anti-Le^b sera, for each specificity one monoclonal (mouse hybridoma; Biotest) and one polyclonal (goat heteroagglutinin; Behringwerke). All the sera were saline reacting.

Results:	Le(a+b-)	Le(a-b+)	Le(a-b-)	Total
Patients	23	66	9	98
Controls	40	142	18	200

Among the 89 patients who produced Lewis antigens 25.8 % were Le(a+b-) and accordingly non-secretors, 74.2 % Le(a-b+) and secretors. Among the corresponding 182 persons of the control group the frequencies were 22 % and 78 %, respectively. Comparing the secretor status of the two groups, a 2 x 2 table gives $X^2 = 0.5003$, 1 d.f., $P \approx 0.48$.
Conclusion: The present study does not support previous reports on an association between meningococcal meningitis and non-secretion of ABH substance.

0538

HUMAN BLOOD GROUP scFv ANTIBODIES DERIVED FROM A V GENE PHAGE DISPLAY LIBRARY

N. C. Hughes-Jones*, B. D. Gorick*, J. M. Bye*, R. Finnern[†], D Voak[†], JD Marks[#+] and W. H. Ouwehand[†$]
*MRC and,[†] Division of Transfusion Medicine, University of Cambridge, UK, [+] SFG Hospital, San Francisco, USA. [$]NIBSC, Potters Bar, U.K.

We have obtained 5 single chain Fv (scFv) antibody fragments specific for the blood group antigens B, Rh(D), Rh(E), Kp^b, and HI. (Marks et al, Bio/technology, 1993, 11,1145-49). The scFv's were isolated from a phage antibody library constructed from the variable (V) region genes of 2 non-immunised humans. All 5 scFv's agglutinated the appropriate red cell phenotype upon addition of a monoclonal antibody which recognises a peptide tag incorporated into the scFv. The anti-B and anti-HI scFv molecules, which recognise high density carbohydrate antigens, spontaneously polymerised and agglutinated red cells directly. None of the antibody fragments showed cross-reactivity with other red cell antigens, with the exception of the anti-E which reacted weakly with E-negative cells. Specific scFv binding was confirmed by ELISA, flow cytometry and radioactive labelling. The anti-D scFv had a Kd of $5.2x10^7M^{-1}$ and a k_{off} of $1.9x10^{-2}sec^{-1}$, and the anti-E scFv $5.3x10^6M^{-1}$ and $2.7x10^{-2}sec^{-1}$. In conclusion scFv's specific for cell surface antigens and with affinities typical of the primary immune response can be obtained from V gene phage-display libraries The results of the serological and kinetics studies are well related with the somatic mutation of the VH genes.

0539

IMMUNOGLOBULIN LIGHT CHAIN EXCHANGE OF A RHESUS D ANTIBODY USING PHAGE DISPLAY TECHNOLOGY: BIAS TOWARDS THE ORIGINAL LIGHT CHAIN VARIABLE DOMAIN SEQUENCE AND IMPROVED BINDING

E. Timmers*, J.M. Bye[¶], H. Sonneborn[†], D. Voak* and W.H. Ouwehand*[$].
[¶]MRC, *Division of Transfusion Medicine, University of Cambridge, U.K., [†]Biotest, Frankfurt, Germany, [$]NIBSC, Potters Bar, U.K.

The heavy (H) chain variable (V) encoding gene segment of a well characterized IgG anti-rhesus D antibody (BS221) was cloned in an antibody fragment display vector containing a human light (L) chain V domain library with a diversity of 10^4. Initial screening of the constructed library showed that 1-2% of the clones had binding activity to papain-treated R2R2 cells in a single-chain Fv haemagglutination assay. A single round of selection of the library on the same R2R2 cells resulted in 20-30% binders. Fifteen positive clones were selected for further analysis. The structure of L chain V gene segments was determined by sequencing. The selected light chain V domains were biased towards sequences that had close homology to the original BS221 light chain V domain. FACS analysis comparing the biding affinity to R2R2, R1r, rr and category VI cells revealed enhanced binding by two scFv antibody fragments, with newly combined L chain V domains, when compared to the original combination of H and L chain V domains of BS221 expressed as a scFv.

0540

A CASE OF "DEFECTIVE" ABO GROUP REVISITED AFTER 30 YEARS

L. Kornstad*, E. Namork*, H.E. Heier**
*National Institute of Public Health, Oslo, ** Ullevaal Hospital Blood Bank, Oslo, Norway.

In 1961 a report was given (Vox Sang. 6:692-697) on a healthy male (B.H.) whose cells behaved as group O, but anti-B was the only detectable alloantibody in his serum. He was a secretor of H but not of A substance. His cells did not absorb anti-A from a group B serum nor did an eluate contain anti-A or $-A_1$.

The renewed studies did not reveal any discrepancies from the previous. However, when group O sera with immune-anti-A were absorbed with the B.H. cells, heat eluates gave positive indirect antiglobulin reactions with A_2 and, more weakly, with A_x cells. Corresponding absorption of group O sera containing immune-anti-B gave eluates with no anti-B or -A activity.

B.H. cells were sensitized with a monoclonal anti-A reacting with all known A oligosaccharides, labelled with 30 nm colloidal gold particles conjugated to anti-mouse IgM, and studied by backscatter electron imaging in a scanning electron microscope. About 2 % of the cells were labelled, some of them very heavily.

We conclude that B.H. is another example of a "weak A" phenotype in which only a minority of the cells express A antigens. The biochemical nature of his A antigen remains to be elucidated.

0541

THE DOMBROCK BLOOD GROUP LOCUS : A LINKAGE ANALYSIS.

G. Coghlan[1], L. White[1], S. Philipps[1], B. Carritt[2] and T. Zelinski[1]. [1]Rh Laboratory, Depts. of Pediatrics and Human Genetics, University of Manitoba, Winnipeg, Canada and [2]MRC Human Biochem. Genetics Unit, London, England.

Dombrock is the only blood group system whose gene has not been chromosomally assigned. In an ongoing linkage analysis of the Dombrock locus (DO) in relation to 105 genetic markers, the only lods which exceed +3.00 occurred with the chromosome 1p marker phosphogluconate dehydrogenase (PGD). The PGD protein polymorphism and DO had peak lods of 5.61 at $\hat{\theta}$ = 0.10 in female meioses and negative lods in male meioses (1). Until now, no second data set has been published to either refute or confirm this possible linkage. In analyzing DO informative families for a restriction fragment length polymorphism of PGD we have observed no evidence of linkage between DO and PGD in female or male meioses. In fact, our results indicate that DO is not within 20cM of PGD (based on lods of -2.00 at a recombination fraction of 0.20). Our results are confirmed by the lack of linkage between DO and a second chromosome 1p DNA marker, PND, which is linked to PGD. Thus the search for DO should continue with consideration given to the fact that its locus has been excluded from approximately 40% of the genome.

(1) Lewis et al., (1983) Ann Hum Genet 47, 49-53.

Work supported by the Medical Research Council of Canada and England and The Children's Hospital Research Foundation.

0542

"RÉUNION"H-DEFICIENT PHENOTYPE. FIRST CASE IN SPAIN.

T.Carrascosa[1], M.A.Pérez[2], M.A.Vesga[2], K.Atucha[1], J.Ojanguren[1], P.Esteban[1], A.Renovales[3], M.A.Basaldua[3]. 1.Hematology Department. Galdakao Hospital, 2.Centro Vasco de Transfusión, 3.Banco de Sangre de Alava. Galdakao. Spain.

INTRODUCTION

We present a non-secretor para-Bombay phenotype whose serological results appear to be similar to those described by Le Pendu as the "Réunion phenotype".

RESULTS

- The patient's red cells reactions were: with Anti-A:-; Anti-B:-; Anti-AB:-; Lectin anti-H Ulex europeaus: w; Lectin anti-H Laburnum Alpinum:-; murine monoclonal anti-H:-; human anti-H made by a person with Bombay phenotype: w; anti-I: 4+.
- The patient's red cells were typed as D negative, M-N+S+s+, P_1+, K-, Le(a+b-), Fy(a+b-) and Jk(a-b+).
- The direct antiglobulin test was negative using polyspecific anti-human globulin reagent and anti-IgG.
- No A, B o H substance was detected in the patient's saliva.
- In the patient's serum was detected a cold reactive antibody of anti-H specificity.
- In the patient's serum were not detected neither N-acetyl-galactosaminyl nor galactosaminyl transferases.
- In the family study we found three brothers group A_2 with decreased anti-H reactivity.

CONCLUSION

This patient has a non-secretor para-Bombay phenotype that fits in the "Réunion phenotype". It is distinguished from a true Bombay phenotype because of its reactivity with Ulex europeaus and anti-H made by true Bombay phenotypes. This is the first case of this phenotype in Spain.

0543

SPECIFICITY OF ANTI-GPA MABS; CHARACTERIZATION OF A NEW MAB THAT IDENTIFIED A NON ERYTHROID SPECIFIC 80 kDa PROTEIN

M. Rasamoelisolo, C. Willem, Y. Petit, M.J. Loirat, W. Dahr, J.Y. Muller and D. Blanchard
Centre Régional de Transfusion Sanguine de Nantes, France.

A series of new mAbs directed against glycophorin A (GPA) have been prepared from splenocytes of Balb/c mice immunized with human RBCs. MAbs without specificity for M or N blood group antigens were characterized by agglutination, agglutination/inhibition tests with peptides and chemically modified glycophorins, and immunoblotting.
MAb NaM26-3F4 (IgG1) recognized the common portion of GPA and GPB (aa residues 6 to 25). MAbs NaM10-2H12 (IgG3), NaM10-6G4 (IgG2a) and NaM16-1B10 (IgM) did not agglutinate trysin-treated RBCs; they recognized epitopes located within aa residues 35-45 of GPA. MAbs NaM13-4E4 and NaM37-5F4 (both IgG1) failed to bind to RBCs but strongly revealed a CNBr peptide (aa 9 to 81 of GPA) on immunoblot, suggesting they bound to aa 60 to 80 of GPA. MAb NaM70-3C10 (IgM) showed atypical properties since it agglutinated trypsin-, chymotrypsin- or ficin- treated RBCs but failed to agglutinate papain-treated cells. Of major interest, this mAb which was inhibited by a synthetic peptide containing aa 50 to 58 of GPA bound a 80 kDa protein expressed by platelets and monocytes. Most probably, the non erythroid specific 80 kDa protein and GPA carry a common epitope.

0544

OVEREXPRESSION OF THE P1 BLOOD GROUP ANTIGEN ON RED CELLS FROM A CDAII PATIENT

D. Bouhours[1], J.F. Bouhours[1], C. Willem[2], E. Planus[1] and D. Blanchard[2]
1Unité INSERM U76, Paris, 2Centre Régional de Transfusion Sanguine de Nantes, France.

BALB/C mice were immunized with RBCs from a CDA II patient (Dub.). Following fusion of splenocytes with SP20/Ag-14 myeloma cells, mAb NaM31-1B11 was selected by agglutination tests. Titers of 4 and 32 were obtained with untreated control P1 and CDAII (Dub.) RBCs, respectively. Trypsin- and papain-treated RBCs were agglutinated with titers of 128 to 512 but no significant difference was observed between control and CDAII cells. In contrast P2 RBCs were not agglutinated.
Immunostaining of glycolipids on thin layer chromatography plates demonstrated that the mAb is specific for the Galα1-4Galß disaccharide present on the Pk (CTH) and P1 antigens. Also, the binding of the antibody to glycolipids could be totally inhibited by the trisaccharide Galα1-4Galß1-4GlcNAc-OEt (P1 structure).
By agglutination test, the overexpression of the P1 antigen was not found on RBCs from two other CDAII samples (KH and MD), suggesting that anti-P1 antibodies might be useful to subtype CDAII samples.
Also, mAb NaM31-1B11 proved to be a specific and potent anti-P1 blood group reagent.

0545

RENAL TRANSPLANT AND KNOPS SYSTEM ANTIBODY

Castañeda A, López R, Cano I, Pinilla J, Martín A, Rubio M, Santacreu M, Ríos P, Ojeda E, García de Bustos J, Ulibarrena C, Jiménez V, Martín MP, de la Cámara C. y Hdez Navarro F
Servicio de Hematología y Hemoterapia. Hospital "La Paz" . Madrid (Spain).

A 48-Year-Old Woman with chronic renal failure three years earlier. Extracorporeal hemodyalisis was begun. Was admitted to hospital a cadaveric renal-transplantation procedure. The patient was treated with Cyclosporin A. The patient's postoperative course was complicate by renal function damaged (microscopical examination of a renal-biopsy specimen showed evidence of light rejection), retroperitoneal hematoma and hypovolemic shock. Seventeen units of packed red cells were transfused in fifteen days.
Her red cells typed as group 0, D negative, probable Rh genotype rr (cde/cde), $M+^{mf}$ N+ S- s+, P_1, Le(a-b+), K-, $Fy(a+^{mf}$ b+), Jk(a+b+), and Kn(a+), Sl(a-) Yk(a-) Cs(a+). In order to obtain patient red blood cells free of recently transfused red blood cells to perform phenotyping, a microhematocric centrifugation separation procedure to harvest reticulocytes was performed. These cells phenotyped as the unseparated sample had, with mixed field reactivity still detected in the M and Fy^a typings. The direct antiglobulin test was negative using polyspecific anti- human globulin reagent. The serum sample, demonstrated microscopic to + in LO-ION AHGT with most cells of panel. The reactivity was similar in ficin testing and all panel cells were reactive in PEG AHGT. Testing of selected cells indicated rectivity was directed at Knops system antigens (Kn^a, MoC^a, Sl^a and/or Yk^a).
In spite of it has been reported a low incidence of alloimmunization in transplanted and immunosupresed patients, we descrive a case of alloantibody to a high incidence antigen in a renal transplanted patient.

0546

A NEW LOW FREQUENCY RED CELL ANTIGEN

JM Jongerius[1], H Rijksen[2], MAM Overbeeke[3], WHJ Derks[2], EF van Leeuwen[1]
[1]Bloodbank Utrecht,[2]Diakonessen Ziekenhuis Utrecht,[3]Central Laboratory of NRC Bloodtransfusion service, Amsterdam, the Netherlands

Introduction: A 60-year-old patient was hospatilized for orthopedic surgery. His transfusion history was unknown. Results of compatibility testing were as follows: Patient bloodgroup A_2 Rhesus D positive, serum screening on irregular antibodies against a 3-cell panel negative, crossmatch with ABO compatible erythrocytes of one of two random donors **positive** at room temperature, 37^0C and in antiglobuline-phase with bovine albumine or polyethylen-glycol (PEG). No anti-A_1- and/or anti-HLA-antibodies were shown to be present. The direct antiglobuline test on concerned donor-erythrocytes (further called VLAAN) was negative. Research on the presence of antibodies directed against a low frequency antigen was initiated.
Results: The antibodies appeared to be of IgG class.
The serum of the patient was positive with red cells of only one of 1068 random ABO compatible donors. This positive reaction showed another pattern in the different assays and appeared to be due to IgM antibodies against another low frequency antigen.
With the assistance of several reference laboratories has been demonstrated that the antibodies in the serum of the patient recognize no known red cell antigen and that the donor VLAAN erythrocytes carry no known low frequency red cell antigen.
Family investigation shows that 2 sisters of donor VLAAN carry the new antigen. Also one of three children of his sister is positive for this antigen. The erythrocytes of his father and 2 nephews are negative. Up till now study of association with Rh, MNS and Duffy system is nonconclusive. The antigen is not associated with sex and ABO.
Conclusion: a new red cell antigen with low frequency is detected. ISBT registration is in process.

0547

EVALUATION OF THE 'BOSS' BLOOD GROUPING MACHINE

A. Patel, E.C. Cullen, R.C. Knight.

North London Blood Transfusion Centre, Colindale London NW9 5BG, UK.

The Menarini BOSS blood grouping machine is designed for ABO and Rh phenotyping at a rate of 60 samples an hour. Disposable racks containing 12 reaction wells are utilised allowing up to 12 reagents to be used.

The test cells are suspended in a bromelin solution and reacted with antisera (supplied from the manufacturer) whilst being stirred; the light transmitted through each well is measured for 45 secs. Transmitted light is plotted on a graph, displayed on a VDU, and the results electronically interpreted as +, - or ?. As cells become agglutinated more light is transmitted

In an initial trial 300 samples were grouped and the results compared to those from existing Kontron Groupamatic machines. No discrepancies were found with a range of samples including selected R_1R_1 (32) R_2R_2 (25) R_1r (32) r'r (31), but 2/9 r"r gave a negative reaction with anti-E on the first run but were E+ on retesting. All 15 weak D samples gave negative results with anti-D on both BOSS and Groupamatic machines. There were no major problems with the machine itself.

0548

MULTICENTRIC STUDY OF BLOOD GROUP REAGENTS ON AUTOMATES OLYMPUS PK 7100 AND 7200

MONCHARMONT P., CHERBY C. AND THE OLYMPUS STUDY GROUP
C.R.T.S. LYON - BP 7015 - 69342 LYON CEDEX 07 FRANCE

Purpose : In aim to determine their quality, a multicentric evaluation was performed with blood group reagents routinely used on immunohematology automates OLYMPUS PK 7100 and 7200.
Methods : ABO, Rh (D, C, E, c, e) and Kell systems blood group reagents of several manufacturers were evaluated with different diluents (Albumin 2 %, Albumine 5 % and NaCl 9 ‰) at different dilutions on erythrocytes by the group members.
Results : In ABO system, 9 out of 13 monoclonal anti-A reagents lots have concordant results in Albumin 2 % at a dilution of 1/200. The performances are lower with polyclonal anti-A (7 lots) (dilution 1/75 in Albumin 2 %). With polyclonal and monoclonal anti-B or anti A+B, data are similar at a dilution of 1/200 in Albumin 2 %. In Rh system, 10 lots of polyclonal and 13 of monoclonal anti-D have good results in Albumin 2 % at 1/50. In the same diluent, good results are also observed with monoclonal and polyclonal anti-C reagents at 1/60 but the polyclonal anti-c was better than the monoclonal. In the other hand, anti-E and anti-e monoclonal reagents were more efficient in Albumin 2 % than polyclonal. Polyclonal and monoclonal anti-K reagents have similar results in Albumin 2 %. In all cases, the values obtained with the reagents are lower in Albumin 5 %. Lastly, with NaCl 9 ‰, the results are either equivalent or lower compared with Abumin 2 %.
Conclusion : Use of dilution of blood group reagents on automates Olympus PK 7100 and 7200 gave better results in Albumin 2 % than in Albumin 5 %.
In some cases, differences are also observed between polyclonal and monoclonal specificities.

0549

Automated microplate ABO and Rhesus D testing with a high speed and simple pipetting protocol

G. Verhoeven, R.C.Schaap, Red Cross Bloodbank Kennemerland, Haarlem the Netherlands

We developed a high speed and simple pipetting protocol for ABO and Rhesus D testing on the Hamilton AT plus Processor.
In the first pipetting cycle monoclonal anti A, anti B and anti D reagents are added to three microplates, each reagent in a different plate. In a fourth plate a 3% redcell suspension is made.
The suspensions are prepared by mixing red cells, aspirated from the samples placed in the testrack, and phosphate buffered solution (PBS).
In the second pipetting cycle the cell suspension is added to the bloodgroupreagent in the three microplates. The total pipetting time of the full plates (96 wells) is only eight minutes.
After incubation on roomtemperature and centrifugation (2 minutes/ 200g) the microplates are read by a Dynatech MR 5000 reader. Sanguin Medusa 2000 software interpretes the results.
Because on every plate there are just agglutinationprofils with one bloodgroup reagent, the software, originally written for the interpretation of elisatests, can be used with only a slight modification. The percentage of mismatches is very low (0,3%) because the high speed of the procedure prevents false positive or negative agglutination patterns. This method can also be used for fenotyping with other monoclonal antibodies (C,c, E,e,Le^a,Le^b,M,P_1,Kell).The batch processing allows fast correction of failures.

0550

STANDARDIZED PROTEINASE ENZYME TECHNIQUE FOR RED CELL ANTIBODY DETECTION USING THE NEW AUTOANALYZER PK7200

T. Mazda[1], R. Yabe[1], K. Nakata[1], K. Fujisawa[1], K. Makino[2] and H. Ohshima[2]
[1]Japanese Red Cross Tokyo Metropolitan Blood Center, [2]Faculty of Pharmaceutical Sciences, Science University of Tokyo, Tokyo, Japan

Enzyme concentrations of papain, bromelin and ficin can be standardized by the casein method for use in red blood cell screening test. The optimal enzyme activity for detecting blood group antibodies using the AutoAnalyzer Olympus PK7200 by the two-stage method for all three enzymes is one casein unit. The optimal enzyme units for the two-stage manual method is however approximately 20-40 casein units. One casein unit of proteinase activity changed the red cell surface charge to a low plateau values as assayed by electrophoretic mobility and sialic acid content, and removed the steric inhibiting structures of surface protein as measured by SDS-PAGE. Therefore we consider that one casein unit is the minimal and yet optimal activity for red cell antibody agglutination screening using proteolytic enzymes.

0551

NEW TECHNOLOGY COMPUTERISED RED CELL ANTIBODY IDENTIFICATION SOFTWARE SYSTEM

R. Benedek[1], D. Cupaníková[2], D. Pavlíková[2]
1ARTMAN-LBM Ltd., 2Central Laboratory of the Slovak Haematology and Transfusion University Clinic

The main purpose of this system is to provide highly professional, accurate and efficient program to support empirical conclusions on Red Cell Antibody Detection.

Features included: detection of up to 5 Red Cell Antibodies simultaneously; nonlimited use of panel combination; flexibility to extend or change the number of panel antigens and tests used.

Furthermore, the programme combines the Quick Non-Quantified Estimation (QNE) and Double Back Coupling (DBC) which are the original software algorithms for sufficient improving the Fisher Exact Test (FET). The final Computer Optimisation simply recommends the user to add, change or create as required the most appropriate panel from specified donor phenotypes. Only Antibodies with a 95-100% level of probability are considered as final results. Incorporation of system output databases to the Lab network, user report generator, quick and precise results, English communication, and user friendliness makes this system internationally attractive.

0552

CONCENTRATED SALINE: AN OPPORTUNITY TO REDUCE PACKAGE DRIVEN ENVIRONMENTAL LOAD

P. Aeby, A. Schumacher, A. Fasel, B. Brick, C. Bläsius, H. Spatz, B. Bircher, S. Müller[1], S. Threin[2]
1 Baxter Diagnostics AG, Düdingen, Switzerland, 2 Baxter Deutschland GmbH, Unterschleissheim, Deutschland

Ready-made phosphate buffered saline (PBS) solutions are being used in many laboratories for the preparation of red blood cell suspensions and cell washing. Commercially available ready-made solutions are packaged in non-reusable plastic or cardboard/plastic containers. Shipment of the saline solution to users means transporting thousands of liters of water over large distances. Ready to use solutions also require vast amounts of storage capacity. A study to reduce packaging, transportation energy and costs, and storage space while not affecting ease of use or performance is described. The following system was developed and evaluated: 500 ml of 20x concentrated PBS solution packed in one-way recyclable bottle is shipped to the final user. A working solution is prepared by mixing the concentrate with 9.5 liters of demineralized water and stored in a re-usable 10 liter container. Careful selection of packaging materials drastically reduced the overall environmental impact. The 500 ml bottle is made of ~ 40 g recyclable, high density polyethylene (HDPE) which is a significant reduction from the ~ 1.25 kg used in a 20 liter container. The bottles are directly printed with heavy-metal-free ink. The 20x PBS formulation was optimized and allows the preparation of a working solution within a defined pH range (7.1 - 7.5). However, the buffer capacity was deliberately limited to provide optimum reaction conditions for pH dependant blood group antibodies. The performance of the reconstituted PBS was compared to a ready-made PBS during a field trial containing antigen typing, antibody screening and compatibility testing segments. Four hundred thirty-five antigen typing tests, involving 22 antigens, 66 antibody screens with 22 different seras and 36 compatibility tests showed no difference in performance between the reconstituted PBS and the ready -made solution. Concentrated PBS packaged in a recyclable bottle represents an environment and user friendly alternative to ready made saline without any performance loss.

0553

EVALUATION OF MONOCLONAL KIDD BLOOD GROUPING REAGENTS

I. Shulman[1], M. Gibson[2], H. Polesky[3], P. Ness[4]
1 LAC/USC Medical Center, Los Angeles, CA, 2 Baxter Diagnostics Inc., Miami, FL, 3 Memorial Blood Center of Minneapolis, Minneapolis, MN, 4 Johns Hopkins Hospital, Baltimore, MD, USA

A monoclonal anti-Jk^a (m-Jk^a) and anti-Jk^b (m-Jk^b), derived from heterohybridoma cell lines, were parallel tested with FDA licensed reagents containing polyclonal antibodies for recognition of Jk^a and Jk^b antigens. The monoclonal reagents were tested by saline tube and microplate methodologies using a five minute room temperature incubation. The polyclonal antisera were used by indirect antiglobulin technique, as recommended by the manufacturer. Red blood cells (RBC) from donors and patients were tested fresh, after storage in a variety of anticoagulants or after frozen storage. Prior to testing with m-Jk^a and m-Jk^b, RBC were either washed with normal saline or unwashed; all RBC tested with the polyclonal reagents were washed. Of 1250 RBC samples tested, 1237 (99%) showed no discrepancy for paired results when using monoclonal versus polyclonal reagents, regardless of anticoagulant, washing of RBC, duration of RBC storage, tube or microplate testing, or donor/patient factors (ABO, age, race, diagnosis). Thirteen (1%) paired test results were repeatably discrepant. All 13 discrepant RBC samples were direct antiglobulin test (DAT) reactive (w+-4+) with anti-IgG and typed as Jk(a+b+) with the polyclonal reagents. In seven cases the monoclonal reagents grouped the RBC as Jk(a+b-) and in the other six as Jk(a-b+). In discrepant cases where previously determined Kidd phenotypes were known, results obtained with the monoclonal reagents matched historical phenotypes. No repeatable discrepancies were observed in samples that were DAT negative. From these data we conclude that the m-Jk^a and m-Jk^b performed at least as well as the FDA licensed polyclonal- derived Kidd grouping reagents and may be more reliable than polyclonal reagents when testing RBC that are DAT positive.

0554

SOLIDSCREEN II-ENZYME: A COMPLEMENTARY METHOD TO SOLIDSCREEN II

L.Sturmfels, S.Hoffmann, H. Uthemann, V.Lenhard
Biotest AG, Dreieich, Germany

An extended application of the solid phase antiglobulin test Solidscreen II consists in the use of enzyme-treated test erythrocytes. Solidscreen II-Enzyme may be performed either as a two-stage papain test or as an one-stage bromelin test. Depending on the enzyme used the red cells (screening- and identification cells as well as autocontrols) are pretreated with papain in tubes, respectively the bromelin is added to the sample preparation of Solidscreen II. In both cases the following test procedure is identical to Solidscreen II. Besides the increased sensitivity in the detection of weak Rh antibodies "real enzyme-reactive antibodies" can be detected.
Comparative studies indicated an increase in sensitivity up to two titer steps, both by using papain-treated cells and by adding bromelin. The two enzyme methods showed comparable results. A total of 818 serum samples and 404 EDTA plasma samples were tested for red cell antibodies. In addition to Solidscreen II 12 antibodies (0.98%) were detected and identified.
Solidscreen II-Enzyme has proved to be an efficient and useful supplement to Solidscreen II. It completes the methods performing antibody screening, identification and compatibility testing in a well established solid phase technique.

0555

A SOLID-PHASE TEST (SPH) FOR ERYTHROCYTE ANTIBODY SCREENING DURING PREGNANCY.

S.Sallander, S.Pegert, A.Shanwell, L.Jakobsson, M. Åqvist, B.Wiechel
Stockholm Blood Transfusion Service, Södersjukhuset, Stockholm, Sweden

We present a semiautomated SPH test for erythrocyte antibody screening suitable for indirect antiglobulin and enzyme enhanced techniques(SPH-IAT and-ENZ)that permit storage of the test cells coated microplates for up to 5 days.
After the test cells been coated on to a poly-L-lysine support surface, areas between the coated test cells were blocked by adding a 1% BSA (bovine serum albumin) solution. After 1 hour incubation at room temperature the microplates were ready to use or to store at +4°C up to 5 days. For screening and identification we used RBC (red blood cells) selected from our own donor pool. The RBC used in the SPH-ENZ were prior to coating treated with papain according to the procedure for 2-stage papain test. Positive screen results were futher investigated using the SPH, manual IAT and 2-stage papain techniques.
Unselected plasma samples of 21376 pregnant women were tested with a positivity of 1.2%. Of the 93 antibodies detected by the SPH-IAT and -ENZ, 71 were detected by the manual tests. SPH-ENZ solely detected 5 anti-E, 7 anti-Jk^a and 2 autoanti-Jk^a. SPH-IAT solely detected 6 anti-M and 2 anti-S. Unspecific reactions in the SPH tests were 0,23% and false positive reactions were 0,46%.
We conclude that the SPH-IAT, -ENZ is an economically favorable test suitable for screening larger sample series of pregnant women.

0556

EXPERIENCE IN THE USE OF A MONOCLONAL POLYSPECIFIC ANTI-HUMAN GLOBULIN REAGENT FOR ANTIBODY INVESTIGATION.

M.K. Moulds, P. Spruell, C. Lomas, J. Chen, K. Champagne, T. Frame, J.J. Moulds.
Gamma Biologicals, Inc., Houston, Texas, U.S.A.

A study was undertaken to evaluate the use of monoclonal vs. rabbit antiglobulin reagents: 1251 samples referred for special investigation were tested. A polyspecific, murine monoclonal anti-human globulin reagent was used. The reagent is a blend of an IgM anti-IgG component derived from the murine hybridoma 16H8, and IgG1 anti-complement components, anti-C3d and anti-C3b, derived respectively from hybridoma cell lines 053A.714 and 055A.305.

Most samples were initially investigated by the referring laboratories using rabbit antiglobulin reagents. The samples contained single or multiple antibody specificities directed at common and high frequency red cell antigens in the major blood group systems, including several uncommon specificities; i.e., anti-Au^b, -Jk3, -Lu12, -LW, -Vel, -Lan, -PP_1P^k, -Cr^a, -Ge, -Hy, -Gy^a, -Ch, -Rg, -JMH, and -Yt^a. All, except five of seven anti-JMH, one of one anti-Rg and two of nine anti-Yt^a, were detected by the murine monoclonal antiglobulin reagent. The anti-IgG component of this reagent is reactive only with IgG1, IgG2 and IgG3 subclasses and not with IgG4 subclass antibodies. Of the eight antibodies not detected (less than 1%), those which were IgG subclassed were found to be only IgG4.

We conclude that this monoclonal antiglobulin reagent is suitable for use in antibody investigations.

0557

USE OF HOME DISULFIDE BONDS-CLEAVING AGENT TO DISTINGUISH IgM FROM IgG ANTIBODIES

N.V.Mineeva,M.A.Matveeva,S.V.Ziuzgina
Research Institute of Haematology and Blood Transfusion,St-Petersburg,Russia.

The efficacy of home disulfide-bonds cleaving agent(DCA) for destroying IgM antibody of anti-A,B and Rh(D) specificity in human blood serum was assessed and compared to that obtained in treatment of the sera by dithiothreitol.

It has been demonstrated that temperature 37°C is optimal for 2-hours inactivating IgM antibodies. After serum treatment by the DCA, the sera were examined in Indirect Antiglobulin Test using monospesific anti-IgG and anti-IgM reagents to determine the immunoglobulin class of the antibodies. To avoid the agglutination of test red cells in the phase of sensitization,the cells were fixed with glutaraldehyde.
It has been shown the absence of IgM antibodies in the DCA treated sera which demonstrates a complete destruction of the above antibodies,while the IgM anti-A,B,D remained intact.

The comparision of the obtained results with data on treatment of sera by dithiothreitol shows the complete similarity of the results.This allows to recommend the method for routine use.

Within last three years the DCA method has found wide application in Russia in determining the immunoglobulin class of antibodies known to be present in a serum.

0558

SEROLOGICAL AND IMMUNOCHEMICAL EVALUATION OF A NEW POLYSPECIFIC MONOCLONAL ANTI-HUMAN GLOBULIN, BLEND OF ANTI-IgG AND ANTI-C_3d MONOCLONAL ANTIBODIES :

MAESTRIA ®

Auteurs : C. BETREMIEUX[2], M. VERSCHELDE[2], L. KEYSER[2], A. GLACET[1] , M .BEOLET[1], L. MANNESSIER[1], D. BOUREL[1].
1 Centre Régional de Transfusion Sanguine de Lille, FRANCE
2 DIAGAST Laboratoires, Lille FRANCE.

Two murine anti-human IgG monoclonal antibodies (cell line 188-33 of IgG class and cell line 188-96 of IgM class) and one murine anti-C3d monoclonal antibody (cell line 120 11 D10 of IgG class) were mixed to prepare a polyspecific anti-human globulin. Characteristics of these monoclonal antibodies were studied :

- Specificity : Tests were performed to define the different subclasses of human IgG recognized by the anti-IgG antibodies - Both antibodies were able to detect human IgG_1, IgG_2, IgG_3 - Additional tests are in progress to define the recognition of IgG allotypes.
  The anti-C_3d monoclonal antibody was studied for the 2nd International Workshop and Symposium, Lund (1990).
  This immunochemical evaluation was completed by serological tests.
- Reactivity (3 steps) :
  1. The monoclonal anti-human globulin was tested in parallel with polyclonal polyspecific anti-human globulins (rabbit anti-IgG and monoclonal anti-C_3d) using sera and plasmas in a tube technique. Several thousand of samples have been tested according to a LISS indirect antiglobulin test. All unexpected antibodies were identified. The majority of these antibodies were known to be of clinical significance.
  2. Direct antiglobulin tests (IgG-type and C_3d-type tests) were performed without discrepancies between the monoclonal and reference antiglobulin reagents.
  3. Phenotyping in saline tube method was performed against weak antigens of the following systems : Kell, Duffy, Kidd, MNSs. Similar results were obtained with both polyclonal and monoclonal anti-human globulins.

All of the above results demonstrated the efficiency of *MAESTRIA* ®, this new monoclonal polyspecific antihuman globulin, for replacing conventional polyclonal anti-human globulins.

0559

QUANTITATION OF ERYTHROCYTE-ASSOCIATED IgG BY COMPETITIVE ENZYME-LINKED IMMUNOASSAY /CELIA/

Ananieva R.,Manolova V.,Toteva Z.
National Center of Clinical and Transfusion Haematology
Sofia, Bulgaria

The competitive immuno-enzyme method (by Kiefel et al 1987) was modified for the quantitation of erythrocyte (Er)-associated IgG. The results of quantitation of IgG were calculated on the basis of prebuilt standard curve by using human standard IgG against rabbit anti-human IgG. Unbound antibodies were determined by using anti-rabbit IgG conjugated with peroxidase. For each probe was calculated % inhibition:

$$\% \text{ Inhibition} = 100 \left\{1 - \frac{OD_{pr} - OD_{bl}}{OD_{max} - OD_{bl}}\right\}$$

The results were presented as fg of IgG on one Er or equivalent number of IgG molecules on one Er.
135 healthy donors were tested who showed IgG under 0,015 fg/Er. Preliminary studies were carried out on 19 patients with AIHA (positive DAT) and their values were in the ranges from 0.1 to 2.5 fg/Er.12 of the patients were studied continuously during the treatment.
The method was highly sensitive, precise and CV was from 1,7 to 9,5. and It gives opportunity for objective estimation of the applied therapy.

0560

MICROWAVE vs ULTRASOUND ELUTION: COMPARISON OF TWO UNCOMMON METHODS.

Yu G[1], Torloni AS[1,2], Sloane T[2] VA Med Ctr[1]. & Univ. of KY College of Med.[2], Lexington, KY

We compared the efficacy of microwave (MW) and ultrasound (US) methods for dissociating IgG from red blood cells (RBC). Direct antiglobulin test (DAT) negative RBCs were phenotyped and coated with human derived unmodified antibodies to A, B, c, D, e, Fy^b, Jk^b and k antigens (DAT w+ to 3+). A minimum of five paired samples for each antigen group were treated by both MW radiation and US, according to described methods[1,2]. Eluates were tested against a panel of phenotyped group O cells and graded by standard methods[3]. The MW method successfully eluted antibody from all samples, while US failed to elute anti-Fy^b. The results of the study are shown in Table 1. The US technique produced significantly stronger eluates for anti-A and anti-B antibodies.

Table 1

N	Antibody	DAT Cells	Eluates MW	Eluates US
5	A	2+	1+	4+
5	B	2+s	2+	4+
5	c	3+	2+	2+
5	D	3+s	3+	1+
7	e	w+	1+	1+
5	Fy^b	1+	w+	0
5	Jk^b	w+	1+	R
5	k	1+s	1+s	w+

MW treatment required less than 50 sec. of irradiation per sample, while US required 120 sec. US consistently produced stronger eluates for anti-A and anti-B antibodies, but did not elute anti-Fy^b from any of the samples. Although both methods offer rapid alternatives to conventional methods of elution, microwaves showed overall more consistent results than ultrasounds.

1) Judd JW, Methods in Immunohematology, p 67-68 1988.
2) Judd JW, Methods in Immunohematology, p 70-71 1988.
3) Technical Manual, AABB, 18th edition 1993.

0561

THE PROTEIN COMPOSITION OF RED CELL ELUATES

H. Sukati, U.J. Dumaswala, T.J.Greenwalt.
Hoxworth Blood Center, University of Cincinnati Medical Center, Cincinnati, Ohio, USA.

The purpose of this study was to elucidate the protein composition of red blood cell (RBC) eluates prepared by the acid and xylene elution methods. Six samples of group 0 R_1R_1 RBCs sensitized with anti-D in vitro and the same RBCs not sensitized were studied. The eluate protein composition was determined by sodium dodecyl sulfate polyacrylamide gel electrophoresis. The immunoglobulin concentrations were established by immunoblotting using horseradish peroxidase conjugated anti-IgG and 3,3' diaminobenzidine. The protein concentrations of the xylene eluates were significantly greater ($p<0.005$) than that of the acid eluates, probably due to the presence of denatured hemoglobin. In all samples the percentage of immunoglobulins (IgG) was less than 0.6% of the total protein content. The acid eluates of the sensitized RBCs contained more IgG than the xylene eluates. The molecular weights of the Coomassie blue stained bands were estimated by comparison with the migration of low and high molecular weight standards. The estimated weights of the proteins in the xylene eluates were 97, 78, 63, 45, 31, 23Kd and in the acid eluates 97, 78, 55Kd. No Schiff-stainable bands were detected. The data indicate that IgG represented only a small fraction of the proteins in the eluates and that the protein composition varied with the elution procedure.

0562

DETECTION OF ABO BLOOD GROUP ANTIGENS USING AFFINITY MEMBRANES OF RED CELL STROMA AND BLOOD GROUP SUBSTANCES BY IMMUNOELECTRODES

K. Furukawa, T. Nakajima, T. Matsuki
Department of Legal Medicine, Gunma University School of Medicine, Maebashi, Japan

Red cell stroma was prepared by the method of Fairbanks et al. (1971) and blood group substances were obtained from human gastric linings. Triacetyl cellulose membrane containing blood group antigens were prepared as follows: triacetyl cellulose 250 mg was dissolved in 5 ml of methylene chloride: ethanol (9:1) and 1 ml of red cell stroma suspension or solution of blood group substance was added and mixed well. For reference membrane without blood group antigens 1 ml of distilled water was added instead of the blood group substances. The mixtures were poured on glass plate and dried at room temperature. Ortho blood typing antisera were used for anti-A and anti-B and eel serum for anti-H. The membrane containing blood group antigens and reference membrane were pasted to make each plastic cell bottom using adhesive and the cells were filled with PBS. The cell bottoms were dipped in plastic well containing PBS. The affinity membrane potential of both cells was measured by electrometer through a pair of saturated calomel electrodes. Antibody binding reaction was detected by the change of affinity membrane potential after the addition of corresponding antiserum to PBS in the well. The change of the membrane potential at the presence of non-reacting antibody was slightly and easy to differentiate with the blood group reactions. The device may be used for the detection of anti-A and anti-B antibodies in the serum using standard membrane containing blood group substances.

0563

AUTOIMMUNE HAEMOLYTIC ANAEMIA WITH AUTOANTIBODY OF ANTI-S SPECIFICITY

J.Fabijańska-Mitek, J.Kopeć, H.Seyfried
Institute of Haematology and Blood Transfusion, Warsaw, Poland

We describe a case with severe AIHA associated with warm autoantibody of an unusual anti-S specificity. On admission blood count in a 21 year old woman M.B.: Hb - 6g/dL, RBCs - $1,1\times10^{12}$/L, reticulocytes - 5,9% and bilirubin - 2,26 mg/dL, serum haptoglobin-0. Twice she developed acute haemolytic reactions at the time of blood transfusions compatible in ABO and Rh blood group system as well as in K antigen, but incompatible by cross-match due to the presence of autoantibody of unidentified specificity in her serum. Then S-negative blood was well tolerated. Utero-vaginal infection by human papilloma virus which might be the cause of AIHA has been detected. Acid/EDTA eluates as well as the presence of S antigen on acid/EDTA treated red blood cells were studied by microtests in gel. Results obtained by this technique showed high affinity of IgG auto-anti-S firmly blocking S determinants on RBCs. The patient was Ss, but in testing by conventional methods she was thought to be S-negative. The patient was under observation for 20 months. Anti-S autoantibody was detected within the period of 18 months. After 20 months very weak anti-U autoantibody appeared.

0564

A COLD AGGLUTININ (ANTI-Pr) IN THE SERUM OF A CARDIAC ENGRAFTED PATIENT

B. David1, D. Bernard1, S. Le Quere1, M. Treilhaud2, D. Blanchard1, J.Y. Muller1
1CRTS Nantes , 2CHR , Thoracic Surgery Unit , Nantes , France.

Case report: A cardiac transplant was performed on May 1993 for a 59-year-old man (H.J.).Because of acute graft rejection , immunosuppresive therapy including Ciclosporin A , High dose Prednisolone , Azathioprine and OKT3 Monoclonal Antibody was done within the tree months after transplant.Two months later , five months after transplant , patient experienced a CytoMegaloVirus infection and severe Anemia(Hemoglobin 70 gr/l).The hemolytic origin of this anemia has been assesed and a potent Cold Agglutinin (CA) discovered.Previous sera were negative for this CA.

The antibody of IgM class was potent (titer : 1024) only at 4°C and agglutinated untreated adult and cord RBCs but failed to agglutinate trypsin- and papain-treated RBCs.After absorption of the serum on Neuraminidase-treated RBCs , titers were lower but remain significant with untreated RBCs.The Cold Agglutinin , witch most probably belongs to anti-Pr , bound to dog RBCs.

The production of an antibody of such specificity has been associated with various viruses-related infection.The coincidence of a severe immunosuppressed status of the patient (almost undetectable CD4 , CD8 , CD3) raise the problem of aberrant immnune responses during severe immunosuppression.

0565

RAPID GENOTYPING OF ABO BLOOD GROUP AS AN EVIDENCE OF ENGRAFTMENT IN BONE MARROW TRANSPLANTATION - A CASE REPORT

C.S.Chang,S.F.Lin,J.C-I.Lee*,T.C.Liu,S.M.Hwang,T.P.Chen
Division of Hematooncology,Kaohsiung Medical College Hospital,Taiwan,*Department of Forensic Science,Central Police College,Taoyuan,Taiwan

Engraftment of bone marrow transplantation can be determined by several methods including cytogenetic analysis for sex, DNA polymorphism (RFLP), blood group analysis, etc. Most methods to determine engraft were time consuming and need complicated procedures. We described a case of acute promyelocytic leukemia with O blood type received marrow transplantation in second remission from his HLA identical, B blood type sibling. DNAs extracted from the leukocytes collected from both the donor and the patient at the various states including remission state before transplantation and early engraftment when peripheral white cell count at the level near 1000/ul posttransplantation were used for PCR genotyping of ABO blood group. Nucleotide 700 of cDNA of A glycosyltransferase were used to distinguish B and O alleles by restriction enzyme, Alu I, digestion of the polymerase chain reaction (PCR) products. The primer pairs used for nucleotide 700 area are:5'primer, 5'-TGGAGATCCTGACTCCGCTG-3' ,located at nucleotide 662 to 682 of the sense strand of cDNA; 3'Primer,5'-GTAGAAATCGCCCTCGTCCTT-3',located from nucleotide 769 to 789 of the antisense strand of cDNA. The result demonstrated the blood type change of this patient from O with uncleavable 128 bp PCR fragment to type B with a 88-bp band visualized in 3 % agarose gel which was the same as his sibling's. This offer an evidence of successful engraftment in this patient. We conclude it's a quick and convenient method to determine the successful marrow engraftment earlier in those patients who received bone marrow transplantation from donors with mismatched blood type.

0566

Ht% VALUE IN AUTOLOGOUS BLOOD SAFE FOR HOMOLOGOUS USE

C.Mazzei,G.Cavagnaro,G.Imberciadori
C.Trasfusionale,Osp. S.Corona Pietra Ligure

Acccording Standards,we accept for donations men and women with Ht > = 41% and 38% rispectively, and patients predepositing with Ht >=33% .In this study we evaluated mean Ht value of 1200 consecutive homologous donors (A) and 893 autologous donors (B),for estimating mean Ht difference between the two groups if we adopt the police of transfusing to other patients autologous blood not reinfused .

Results:

Age		N	A (Ht%)	N	B (Ht%)
<18	M	–	–	56	41.4
	W	–	–	102	39.2
>18 <65	M	843	43.6	205	42.8
	W	377	40.5	280	40.1
>65	M	–	–	50	43.2
	W	–	–	200	39.9

We didn't found significant differences in the two groups .Men and women are expressed in different rate in homologous and autologous donors being women prevalent in B and men in A. Mean Ht values satisfy Standards also in autologous group and we conclude that it ,if not reinfused and safe for homologous use,can be transfused to others.

0567

SEMI-AUTOMATED BLOODCOMPONENT PRODUCTION: A GUARANTEE FOR A PRODUCT OF CONSTANT QUALITY.

J. Vermeij, D.J. van Rhenen, G.V. Kruit, Red Cross Blood Bank Rotterdam, The Netherlands.

In 1989 the Blood Bank Rotterdam started with the semi-automated Optipac™/Optipress™ bloodcomponent preparation system. One of the aims was to guarantee a constant quality of blood products for the patients. In 4 years time the composition of 3940 (> 1%) units of produced red cells (EC), plasma (FFP) and buffy-coats (BC), was analysed with a quality control system. The product quality was compared with the product criteria, defined before starting the control system. Constant quality was defined if over 95% of the control results met the criteria.

Production and control criteria:

	vol. ml	RBC 10^{12}	free HB mg	WBC 10^9	PLT 10^9	HT %
EC	>255	>1.5		<1.2	<10	53-63
FFP	>260		<20	<9	<5	
BC	50-60	<0.36		>2.0	>80	50-60

Results: 97-100% of the EC's met the criteria; 91% of the FFP's met the PLT criterion; 96-100% met the other criteria; 95% of the BC's met the volume criterion, but 79% met the PLT, 82% met the RBC, 89% met the Ht and 93 % met the WBC criterion.

Conclusion: The Optipac™/Optipress™ system makes it possible to produce highly constant EC and FFP. Only in the BC product the existing biological variation is present.

0568

COMPARISON OF BLOODPROCESSING WITH TOP- AND BOTTOM-SYSTEM AND CONVENTIONAL 4-BAG SYSTEM

H.J. Geerligs, H.J. Bos, G.C. van der Plas
Red Cross Bloodbank Arnhem, The Netherlands

We compared the conventional 4-bag system with the combination of the Top- and Bottom-system (TB) and Optipress bloodprocessingdevice of Baxter. In both methods the separation of whole blood into plasma, buffy-coat and red cells takes place within 6-18 hours post-donation after an 8 min. spin at 6000 xg.

	TB (n=94)		**4-bag (n=81)**	
Packed cells (PC)	**Mean**	**SD**	**Mean**	**SD**
Leukocytes x 10^9	0.4*	0.3	0.8	0.4
Thrombocytes x 10^9	2*	1	14	13
Heamatocrit (1/1)	0.59	0.03	0.60	0.03
Removal % (Whole blood-PC)				
Leukocytes	83*	10	67	11
Thrombocytes	98*	2	86	13

* $p < 0.01$; Wilcoxon test.

The TB-system of Baxter used in combination with the Optipress device reduces the variation in produkt specification and shows a significant better leukocyte and thrombocyte removal from the packed cell.

0569

THE PREPARATION OF POOLED THROMBOCYTE CONCENTRATES FROM BUFFY COATS OBTAINED WITH THE TOP- AND BOTTOM-SYSTEM AND OPTIPRESS BLOOD-PROCESSINGDEVICE

H.J. Geerligs, H.J Bos, G.C. van der Plas
Red Cross Bloodbank Arnhem, The Netherlands

Using the Top- and Bottom-system (TB) and Optipress bloodprocessingdevice from Baxter, whole blood was after centrifugation separated in plasma, buffy coat and red blood cell concentrate. Pooled thrombocyte concentrates (PTC) were made from six buffy coats and one unit fresh plasma. After centrifugation at 2250 xg for 4 minutes, the PTC were collected and stored in a shaking incubator at 22°C in a Baxter PL732 tissue culture flask until use.

Data of PTC at day 1 and day 5 after donation

Data per PTC	day 1 (n=535)		day 5 (n=40)	
	Mean	SD	Mean	SD
Volume (ml)	264	29	ND	ND
Thrombocytes x 10^9	373	63	369	65
Leukocytes x 10^6	10.5	12.9	ND	ND
pH	7.1	0.1	6.8	0.3
Swirling (1=little, 3=much)	2.9	0.3	1.5	0.9

ND=Not done

The PTC made from buffy coats prepared with the TB-system and Optipress, have a good quality (pH, Swirling and leukocyte count) and can be succesfully stored for a period of 5 days.

0570

PLATELET CONCENTRATES PREPARED FROM OPTIPAC™ BUFFYCOATS: A PRODUCT OF CONSTANT QUALITY.

J. Vermeij, D.J. van Rhenen, G.V. Kruit and M.H.J. Molijn
Red Cross Blood Bank Rotterdam, The Netherlands.

With the introduction of the Optipac™/ Optipress™ system in 1989, a simple, fast and flexible preparation method was developed to prepare platelet concentrates (PC) of constant quality.
Six buffy-coats (55 ml, Ht 55%) prepared from stored blood (16-20 hour at 22°C) and ± 250 ml homologous plasma are sterile pooled into the transferbag of a poolingset. After a soft spin (2282g, 3 min, code 25), platelet rich plasma is slowly pressed off.
Initially the total number of platelets was stored in one PL-732 bag. However, because of the large quantity of cells the PH dropped on day 4 to 6.5. For this reason the PC was subsequently stored in two bags (2/6 in a pl-2209 plasma bag and 4/6 in the PL-732 bag) that were still connected and before transfusion both parts were united again.
In 4 years time the composition of 1,450 units was analyzed in a quality control system. Product quality was compared with the following quality criteria; Volume > 240 ml, free Hb< 30 mg, PLT > 3.3 x 10^{11}, WBC < 1.2 x 10^8 and pH day 4 > 6.5 later > 6.8. Constant quality was defined if over 90% of the controle results met the criteria.
The PC's met the criteria with the folowing percentages; volume 95%, free Hb 98%, PLT 92%, WBC 94% and pH 77% later 100%.
In conclusion: A reliable production method offered a high quality transfusion PC product.

0571

COMPARATIVE STUDY OF TWO SYSTEM FOR AUTOMATED BLOOD COMPONENTS PREPARATIONS

Pinilla Ibarz J, Martín Recio A, Cano I, Castañeda A, López López R, de la Cámara C, Pérez Piñó T, Arrieta R, Santacreu M, Rubio M, Jiménez V, Martín MP, Ríos P, Ojeda E, Hdez Navarro F.
Servicio de Hematología y Hemoterapia del H. "La Paz".

The use of system for automated total blood component preparations is increase in blood banks. The aim of this paper is to evaluate two of system usually more employed in our country: Compomat ® (Menarini) and Optypress® (Baxter)
Material and Methods. Study and fractionated a minimum of 30 units of total blood for each system. In all donors to perform a previous complete hemogram, furthermore automated counts of different components were obtained and weight of each component.The time and speed of centrifugation were adjust for each system. Anova was statistical test used for the comparations.

Results

	Plat N° x10^{10}	% Plat Rec	Leu N° x10^8	%Desl RBC	N°LPC x10^7
C	6,3±2,1*	56±9**	5,1±4	85,3±10	3,6±5,4*
O	7,3±1,4*	69±12**	4,1±2	85,9±9	7,4±6,5*

* $p < 0.05$ ** $p < 0.001$ CH: red blood cells. PC: platelet concentrate.
%Plat Plat: platelet recuperation. % Desl CH: leukocytedeplection N°LPC: leukocyte PC.

Conclusions.
More number and percentage of platelet recuperation were obtained with Optypress system, moreover two system were above on recommended standard of AABB. Leukocyte number in platelet concentrate was lesser with the Compomat system. In RBC were obtained more yield with the Compomat system and leukocytedeplection was similar in both system

0572

QUALITY CONTROL OF RED BLOOD CELL CONCENTRATES(RBCC).

A. Rapaille, D. Sondag-Thull
Blood Transfusion Centre, Liège, Belgium

We present the results of a quality control of the three types of RBCC, with additive solution, SAGM. Blood samples were counted by Sysmex 5000 and Cell-dyn 3000.

For the RBCC prepared by high speed (hs) centrifugation (n=161), the mean of the hematocrite (hc) is 59.1% with 11 RBCC >65% and 24 <55%. For the RBCC prepared by low speed (ls) centrifugation (n=115), the mean of the hc is 51.9% with 5 RBCC >60% and 42 <50%. For the leukocyte-poor RBCC prepared by a manual technique (n=83), the mean of the hc is 49.6% with 47 RBCC <50% and the mean of residual leukocytes is 0.93 10^9 with 13 RBCC > 1.2 10^9.

The hc of RBCC hs is suitable. Concerning the two others, the hc is too often weak. Nevertheless, an other important point is the preparation of Platelet Concentrates (PC) using these technics. We obtain PC with a good yield of platelets (> 0.6 10^{11} for 75% PC). And the number of residual leukocytes in leukocytes poor RBCC is also appropriate. Then we don't change any parameter of centrifugation.

0573

EFFECT OF COLD EXPOSURE ON PLATELET SIZE DISTRIBUTION INDICES AND HYPERAGGREGABILITY

Pranee Krailadsiri[1], Jerard Seghatchian[2]
1 Department of Laboratory Medicine, Chulalongkorn University Hospital, Bangkok, Thailand, 2 Quality Assurance Laboratory, North London Blood Transfusion Centre, London, England

Response of platelets to cold exposure was determined: firstly by calculating the difference in cellular indices of paired samples of platelet concentrates, held overnight at 4°C, and 22°C; secondly by evaluating the effect of ageing - induced disc/sphere conversion or EDTA-induced pseudopod formation on cold-induced platelet shape change; thirdly by assessing disparity between leucocyte peroxidase/basophil count (WBCp/WBCb) as index of aggregation states. Upon cold exposure the mean platelet volume (MPV) increased by 1.5 - 2.0 fL with a shift to right in size distribution pattern and concomitant decrease (12-13%) in platelet width. Disc/sphere conversion was associated with a shift to the left, with decrease (0.2 - 0.5 fL) in MPV at day 5 and reduced response to cold. EDTA treated samples also responded to a lesser extend (0.5 - 0.8 fL) to cold shock. Moreover cold exposure enhanced disparity in WBCp/WBCb. These results, using a new generation technology (Technicon H*1), confirm that platelet are highly sensitive to changes in microenvironment during, processing and storage, undergoing rapid cellular injuries. These can be easily monitored, on quantitative basis, by changes in cellular indices of paired samples, providing a new quality index for platelet functions.

0574

QUALITY CONTROL OF PLATELET CONCENTRATE USING THE FLOW CYTOMETER: A PILOT STUDY

RL McShine, A Heethuis, PC Das, CTh Smit Sibinga. RC Blood Bank Groningen-Drenthe, Groningen, NL.

Quick and reliable quality control testing of platelet concentrate (PC) is still highly desirable in blood banking. The quality of donor platelets in whole blood before (WB-b) and after (WB-a) platelet apheresis and in the platelet concentrate (PC) was monitored. The increase of platelet-bound fibrinogen after adenosine diphosphate (ADP) induced activation was measured in the Ortho Cytoron Absolute using monoclonal anti-fibrinogen-fluorescein isothiocyanate (FITC), and platelet size estimated after calibration with polystyrene microspheres. Mean platelet volume (MPV) was measured by Sysmex F-800 haematology counter.

RESULTS:

Product n=6	MPV (fl)	plat size (μm)	plat activ (%)
WB-b	9.1±0.82	2.18±0.04	78.3±2.91
WB-a	9.1±0.99	2.18±0.05	77.6±2.37
PC	8.9±1.24	2.25±0.06	69.0±5.76

Student's paired t test: WB versus PC-platelet size ($p<0.001$), - platelet activation ($p<0.01$), both cases significant.

CONCLUSION: It seems as though a qualitatively different population is collected in the PC.

0575

COMPARISON OF PH DETERMINATIONS AT 22°C AND 37°C IN PLATELET CONCENTRATES.

J.de Wildt-Eggen, M.Bins
Bloodbank Zwolle, the Netherlands

For pH-determinations in whole blood it is reckoned that per °C pH falls by 0.0147 (Kelman and Nunn formula). We studied the influence of temperature on pH of platelet concentrates (PC) at 22°C and 37°C . In 68 PC immediately after preparation pH was determined, at 22°C using a glass electrode (Radiometer) and at 37°C using a 634 micro pH analyzer (Ciba-Corning). Of 20 outdated PC pH was determined in the same way at day 6. Determinations were performed immediately after each other. Prior to the determinations both apparatuses were compared in a pH7.00 buffer.

Results.

	day 0		day 6	
	pH22°C	pH37°C	pH22°C	pH37°C
n	68	68	20	20
mean	7.27±0.05	7.13±0.03	7.11±0.12	7.00±0.11
range	7.16-7.37	7.06-7.18	6.84-7.29	6.74-7.14
pH/°C	0.0088		0.0073	

Conclusion: The influence of the temperature on pH was considerably smaller in PC than in whole blood (0.009°C vs. 0.015°C), but still sufficient to advise the pH of platelet concentrates to be determined at a fixed temperature. Of the 20 platelets studied here 1 met the pH-criterium at day 6 (pH>6.8) at 22°C but would have failed to do so at 37°C.

0576

SWIRLING EFFECT OF PLATELET CONCENTRATES AND pH

R.N.I.Pietersz, W.J.A.Dekker, A.M.Joustra-Dijkhuis, H.W.Reesink. Red Cross Blood Bank Amsterdam, Amsterdam, The Netherlands.

Quality checks of platelet concentrates (PC) prior to issue are difficult to perform. Discoid morphology has been found to correlate well with survival in vivo. The presence of discs in a PC can be estimated by judging the 'swirling effect' induced by light reflection

Aim: To assess whether the absence of swirling in platelet concentrates (PC) would be predictive for a pH value below 6.8.

Method: Pools of PC were prepared by mixing 4 units of 50 ml-BC with 200 ml plasma from 1 of the donors. Following centrifugation for 7 min at 1,250 rpm the platelet-rich-plasma was transferred into a 1,000 ml PL 732 (Baxter) bag and stored at 20 - 24°C for up to 6 days with gentle agitation. Prior to issue (day 4 or 5) or discard (day 6) swirling effect was judged and scored as excellent; present or absent. pH was measured at 37°C.

Results: the median age of the PC (n = 123) was 5 days (range 4 to 6 days).

swirling	excellent	present	absent
pH < 6.8	4	9	16
pH > 6.8	58	19	17

The number of PC without swirling was significantly higher in the pH < 6.8 group (p < 0.001). The number of PC with excellent swirling was significantly higher in the pH > 6.8 group (p < 0.001).

Conclusion: absence of the swirling phenomenon in PC predicts in 55% a pH < 6.8, whereas presence of swirling predicts in 82% a pH > 6.8.

0577

AN INTEGRATED QUALITY ASSURANCE APPROACH FOR BLOOD IRRADIATION PRACTICE

S.A. Papoulias, D.F. Lewis, J.M. Donahue, R.M. Fairman, International Specialty Products, Wayne, NJ, U.S.A.

As the practice of blood irradiation is rapidly growing to account for 10-15% of all transfusions, there is increased emphasis to address the safety and quality assurance (QA) of irradiated blood components. The three necessary elements of an effective QA program are proper radiation dose, equipment calibration/ validation and irradiation indication. A 25 Gy central dose and a 15 Gy minimum dose at any point in the irradiation field are recommended for proper treatment of irradiated blood products. Irradiation equipment can be calibrated using either discrete thermoluminescent dosimeters (TLDs) or continuous radiochromic films (DOSE-MAP™) that validate irradiator performance at 10% and 5% accuracy, respectively. The use of a positive visual indicator on each blood unit is the final QA element to verify proper irradiation treatment of each individual blood component before it is issued for transfusion.

0578

QUALITY OF PLASMA COLLECTED DURING PLASMAPLATELET APHERESIS (PPA) WITH AUTOPHERESIS - C AND MCS

G Baldini,M Mariano,R Roncaglia,G Montagnani,S Roncaglia
Blood Transfusion Service.Policlinico of MODENA-ITALY

Plasma collection in PPA offers a relevant economical advantage.We assessed platelet poor plasma (PPP) quality by evaluating before freezing the degree of platelet (PLT) contamination with direct PLT count, and the levels of plasma stable proteins by electrophoresis. F VIII levels were measured after freezing of PPP in cold ethanol bath and storage at -30°C for 1 month. RESULTS (mean value)

	AUTOPHERESIS PPP (n=11)	MCS PPP (n=11)
PLT x10e9/L	1.0	7.4
Total Protein g/dl	6.72	6.16
Albumin g/dl	3.94	3.71
Immunoglobulin mg/dl	1484	1429
F VIII %	105	85

All PPP units fulfilled quality requirements established by Italian law and Council of Europe recomendations. PLT contamination in MCS-PPP was related to the number of PLT processed during PPA ($r=0.78, p<0.05$) and resulted higher than in Autopheresis PPP ($p<0.001$). Total protein concentration and F VIII levels were higher in Autopheresis PPP ($p<0.001$ and $p<0.02$ respectively) than in MCS PPP. The higher amount of ACD used by MCS (1/10) respect with Autopheresis (1/16) may explain the observed differences , when considering the dilutional effect of citrate on plasma components.

0579

EVALUATION OF V AND VIII CLOTTING FACTORS AS QUALITY CONTROL OF FRESH FROZEN PLASMA

Alvarenga, M.; García - Villaescusa, R. y Roig, R.

GALICIA REGIONAL BLOOD TRANSFUSION CENTER. SANTIAGO DE COMPOSTELA (SPAIN)

In this Center the Quality Control Laboratory realizes the screening of about 8 to 10 per cent of the whole blood donor units to evaluate the V and VIII clotting factors by a chromogenic substract technique in order to determinate the quality control of fresh frozen plasma (FFP) and their percentage of unitary activity.

MATERIAL AND METHODS.- In this work we have studied 728 and 424 samples, respectively, for V and VIII clotting factors. To evaluate the activity of these clotting factors we used a crhomogenic substract technique with the authomatic device Electra 1000 C.

RESULTS- 1) Factor V: we have studied 728 samples with an average of 101.0093 % clotting factor activity. 2) Factor VIII: there are 424 samples studied with an average of 90.4318 % clotting factor activity.

CONCLUDING REMARKS.- 1) The clotting factors evaluated were in the useful rank for FFP according to the standars of EEC, FDA and SSBT. 2) The systematics used in our quality control laboratory is a useful method to evaluate the quality of FFP.

0580

Sobuble CD4 and CD8 molecules in commercial blood Products.

K.Komuro[1), K.Okuyama[1), S.Furukawa[2) , K.Okumura[3), K.Imai[4).
National Inst. of Health[1), Ymamaguchi Uni.[2)
Juntendo Uni.[3), Sapporo Med. Colledge[4).

Soluble forms of CD4 and CD8 molecules in the immunoglobulin and albumin preparations were analysed by enzyme immuno-assays.
We measured 28 immunoglobulin preparations and 4 albumins made by 6 different manufacturers.
11 immunoglobulin preparations contained detectable CD4, and 19 had solubles CD8 in varying amounts.
Immunogloblin preparations made by plasma collected by plasmapheresis did not contain soluble CD4 and CD8 molecules, but source plsama collescted from whole blood contained high amount of soluble CD4 and CD8.
Methods to collect the source plasma may be the main factors of contaminant of soluble CD4 and CD8.

0581

CONTAMINATION OF IMMUNOGLOBULIN PREPARATIONS WITH PLASMA KALLIKREIN AND OTHER PROBLEM PARAMETERS

W. Heller, H.P. Wendel
Dept. of Thoracic- and Cardiovascular Surg., Univ. of Tuebingen, Germany

Immunoglobulins fulfill a partial task during antigene resistance. However, the intravenous injection of 7 S-immunoglobulin preparations result in incompatibility reactions. In order to register the respective side-effects, gammaglobulin preparations were examined for contamination by inhibitors and enzymes of the coagulation system. Besides the determination of coagulatory physiological substances the present study also investigates the fluctuations of individual immunoglobulin concentrations in various batches. Ten 7S-immunoglobulin preparations in clinical use were investigated. From each manufacturer 10 bottles of the same batch number were tested for the most relevant haemostaseological parameters. The parameters of the kallikrein-kinin system (prekallikrein, kallikrein-like activity) as well as kallikrein inhibition were determined by means of chromogenic substrates. The determination of C1-inhibitor, alpha$_2$-macroglobulin and IgG was conducted immunologically.

The normal value of IgG concentration of 5000 mg/dl as targeted by the manufacturers is approximated only in immunoglobulin preparation 7 and 8. The IgG concentrations of IgG preparations 1 and 2 lay below the normal level, those of products 3 to 6 beyond that level. A comparison of the batches revealed a significant difference in the IgG concentrations for all manufacturers.

The measured values lay clearly below the norm. It may be assumed that in the case of a patient suffering from a disease characterized by an increase of the plasma kallikrein level and thus dependent on immunoglobulin infusions, the slightest amount of kallikrein contained in the IgG preparation, results in an interference in metabolic processes. The varying values during the kallikrein determination could be the result of the different production methods.

0582

A QUALITY ASSURANCE PROGRAM FOR BIOLOGICAL ASSAYS AND ITS USE FOR MONITORING THE FACTOR VIII POTENCY ESTIMATION IN AN 80° HEAT TREATED F-VIII CONCENTRATE

A. Knevelman*, M. Imholz**, H.J.C. de Wit*
Red Cross Bloodbank Friesland*, Leeuwarden and Red Cross Bloodbank The Hague**, The Netherlands.

Introduction: Since july 1991 seven Dutch bloodbanks are involved in the production of a small pool, 80°C dry heated factor VIII concentrate. The laboratory departments of six bloodbanks are responsible for the quality control of this product. In order to evaluate the quality of the potency estimation of factor VIII:C, a quality assurance program was started in 1992. The current approach dates from Januari 1993.

Method: A bulk solution was produced by dissolving the contents of a large number of vials containing heat treated factor FVIII concentrate in 10 ml of water (normally 15 ml) and pooling. From this concentrated solution 4 diluted solutions in freeze drying buffer were produced. The 5 solutions were dispispensed in plastic, randomly numbered tubes (1 or 2 ml), frozen (-70°C) and transported to the participating laboratories on dry ice. During each run, the participants determine the potency of the sample in one tube. In September 1993 a survey of the results (tube numbers and potency) was send to the coördinator of the program.

Results: The number of observations varied from 5 to 21. Low numbers of observations are caused by a late start, not measuring a sample during each assay run or missing tube numbers. In all cases the linearity of the potency vs dilution factor plot was good (R^2 0.95-0.98). The values reported by 5 out of 6 laboratories did compare well. The results of one laboratory showed a deviating regression coëfficient and an abnormal intercept of the potency vs dilution factor plot.

Conclusion: The new approach yields continuous information on the assay performance in a broad potency range. The results of 5 participants did compare well. One participant had to revalidate the assay. Future developments involve a better motivation to participate on a regular basis, an independent estimation of the potency of each solution and advanced methods for statistical analysis

0583

REGIONAL QUALITY ASSURANCE PROGRAM FOR CLOTTING ASSAYS IN HOSPITALS WITH A BLOOD BANK DERIVED STANDARD PLASMA POOL

De Wit HJC, Lerk ME*, Alderkamp GHJ, Potstra P, Bakker AJ*, Red Cross Bloodbank Friesland, *KCL, Leeuwarden, The Netherlands.

Introduction: The Bloodbank Friesland produces a pooled normal control plasma that is distributed in a frozen state to local hospital labs as part of a quality assurance program for Activated Partial Thromboplastin Time (APTT), Prothrombin time (PT) and fibrinogen assay. Since 1990 this standard plasmapool is distributed in a much larger area: The northern part of The Netherlands.

Method: 40 healthy bloodbank donors are randomly selected and 500 ± 10 ml blood in 70 ml CPD is collected. Within 1 hour the blood is centrifuged at 28000 gmin and the separated plasma is spun hard again. 40 units of plasma are pooled in a 15 liter pvc bag. Within 4 hours 12000 polystyrene tubes, 1 ml each are filled, frozen in alcohol (- 45°C) and packed in paper boxes, each containing 23 tubes. Storage is at -80°C. The plasma standard is distributed in a frozen state with a frequency of 1 - 2 times a month, if necessary by a neighbouring bloodbank. Production is one batch a year.

Results: The reproducability of APTT, PT and fibrinogen did not change in 4 labs during the first year. For APTT and fibrinogen the mean values converged and for 12 labs the range of assay data improved in one year from 7,03 sec to 5,03 sec (APTT) resp. from 0,82 g/l to 0,35 g/l (fibrinogen).

For all labs the mean assay results are very stable, even when a new batch of poolplasma is used. The pool plasma is stable for at least 1,5 years at - 80°C. A frozen control plasma is judged to be userfriendly and accurate because reconstitution with water is not necessary.

Conclusion: A regional quality assurance program with a blood bank derived frozen standard plasma pool improves control of clotting assays in hospital labs. The plasma pool is stable and userfriendly.

0586

CRYOPRESERVATION OF PERIPHERAL BLOOD STEM CELLS (PBSC) : EXPERIENCE WITH TWO DIFFERENT METHODS OF CELL MANIPULATION.

G.Adorno , A.Bruno , M.Silvi , L.Cudillo, T.Dentamaro,A. Rainaldi T. Caravita , G.Del Poeta , E.Stipa , M.Masi, M.Tribalto and G.Papa
Haematology - Rome "Tor Vergata" University - S.Eugenio Hospital

We report here the experience on cryopreservation of PBSC collected from 69 leukaphereses performed on 22 patients affected by Multiple Myeloma (14), High-Grade Non-Hodgkin Lymphomas (6), Acute Leukemias (2). Three-four consecutive procedures were performed for each patient,using a CS-3000 blood cell separator; program 3 (8 pts) or program 1 -modified (14 pts) were used : in the first case sedimentation with HES was necessary to reduce red blood cell contamination. Cryopreservation was performed using a computer controlled rate of freezing. The results are shown in the following table:

	Apheresis	HCT %	WBC / mmc	PLTS / mmc
		(m e a n	v a l u e s	)
Prog. 3	53	2 , 5	35. 600	432. 900
Prog. 1 - Mod	16	5 , 3	56. 100	325. 000

All patients were reinfused; 11 received PBSC+BM, 11 PBSC alone:all engrafted well. It is author's opinion that the referred data would be of some interest because of the evidence that cryopreservation may be safely performed using a wide range of WBC concentration and HCT value.

0587

COLLECTION OF CIRCULATING HEMATOPOIEIC PROGENITORS AND EVALUATION ON THE SIMPLE FREEZING PROCEDURES

Y.Amemiya, T.Suzuki, K.Muroi, K.Kishino, K.Minamiru, Y.Nakagi, Y.Miura
Division of Transfusion Medicine, Jichi Medical School Hospital, Tochigi, Japan.

Peripheral blood stem cells(PBSCs) harvest required numerous leukapheresis to collect adequate numbers of cells. This study was desigend to investigate the efficient and lavor-saving collection, storage, and to analyze the kinetics of PBSCs.
The PBSCs collection was evaluated in normal healthy donors and hematologic malignancy. The cells were suspended in autologous plasma, and cryopreserved using a mixture containing 5% DMSO and 6% HES.
As simple as such, the cells were frozen and stored in a deep freezer at -80 degree C.
Before freezing and after thawing, each sample of PB SCs collection was assayed for its content of RBCs, nucleated cells, and CD33, CD34, CD13, CD38, HLA-DR cells, and also hematopoietic progenitors, including CFU-Mix, BFU-E and CFU-GM, were assayed. From the bone marrow cells and PB in some cases, CD34 cells were purified by immunopanning technique.
The absolute recovery of CFU-GM was estimated as less than 40% at the 6 month. Purified CD34 cells from PB in healthy donors contained same numbers of CFU-GM and BFU-E, and more than 90% of CD34 cells expressed CD13, CD33, CD38, HLA-DR. These characteristics could distinguish the nature of PBSCs from the stem cells in bone marrow. However, a little differences was observed on PBSCs in the patient who underwnt marrow suppresive therapy and G-CSF.

0588

EXPERIENCE OF CRYOPRESERVATION OF BONE MARROW (BM) FOR AUTOLOGOUS BONE MARROW TRANSPLANTATION (ABMT).

AbdulKadirov K.M., Moiseev S.I., Grycaev S.V., Ganapiev A.A., Balashova V.A.
Russian Institute of Hematology and Transfusiology, St.-Petersburg, Russia.

In period 1991-1993 years 20 BM samples were prepared and cryopreserved for ABMT. 11 samples of BM were freezed with new cryoprotector "Gecmolyt"(group 1) and 9 were freezed with 10% DMSO (group 2). In group 1 the rate of freezing was 1°/min from +4°C to -15°C, 10°/min from -15°C to -40°C, 20°/min from -40°C to -140°C. In group 2 the rate of freezing was 1°/min from +4°C to -20°C, 2°/min from -20°C to -80°C, 20°/min from -80°C to -140°C. BM was stored at -196°C at 6-246 days. The cryopreserved BM were thawed in water bath at 38°C in group 1 and at 39°C in group 2. BM after preparing, cryopreservation and thawing were with a nucleated cells recovery of 56,4±3,8% and 82±2,8%, mononuclear cells recovery of 66,5±18,9% and 85,7±16,8%, CFU-GM recovery 14,3±8% and 65±5,1% in group 1 and group 2 accordingly. The rates of engraftment in patients undergoing ABMT were 16-44 days in group 1 and 19-32 days in group 2. We conclude that DMSO is more preferable for cryo-preservation BM in cases with more myelo-ablative preparative regimens for ABMT than "Gecmolyt"

0589

WAYS OF IMPROVEMENT OF BONE MARROW CRYOPRESERVATION (CRP) WITH 10% DMSO.

Moiseev S.I., Grycaev S.V., Golubev A.E.
Russian Institute of Hematology and Transfusiology, St.-Petersburg, Russia.

One of main steps of autologous bone marrow transplantation is CRP of bone marrow cells (BMC). We studied the cryoprotective effect of 10% DMSO on BMC depending on conditions of the CRP process. 25 samples of BMC of patients with acute leukemia were freezed with employment of the next program: 1°/min from +4°C to -20°C, 2°/min from -20°C to -80°C, 20°/min from -80°C to -140°C. BMC after CRP and thawing were with nucleated cells recovery of 56-100%, mononuclear cells recovery of 54-100%, CFU-GM recovery of 1-112%. The viability of BMC was depended from duration and intensity of process of crystalization (PC), from time of first step of freezing, from t°C of beginning of PC. The duration of PC and t°C of beginning of PC were in straight depending of cellularity of BMC suspension before CRP and difference of t°C between freezer and imitator in during of process of CRP. Best conditions for CRP of BMC are the end cellularity of BMC suspension not more than $20x10^9$/l, dilution of BMC and DMSO by autologous blood serum, 20° difference of t°C between freezer and imitator in during automatic process of CRP or manual extingushing of heat in during PC, small rate of freezing on the first step. It is allow to receive 96±3% viable BMC after CRP.

0590

HAEMONETICS MCS RED CELL/PLASMA DONATIONS: DONOR SAFETY AND ACCEPTABILITY

C A Ribbons, G Bremner, S Brown, J Gillon
Scottish National Blood Transfusion Service, Edinburgh & South East Scotland Blood Transfusion Centre, Royal Infirmary, Edinburgh EH3 9HB

The Haemonetics Red Cell/Plasma procedure uses an modified MCS 3 pump to obtain a single unit of red cells in SAG-M and approximately 450 mls plasma in around 20 minutes using a single vein. Studies are under way to assess the quality and sterility of the products. We report here on the attitudes of regular whole blood donors recruited to this procedure de novo, and on the incidence of adverse events. 57 regular whole blood donors and 3 plasmapheresis donors have been studied, 45 males and 15 females (mean age 32.1 years, mean previous donations 21.8) and 3 plasma donors. 4 (7%) of procedures were aborted because of failed venepuncture, 7 (12%) others had slow flow. 2 donors (3%) felt faint and 2 felt mildly unwell. 83% of donors expressed a liking for the procedure and 90% said that the extra time required did not matter. 77% would be willing to donate in this way every time, and 17% only if required. No donor would refuse to give again.

In summary, the procedure was popular with donors, was well tolerated and had an acceptable level of adverse events. The high rate of difficulty with venous access may be a problem in previously unselected donors.

0591

EARLY DIAGNOSIS OF VIRAL AFFECTION OF THE BLOOD SYSTEM

V.Rugal, V.Ponomarenko, K.Abdulkadyrov, V.Shabalin
Institute of Hematology and Transfusiology, St.Petersburg, Russia

Ultrastructural study of the hemopoietic microenvironment cells in fragments of the iliac bone has shown 3 types of intranuclear virus-like inclusions in patients with aplastic anemia, myelodysplasias and immunodeficiency states. The first type inclusions had a loose fibrillar-granular structure which differed considerably from the nuclear chromatin structure by a lower electron translucence. The 2nd type showed the fibrillar structures arranged in circles with dense granules and the envelope made of fibrillar circles. There were virus-like bodies identical, in their structure, to the mature viruses in the cytoplasma of cells of microenvironment. Thus the slowly repopulating cells of stromal microenvironment can be a place of prolonged persistence of viruses in hematologic diseases and immunodeficiency states. Study of microenvironment opens the possibility of an early diagnosis and prognosing of the viral affection in man.

0592

SUCCESSFUL PARTNERSHIP BETWEEN A BLOOD CENTER AND A UNIVERSITY HOSPITAL IN COLLECTION OF PERIPHERAL BLOOD STEM CELLS FOR AUTOLOGOUS TRANSPLANTATION

R.L. Reddy, L. Thoreen
American Red Cross Blood Services, Midwest Region, Omaha, Nebraska, USA.

American Red Cross Blood Services, Midwest Region is the sole provider of blood components to over 90 hospitals in the area and also provides therapeutic apheresis services at all metropolitan hospitals in Omaha, a city of 650,000 population. Because of the availability of apheresis equipment and trained staff, collection of Peripheral Blood Stem Cells (PBSC) is a logical extension of apheresis activity. We participated in the research and development phase of PBSC transplantation with the University of Nebraska Medical Center starting in 1984 and entered into agreement for collection of PBSC in 1986. The Oncologist, Blood Bank Medical Director and the Blood Center Medical Director were designated as the co-directors of the PBSC Collection program. The hospital Blood Bank processed and stored the Stem Cells. The collection and transplant protocols were modified 14 times to date and we have performed more than 5,000 PBSC collections for about 350 patients without serious complications. With planning and cooperation, a Blood Center can successfully support a stem cell transplant program not only in providing required blood components, but also providing PBSC collections.

0593

COMPARISON OF TWO CFU GM ASSAYS IN VIEW OF A STANDARDIZATION

Boccaccio C.,Merlin L., Leblond V.,Fournel JJ.

Peripheral blood stem cell(PBSC) autograft is now extensively used.Ability of cytapheresis product to restore hematopoiesis is evaluated by flow cytometry(number of CD34 positive cells) and /or CFU GM assay.There is a considerable interlaboratory variation in the results.The aim of this study was to compare two kinds of CFU GM assays to allow a standardization.6 bone marrow(BM) and 15 PBSC samples were cultured under different conditions:our standard laboratory medium (agar,FCS,human placenta conditioned medium,10^5 cells per dish) and a commercially available medium (methylcellulose,FCS, EPO,GCT,10^4 cells per dish).Results were expressed in term of CFU GM number /dish.Median CFU GM growth for 2 10^5 cells was following:BM 44.1$\pm$13(agar);79.7$\pm$35(Gibco)
PBSC 30.2$\pm$29(agar);141.4$\pm$63(Gibco)
Cloning efficiency was better with Gibco medium which is easy to use,reliable but expensive.Further tests are necessary and other media must be tested in view of a standardization.

0594

CORRELATION OF PCR FINGERPRINTING OF HLA DRB AND MLC RESULTS IN BONE MARROW RECIPIENTS AND RELATED DONORS

E.Brojer, M.Sankowska,J.J.Stańczak, A.Gronkowska,B.Stępień-Sopniewska*, A.Górski*,B.Żupańska
Institute of Haematology and Blood Transfusion,Warsaw,Poland
*Institute of Transplantation,School of Medicine, Warsaw, Poland

PCR fingerprinting of HLA DRB genes' amplification products was applied in order to find a potential family related bone marrow donor. For 29 patients at least one HLA class I identical donor was found. In all recipients and donors PCR fingerprinting was performed. In 18 pairs, the MLC was also done.Compatibility in PCR fingerprinting and MLC was observed in 60% and 65% respectively. A high correlation between both tests was found.In 9 pairs both tests showed HLA compatibility and in 5 - incompatibility; in two cases PCR fingerprinting was compatible but MLC positive, while in two others - the opposite.The bone marrow transplantation is in progress and the outcome will be discussed in comparison with the data hitherto presented.

0595

IMMUNOHAEMATOLOGICAL ASPECTS OF TRANSFUSION SUPPORT FOLLOWING ALLOGENIC RED CELLS MISMATCHED BONE MARROW TRANSPLANTATION

O.Volkova, L.Fregatova, G.Platonova, B.Afanasiev

Clinical Centre of Advanced Medical Technologies, Petrov's Institute of Oncology, St.-Petersburg, Russia

Immunohaematological monitoring of patients after allogenic red cells (RBC) mismatched bone marrow transplantation (BMT) was developed. It has been investigation for correct transfusion support of these patients.
Both RBC typing and antiglobulin test were performed by standard techniques. Posttranplantation ABO antibody titers were realized using our new latex test-systems with synthetic A and B antigens. RBC from bone marrow graft were removed by our modification of buffy coat and "self" sedimentation method without automated cell processor.
22 RBC mismatched BMT have been observed. Data of immunohaematological assay have made possible to choose modification of bone marrow processing. Patients'antibodies were not removed before BMT. Posttransplantation transfusion therapy was corrected by immunohaematological monitoring of these patients. We reached a conclusion that indication "mixed chimera" allows to use donor type RBC transfusion.
Due to such tactics of transfusion therapy we avoided any cases of hemolytical complications.

0596

IMMUNOHAEMATOLOGICAL RESPONSE OF RECIPIENT ON AN INCOMPATIBLE BONE MARROW TRANSPLANTATION

D. Cupaníková, D. Pavlíková, M. Hrubisko
Institute of Haematology and Blood Transfusion, University Hospital, Bratislava Slovakia

After ABO and Rho (D) incompatible bone marrow transplantation (BMT) all recipients acquired blood group characteristics of the donors apart from the secretory status of A,B,H antigens which remained the same as before the BMT.

Rho (D) negative recipients have not developed antibodies against Rho (D) positive donor erythrocytes. We have not observed any signs of haemolytic anaemia in recipients of incompatible BMT.

Incompatible anti A and/or anti B agglutinins were undetectable probably as a consequence of the neutralisation by tissue glyco and lipoprotein antigens of the recipients.

Recipients did not acquire secretory status of the donors. There was no dependence on the acquired donor's blood group.

It should be proved that Lewis system antigens are produced by some types of bone marrow cells probably other than haemopoetic cells.

0597

BONE MARROW TRANSPLANTATION (BMT) THROMBIN ACTIVATION AND THE ROLE OF THE NATURAL ANTICOAGULANT SYSTEMS. M. Charania, A. Duncan, R. Emmens, J. Boysza, C.D. Hillyer, J.Wingard, Emory University Hospital, Clifton Road, Atlanta, Georgia. 30322. USA

BMT is complicated by Hepatic veno-occlusive disease (VOD). Recent evidence suggests that deficiencies in the natural anticoagulants ATIII and Protein C (PC) may occur in these patients. We initiated a pilot study to investigate thrombin activation and the responses of the natural anticoagulants in 11 pts (5 allogeneic: 6 autologous) from day 0 to d-20 post BMT. Six pts > 40d post BMT served as a comparison group. The study also evaluated the variability of the test parameters in the acute transplant phase to establish their discriminant power. ATIII, Fibrin Monomer (FM), PC & Protein S (PS) activities, Prothrombin Fragment 1.2 (PF1.2) & Thrombin: antithrombin complexes (TAT) were quantitated with commercial kits (Biopool, Behring & Stago) The six late phase patients had only isolated abnormalities in their data..

DATA: Results expressed as % difference between mean day O and mean of nadir values post BMT.

% CHANGE	ATIII	PC	PS	FM	PF1.2	TAT
ALLOGENEIC	-14%	-15%	-21%	+320%	-4%	+118%
AUTOLOGOUS	-11%	-48%	-6%	+200%	0%	+80%

This small study suggests that increased thrombin generation occurs after BMT with a decrease in the natural anticoagulants. A role may exist for monitoring and therapeutic support of the natural anticoagulants in BMT. Whether this increased procoagulant activity is related to the occurrence of VOD, will require further studies.

0599

Possible involvement of a HLA-DP mismatch in the development of graft versus host disease in bone marrow transplantation.

H.R. Lang[1], A.A. Fauser[2], H. Beeser[1]
Albert-Ludwigs University, Freiburg, 1Transfusion Medicine, 2Centre for Transplantation, FRG

For allogeneic bone marrow transplantation (BMT) of unrelated donor and recipient matching of HLA-DR subtyps is required. HLA-DQ and HLA-DP testing is recommended but not obligatory. Further analysis are important in order to provide data on HLA-DP combinations that might be involved in the development of a graft versus host disease.
Here we report a case in which we anticipate the involvement of a HLA-DP mismatch in a severe graft versus host disease (GvHD). Patient E.R., female, 36 y, CML, (chronic phase) was typed A1, A3, B51, -, Cw1, DRB1*0101, 1501, DQB1*0501, 0602, DPB1*0301, 1801. A unrelated donor with HLA type: A1, A3, B51, x, Cw1, DRB1*0101, 1501, DQB1*0501, 0602, DPB1*0401, 0402 was choosen for BMT.
The mixed lymphocyte culture (MLC) that is regularly done for pre-transplantation testing in our laboratory was repeatedly uninterpre-table because of a high spontaneous proliferation of the patient's cells. Since the HLA- type of the patient and the donor is considered a good match, a bone marrow transplant was performed.
Within days the patient developed a severe GvHD.
Although we did not established HLA-DP-specific T cell clones, and thus can not exclude the involvement of other antigens, it is suggested that this DP mismatch might be responsible for a GvHD in this patient, and therefore we consider this particular DP mismatch critical. Additionally, from this experience we recommend to do cellular compatibility tests that may indicate incompatible HLA types of bone marrow donors and recipients.

0600

EVALUATION OF DIFFERENT LYSING PROCEDURES FOR FLOW CYTOMETRIC STEM CELL DETECTION IN UMBILICAL CORD BLOOD

U. Cassens, I. Ganschow, H.P. Benn, K. Gutensohn, R. Dittmer, P. Kuehnl,
Dept. of Transfusion Medicine / Transplant. Immunol., University Hosp. Hamburg, FRG

Since umbilical cord blood is a potential source of stem cells, we tested 3 different lysing reagents for their ability to lyse whole cord blood and achieve a reliable detection of (CD34-positive) stem cells.
The lysing reagents from BECTON DICKINSON® (BD), IMMUNOTECH® (IT) and ORTHO DIAGNOSTICS® (OD) were applied to the same 14 samples (in duplicate). The leukocytes were tested for the expression of the stem cell marker CD34 and the co-expression markers CD33, CD38, HLA-DR by flow cytometric analysis (Facs scan BECTON DICKINSON®).
The lysis by the IT reagent yielded an average of 0.46% CD34-positive cells compared with 0.42% by the OD lysis and 0.31% (BD lysis). There was no significant difference in the distribution of the expression of CD33, CD38 and HLA-DR on CD34-positive cells. Overall, the IT- and BD-lysis showed a more homogeneous distribution of subpopulations in the scatter properties.
Consequently, the 3 lysis reagents showed distinctly different CD34 counts. We conclude that the quantitation of peripheral blood stem cells needs to be further investigated and standardized.

0601

CORD BLOOD PLASMA-MEDIATED *EX VIVO* EXPANSION OF HEMATOPOIETIC PROGENITOR CELLS.

F. Bertolini, L. Lazzari, E. Lauri, C. Corsini, G. Sirchia. Centro Trasfusionale e di Immunologia dei Trapianti, Ospedale Maggiore, Milan, Italy

We investigated the effect of cord blood (CB) plasma, maternal blood (MB) plasma, peripheral blood (PB) plasma and fetal calf serum (FCS) *per se* and in association with stem cell factor (SCF), IL-3 and IL-11 in liquid cultures of low density cells (n=8). In cultures of CB cells supplemented by CB plasma but without cytokines, we observed a 2.8±0.3 fold expansion of the number of CFU-GM (peak on day 2), while BFU-E were stable and CFU-Mix decreased. Addition of MB plasma to CB cell cultures resulted in a 1.8±0.2 fold expansion of CFU-GM. In absence of cytokines, CFU-GM expansion did not occur in CB cell cultures supplemented with PB plasma or FCS and in BM cell cultures supplemented with CB, MB or PB plasma or FCS. When SCF, IL-3 and IL-11 were added to liquid cultures, an expansion of CFU-GM was observed in CB and BM cell cultures supplemented by either CB, MB or PB plasma or FCS. Nevertheless, progenitor cell expansion was significantly superior in CB cell cultures in presence of CB plasma (8.7±0.7, 2.4±0.3 and 2.6±0.3 fold expansions on day 10 for CFU-GM, BFU-E and CFU-Mix, respectively). In conclusion, an unknown factor(s) present in CB plasma, probably capable to cross the placenta, can support expansion of CB-derived progenitors. The synergistic action of CB plasma, SCF, IL-3 and IL-11, moreover, has promise for expansion of CB-derived progenitors and preservation of multipotential cells.

0602

PRESERVATION OF RED BLOOD CELLS IN THE SOLUTION OF GELATINE WITH ADENINE AND PHOSPHATE ADDED

E.A.Selivanov, V.N.Melnikova, V.T.Pleshakov, I.N.Degtereva, I.M.Krivtsova
Russian Research Institute of Hematology and Transfusiology, St.Petersburg, Russia

Adenine and phosphate were added to the preservative ("Modegelum-AP") in order to improve the characteristics of the preservative used for red blood cell (RBC) storage.
RBC suspended in the preservative (1:1) retained their morphofunctional characteristics at 4°C storage for the period of 42 days. By this time the ATP level in the cells was 82.5±2.8% of the initial one.
As distinct from the known glucose-saline preservatives, the new one is a colloid plasma substitute. RBC suspended in the preservative transfused for shock or blood loss had hemodynamic, rheologic, and detoxicating effects and improved the microcirculation.

0603

AUTOMATED BLOOD COMPONENT DONATION WITH MCS-3-P IMPROVES RED CELL QUALITY

G. Matthes[1], I. Pawlow[1], K.-P. Krause[1], U. Tofoté[1], W. Kucera[2], D. Lerche[2]

[1]Institute of Transfusion Medicine, [2]Institute of Medical Physics and Biophysics, Humboldt University Berlin, Germany

With the cell separator MCS-3P two different programmes were used for the erythroplasmapheresis: RBCP (collection of one unit of red cells and two units of plasma) resp. RBCPS (one unit of red cells and one unit of plasma). The quality of the red cells during the storage of 42 days was measured by biochemical and rheological parameters. The donation time at 53 donors was 20 min for 355 ml RCC-SAGM and 440 ml plasma resp. 7 min for 335 ml RCC-SAGM and 239 ml Plasma. The donor tolerance was analogous to during plasmapheresis. The results for red blood cell storage are better (ATP, 2,3 DPG, p50, hemoglobin derivatives, filtration/rigidity index) or at least as good as with standard collection (free hemoglobin, free potassium, glucose, lactose, hemolysis) du to prevention of collection lesion. All blood preparations were steril after storage.
The automated blood component donation with MCS-3P can be especially recommended for application in an autologous blood programme because the consequent application of autologous blood donation in hospitals is often limited by missing preconditions for component separation.

0604

BLOOD BAG CAPACITIES - WHAT DO THEY MEAN ?

RJ Hawker.
West Midlands Blood Transfusion Centre, Vincent Drive, Edgbaston, BIRMINGHAM. B15 2SG. U.K.

The optimal storage of platelets depends on many factors including platelet concentration, volume of the platelet concentrate, blood bag polymer and surface area. The latter two are controlled by the blood bag manufacturer with individual laboratories favouring different sources. Often the blood bag has a specified volume printed on the label and this figure, from the manufacturer, is regularly quoted in the sales literature and in research publications. These volumes rarely relate to the actual capacity of the bag and bear no relationship to the volume of platelet concentrate it will support during storage. For example a typical trimelliate plasticised-PVC "400mL extended platelet storage transfer pack" has a capacity of 626mL and 380cm^2 surface area but will only support platelets at a concentration of $1.4x10^6/\mu L$ in a volume of 55mL ie $7.7x10^{10}$.

The maximum capacity and surface area of blood bags from seven manufacturers were computed from dimensions. Laboratory experimentation confirmed the theoretical results. Of the bag types studied, the majority had quoted volumes 50% less than their actual capacity. For plasma or whole blood the maximum safe working capacity is important and may explain the generally low quoted figure for bag capacity. Computer modelling of surface area(SA) to volume(V) is important for platelets. The platelet storage capacity of a bag can be described for each plastic film, of which there are limited licenced formulations, based on platelet concentration, plasma volume and surface area. It can be calculated that to maintain platelet viability for 5 day storage PVC (TEHTM) should have a SA/V of ≈ 7.0 and PVC(BTHC) and polyolefin of ≈ 3.0. These figures appear to relate to the available area of gas permeable plastic film surface area excluding the area covered by labels.

It is recommended that manufacturers note these observations and, prescribe the maximum (and minimum) platelet concentration and plasma volume for storage to five days for each container based on the best research data available and/or provide the "maximum safe (recommended) working capacity"

0605

LONG-TERM LIQUID PRESERVATION OF PLATELET CONCENTRATES IN A DOUBLE-BAG SYSTEM

T.A. Takahashi[1], C. Yakushiji[2], Y, Kino[2], S. Sekiguchi[1]
[1]Hokkaido Red Cross Blood Center, Sapporo, [2]Kawasumi Laboratories Inc., Tokyo, Japan.

We have developed a double-bag system to extend the storage period of platelet concentrates (PC) in liquid form. The double-bag system consists of two compartments in which the inner compartment is separated from the outer one by a semipermeable membrane. One hundred milliliters of PC prepared by platelet apheresis was put in the inner compartment and 500 ml of the synthetic medium for platelet storage developed by Holme et al. was put in the outer compartment. To adjust the colloidal osmotic pressure, 2.5% w/v dextran was added to the platelet storage medium. The double-bag was vertically rotated at 5 rpm at an angle of 45° in a 22°C incubator under a normal air atmosphere. The medium in the outer compartment was not changed during the storage period. As a control, the same volume of PC was put in polyolefin containers and stored on a horizontal agitator at 22°C.

The PC stored in the double-bag system could maintain platelet count and mean platelet volume as well as those preserved in the polyolefin containers. In contrast, morphology, membrane glycoproteins such as GPIb, hypotonic shock response and aggregability of platelets were much better preserved when platelets were maintained by this new system than when stored in the polyolefin containers at the 10th day of storage, and platelet functions were retained even after 21 days.

0606

***IN VITRO* & *IN VIVO* STUDIES OF PLATELET CONCENTRATES STORED IN PL-2209 AND PL-1240**

VS.Turner, SG.Mitchell, SK.Kang, RJ.Hawker
West Midlands Blood Transfusion Centre, Vincent Drive, Edgbaston, BIRMINGHAM. UK

BTHC plasticised PVC has been shown to have advantages in blood component storage. Two studies were carried out to compare platelet concentrates (PC), mean volume 69.7±11ml., mean plt. conc. $10^6/\mu l$ stored in PL-2209 (PVC-BTHC) or PL-1240 (PVC-TEHTM) 600ml packs. In an *in vitro* study, five pools of four donations were divided equally into PL-2209 and PL-1240 packs and processed to PCs. PCs were stored and assayed on days 1, 3 & 5. In a paired study, 10 volunteers gave whole blood donations on two separate occasions and derived PCs were stored in PL-2209 or PL-1240 packs. On day 5 stored PCs were labelled with ^{111}Indium and an autologous sample reinfused. Remaining platelets were assayed *in vitro*. *In vivo* recovery and survival were determined from sequential blood samples.

***In Vitro* Study**

Paired Statistics PL-2209 v PL-1240

Assay Day	1	3	5	max.mean diff	Higher Value
Hypotonic Shock Rec.	*	*	**	13.53%	1240
ADP Aggregation 3.2μM	***	**	*	9.66%	2209
ADP Aggregation 32μM	***	***	*	10.63%	2209
Coll.+ Epi.Aggregation	NS	NS	**	10.28%	1240
pH	***	NS	NS	0.07	2209
pCO_2	***	**	*	1.67KPa	1240
LDH release	***	***	***	4.20%	1240
Platelet ATP	NS	NS	**	10.96nmol/10^9	1240
Lactate	**	***	***	2.04mmol/L	2209

*** $P<0.001$ ** $P<0.01$ * $P<0.05$ *NS = Not Significant*

Data derived from Day 5 assays of the *in vivo* study showed similar results. Gaseous exchange was higher in PL-2209 which was reflected in a maintained pH and lower pCO_2 (3.5 v 5.3 KPa). There were no significant differences in the recovery (43.5%) and "multiple-hit" survival (116.7hr.) of platelets stored in the two plastics. We conclude that PL-2209 is at least as good as PL-1240 for the 5 day storage of PCs at 22°C with agitation.

0607

BUFFY-COAT DERIVED PLATELETS USING 0.5CPD AND CPD AS ANTICOAGULANTS AND THREE PLATELET ADDITIVE SOLUTIONS

H.G.T. Gulliksson[1], L. Eriksson[2], and C.F. Högman[2]
1 Stockholm Blood Transfusion Service, Stockholm, and
2 Department of Clinical Immunology & Transfusion Medicine, University Hospital, Uppsala, Sweden

CPD with half-normal concentration of citrate (0.5CPD) improves factor VIII stability and red cell quality (Vox Sang 1993;65: 271-278). Platelet concentrates (PCs) were prepared from blood collected in 0.5CPD and CPD; pools of 4 or 6 buffy coats (BCs) were suspended in either saline, a platelet additive solution (PAS-1, Vox Sang 1990;59:140-145), or acetate-containing PASs. Blood gases, pH, bicarbonate concentration, ATP, total adenylates, BTG- and LDH-release were tested. Earlier findings (Transfusion 1993;33:301-303) were confirmed that a low citrate concentration (8 mmol/l) is beneficial (40% plasma in saline); lower concentration than that could cause clotting problems and should be avoided. The presence of acetate in the PAS reduced the lactate formation when the citrate concentration was higher than 8 mmol/l; 30 mmol/l acetate (PAS-2) was optimal. Acetate had also the benefit that it promoted bicarbonate formation and thereby the buffering capacity of the diluted plasma; pH was thus better maintained in 30% plasma/ PAS-2 than in 40% plasma in saline. In PCs with undiluted 0.5CPD plasma enough bicarbonate remained at the end of 9-day storage to avoid a decrease in pH. We conclude that platelets can be prepared from 0.5CPD-BC as well as from CPD-BC. PAS-2 was superior to saline and PAS-1.

0608

RANDOMISED, PLACEBO-CONTROLLED, DOUBLE-BLIND IN VITRO STUDY ON THE EFFECT OF THROMBOXANE A_2 RECEPTOR ANTAGONISTS AS AN ADJUNCT TO PLATELET CONCENTRATES TO IMPROVE THE QUALITY OF STORED PLATELETS.

Beate Kehrel, Joachim Kardoeus, Birgit Fehmer, Barbara Bettin-Wille(1), Jürgen van de Loo, Norbert Müller(2). Dept. of Internal Medicine and (2)Inst. for Transfusionmedicine, University of Muenster, Germany; (1)Boehringer Mannheim GmbH, Mannheim, Germany.

The storage of platelet concentrates results in a decline in platelet function and integrity. Platelet activation plays a major role in the development of this storage lesion. The thromboxane A_2 receptor antagonists solutroban and daltroban have been proved to be effective drugs in preventing platelet activation in vitro and vivo. Both drugs have a competitive mode of action. Therefore the effect of the drug in the platelet concentrate might be antagonized by TXA_2 formation in the body when the concentrate is applied.
Platelets from 30 healthy normal donors were collected on a Haemogenetics blood cell separator and stored at 22°C continuously agitated for ten days. Solutroban (8 mg / 400 ml), daltroban (0.8 mg / 400 ml) and placebo were added in a volume of 80 µl to 10 platelet concentrates (400 ml) respectively. Small samples were taken every 24 hours and changes in structural integrity using a morphology score (Kunicki et al, 1975), loss of aggregability in response to collagen, ADP and epinephrine, decrease in pH, increase in lactate and the expression of markers for platelet α-granule and lysosome degranulation were measured.
All platelets lost their aggregability in the first four days of storage. The pH decreased from pH 7.2 to pH 6.8 and correspondingly lactate concentration increased. The expression of GMP140 and CD63 slowly increased from day 0 to 5 with an even stronger increase till day 9. On day 0 13±6 percent of the platelets were positive for GMP140 and 17±5 percent for CD63. This increased to 59±20 percent for GMP140 and 47±14 percent for CD63 on day 9. There was a strong linear correlation between morphology score and activation marker expression. No statistical significant difference was observed between the placebo, solutroban and daltroban treated platelets.
We postulate that blockade of the TXA_2 pathway is not sufficient to prevent platelet storage lesion.

0609

SPLITTING DOUBLE-DOSE APHERESIS PLATELET UNITS

A. van den Bos, H. Olthuis, B. van Dijk, B. Bär, V. Kunst
Blood Transfusion Department University Hospital;
Red Cross Blood Bank, Nijmegen, The Netherlands.

There is concern about the quality of stored apheresis platelets. The growing practice of storing apheresis platelets is the result of the advancement in platelet apheresis procedures, by which a high number of platelets in one collection procedure can be obtained.
In the collection procedure we try to obtain a double-dose unit which is defined as a unit containing more than 500.10^9 platelets. Leukocyte poor ($<2.10^7$ leukocytes) units containing more than 500.10^9 platelets, are splitted and stored up to 4 days.
In patients with hemato-oncologic diseases platelet counts are measured before and 24 hours after platelet transfusion and the Corrected Count Increment (CCI) is calculated. In the table listed below the results are shown.
We conclude that stored apheresis platelets can be transfused up to four days after collection from the donor. This finding supports our method to obtain and to split double-dose apheresis platelet units.

days	0	1	2	3	4
CCI-24 h	10.0	6.8	6.0	6.2	7.0
number (n)	10	18	21	12	13

Table: random single donor apheresis platelet units: mean Corrected Count Increment after 24 hours (CCI-24 h) related to days of storage

0610

IN VITRO TESTING OF PLATELET FUNCTION IN STORED CPDA-1 WHOLE BLOOD (WB) OVER A STORAGE PERIOD OF 34 DAYS

R. Grunenberg, P. Freischem, J. Krüger
Institute of Transfusion Medicine, University of Cologne, D-50924 Cologne, Germany

Acute massive blood loss is still treated with WB. In contrast to single component therapy it does not double or treble the risk of transfusion-transmitted disease. Storage conditions of WB require only a 75% recovery of RBCs at 24 hours after transfusion, viability and function of leucocytes or platelets are disregarded. The in vitro functional capacity of platelets after storage up to 34 days is therefore of interest and was investigated. Response to hypotonic stress (A), ADP- and collagen-induced maximal aggregation (B and C) and spreading capacity on plastic surfaces (D) were used for the evaluation of stored platelets in 20 units of WB. The median number of platelets decreased from $2.03 \times 10^5/\mu l$ to $0.96 \times 10^5/\mu l$ after 34 days. The median values of the functional tests are given below.

tests	days of storage										
	0	1	2	3	4	6	9	13	18	24	34
A [%]	49	50	53	53	49	45	38	26	14	6	0
B [%]	60	65	63	61	56	49	38	29	23	16	12
C [%]	56	37	29	27	26	18	13	12	8	4	1
D [%]	80	69	66	63	61	52	43	25	21	8	1

These data indicate that during the initial period of storage a fair amount of functional platelets are available. Their functional profiles are compared with the storage lesion of polymorphonuclears and T-lymphocytes.

0611

EFFECT OF EXPOSURE TIME TO TEMPERATURES BELOW 20°C ON LOSS OF PLATELET DISCOID SHAPE DURING 5-DAY STORAGE AT 22°C. S.Holme, A.Heaton, J.Sweeney,S.Sawyer.American Red Cross,Norfolk,VA,USA.

Exposure of platelets to temperatures below 20°C is related to loss of discoid shape and viability. In this study, the limitations of exposure time of platelets to cold was systematically investigated. Six units of day 1 standard PC were mixed, split, and returned to single containers. Five were then stored unagitated at various temperatures (4°, 12°, 16°, or 18°C) for up to 24 hours, after which they were stored at 22°C (test units) for a total of 5 days. The sixth unit acted as control with storage at 22°C for 5 days. 93 PC were studied. Loss of platelet discoid shape was determined photometrically by the extent of shape change assay (ESC), as an increase in apparent platelet size by impedance, morphologically using phase microscopy, and by "swirling" as determined visually and by a light scatter device (NAPSAC). Test unit results were expressed in percentage of control. High correlations ($r > 0.55$-0.70) were found between various assays of platelet shape. A mathematical model was developed by nonlinear regression based on observed loss of the platelet discoid shape as a function of exposure temperature and time. High correlations were found between values predicted by the model and actual measured values ($r = 0.70$-0.82 for the various assays). Previous studies have suggested that a 20% decrease or more in % discoid shape (by ESC) represents a clinically significant loss in platelet viability. The model ($ESC = 100 + 0.18 \cdot temp \cdot time - 4.1 \cdot time + 0.07 \cdot temp$) predicts that this occurs at 16°C for 16 hours, 12°C for 10 hours, or 4°C for 6 hours, while exposure to 18°C for up to 24 hours does not reach this level.

0612

MEASUREMENT OF GMP140 IN PLATELET CONCENTRATES

S. Stienstra, R. Laport, H.P. Olthuis
Red Cross Blood Bank, Nijmegen, The Netherlands

Preactivation due to ageing of platelets in a platelet concentrate can be recognized by the presence of GMP 140 antigens (CD62, PADGEM) on the outer membrane of platelets.
With a Coulter Epics Profile II flow cytometer we measured the presence of GMP 140 on the platelets and microvesicles with PE-labelled monoclonals directed against GMP 140. To identify the measured fluorescent particles as originating from platelets, a FITC conjugated monoclonal antibody, directed against the specific platelet antigen GPIb (CD42b), which is present in both resting platelets and activated platelets in the same content, is simultaneously used. This second antibody is also a check, which excludes the possibility that activated platelets have aspecific binding to the used monoclonal antibodies.
We have seen both in flow cytometry and microscopy a correlation between the moment of the platelet shape change and the GMP 140 presentation on the membrane. The technique was applied on fresh platelets and 5-days old platelets, which were prepared by the buffy coat method or by aferesis. Older platelets had more reactivity with the GMP 140. 64% of the fresh platelets showed red fluorescence with a mean fluorescence intensity of 3.06 and 85% of the 5-days old platelets presented a red fluorescence with a mean fluorescence intensity of 7.39. Thrombin activation of fresh platelets resulted in 95% fluorescence with a mean fluorescence intensity of approximately 10. The described method is an objective method to measure the activation state of the platelets in a platelet concentrate.

0613

SEROTONIN UPTAKE IN PLATELET CONCENTRATES

H.P. Benn[1], I. Ganschow[1], R. Fischer[2], B. Dresow[2], U. Cassens[1], R. Dittmer[1], and P. Kuehnl[1];
[1]Transfusionsmed., [2]Med. Biochemie, UKE, Hamburg, FRG.

The platelet-plasma serotonin exchange in different apheresis products and platelet concentrates from buffy coats (PCs) was studied for quality control over a period of 7 days.
Measurements of serotonin (5-HT-ELISA; IBL Hamburg) in platelets and suspension medium (plasma) were done with and without the 5-HT pump inhibitor imipramine together with platelet counts, mean platelet volume, and pH.
RESULTS: The initial concentration of 5-HT in platelets correlated with platelet counts ($r=0.65$, $p<0.001$), irrespective of the product or container. In PCs with rapidly decreasing pH values due to inappropriate gas exchange, the platelet 5-HT concentration increased significantly (>10% positive netto uptake) during the first day of storage. Thereafter, at pH < 6.5 platelet serotonin dropped with $t_{1/2}=1d$, but platelet counts were constant and 5-HT uptake was inhibited concomitantly. The plasma 5-HT increased as pH decreased. This can be enforced by competitive inhibition of serotonin uptake due to imipramine. However, in platelet concentrates with stable pH the 5-HT pump kept steady-state conditions up to 7 days.
CONCLUSION: As transfer rate constants are functions of the actual pH (range: 8.0 - 6.5) the active transmembrane shift of 5-HT in either direction can be induced ex vivo. Thus, the serotonin platelet / plasma ratio serves as an additional platelet viability parameter.

0614

NERVE GROWTH FACTOR STIMULATION OF HUMAN PLATELETS

Vadim Yu. Prokudin[1], Oleg S. Brusov[1], Dirk de Korte[2]
[1] National Mental Health Research Center, Moscow, Russia. [2] Central Laboratory Netherlands Red Cross Blood Transfusion Service, Amsterdam, the Netherlands

The influence of nerve growth factor (NGF) on human platelets was studied. NGF stimulation of human platelets in a dose from 100 nM to 500 nM resulted in a very weak shape change reaction. NGF stimulation of human platelets did not result in changes of adenosine and guanosine nucleotides but evoked an increase of intracellular IMP levels (from 0.9 ± 0.22 to 2.1 ± 0.71 pmol/10^6 platelets at 128 nM NGF) reflecting the energy consumption during this stimulation. NGF induced a considerable elevation of the intracellular calcium concentration from 28 ± 6.6 nM to a maximal value of 675 ± 123.4 nM in the presence of 16 nM NGF, with an EC_{50} of 11.8 ± 0.61 nM. It was shown that the basic source of calcium used during NGF stimulation was extracellular calcium. These data reveal an active reaction of human platelets on NGF, with a discrepancy between aggregation response and calcium mobilization. This will promote further investigations on the mechanisms of human platelet activation by various ligands, including NGF.

0615

HYDROXYETHYL STARCH(HES) CRYOPRESERVATION OF RED CELLS

M J G Thomas, S H Bell, ABSD, Aldershot, GU11 2AF, UK

In war or major disasters there is a need for large volumes of blood. Stockpiling with fresh blood, having a shelf life of 35 days, is impractical. Various methods of cryopreservation have been investigated, most using glycerol, which has to be removed prior to transfusion. This process is expensive in manpower, requires sophisticated equipment and the product is microbiologically incompetent, with a post-thaw shelf life of 24 hours. The British Army requires a rapid, simple process which yields a microbiologically competent product with at least a 7 day shelf life. The cryoprotectant HES is non toxic and does not require removal prior to transfusion. The absence of a washing process requires haemolysis to be kept to less than 3%. Using a sterile connecting device, 200mls of WBC depleted red cells, PCV > 90%, are introduced into the freezing bag to which 35mls of a 40% solution of HES is added. The bag, manufactured by NPBI, is placed in a slightly curved freezing frame keeping the maximum thickness of the blood film less than 4mm. The frame is plunged into liquid nitrogen, -196°C, the blood is snap frozen within 30 seconds, and is then stored in the vapour phase, -150°C or in a mechanical freezer <-90°C. The units are thawed in a water bath at 43.5°C for 10 minutes after which the blood is ready for transfusion. Red cell recoveries (n=108) average 99.1% SD=0.12%, 30 minute saline stabilities average 91.0% SD=0.75% and 24 hour post transfusion survivals (n=10) average 89.4% SD=2.1%. 2,3 DPG and p50 are unaffected. ATP and haemolysis levels post thaw remain acceptable for 14 days when the blood is stored at 4°C.

0617

Studies of the effective utilization and the desirable supply of Red Cells products in Kyoto Red Cross Blood Center

S. Yokoyama, T. Matsuura

Kyoto Red Cross Blood Center

Purpose: The purpose of this study is to evaluate the effective utilization and the desirable supply of Red cells stored in MAP additive solution (RC-MAP, Japanese Red Cross) in order to avoid the risk of transfusion-associated Yersinia enterocolitica sepsis. Method: Since October 1992 we replaced Concentrated CPD Red Cells with RC-MAP, and surveyed the effective utilization of RC-MAP reviewing the number of RC-MAP products supplied and finally discarded because of outdated in each month. At the same time, we monitored the number of days each product was stored prior to distribution to hospitals. Results: Whole blood collection of 400ml and 200ml units was carried out according to the monthly collection plan based on clinical demands. From October 1992 to June 1993, approximately 11,300 units was distributed each month. Almost all of the products were transfused. As for the results, the monthly discard rate was under 10%(0.8-9.4%). In addition, it was possible to supply about 95% of RC-MAP products within 25 days of collection. Conclusion: We concluded that an accurate monthly blood collection program according anticipated clinical demands is necessary for effective utilization and desirable supply of RC-MAP products.

0618

BLOOD COMPONENT THERAPY IN WAR

M. Radović, J.Taseski

Institute of Transfusiology of MMA
Belgrade, Yugoslavia.

There have been notable scientific and technical developments in transfusiology, resulting to the introduction of modern blood component therapy in war time. According to previous results, in addition to whole homologous snd autologous blood, for medical treatment of war casualties have been used: red blood cells (RBCs), concentrated platelets, albumin, plasma protein fraction, fresh frozen plasma, cryoprecipitate depleted plasma, native plasma, cryoprecipitate, fibrinogen for i.v. use, standard immunoglobilins for i.m. or i.v. use, antitetanus immunoglobulins, and fibrin glue (homologous and autologous). For appropriate therapy of acute blood loss and urgent resuscitation in severe hypovolemic casualty, of great significance have been RBCs (rapid increase of oxygen carrying capacity) and albumin (first line acute expander applied to restore circulating blood volume). Together with surgical-reanimation measures, those two blood products have been most valuable for survival of war casualties. It is clear that war time availability of blood products depends on clinical use of RBCs in peace time, primarily. The ready availability of blood products, adequate to supply the requirements of war casualties, must be feasible at field hospital level.

0619

FREQUENCY OF INABILITY TO FIND OUT COMPATIBLE BLOOD DONORS

J. Georgopoulos, N. Vgontza, E. Digenopoulou, J. Spiliotopoulou, L. Dadiotis, K. Maragos, Ir. Kontopoulou
1st R.T.C "Hippocration" Hospital, Athens, Greece

The patients with incompatibility during cross matching due to clinicaly significant alloantibodies increase continiously because of the extent use of blood. We present the incompatibility problems, we faced during the last five years in a tertiary University hospital. During the last five years 144.135 compatibilities have been performed and 60.879 units have been transfused to 17.905 patients. In 119 patients we had incompatibility due to clinicaly significant alloantibodies, all indetified except one. 96 cases had one alloantibody while 23 had 2 to 4 alloantibodies. The alloantibody's frequency was anti-E>K>$\bar{c}$>JK^a>Fy^a the other following. All patients, except three, were transfused without delay through the available panel of typed blood units of our center. In two cases with antibodies of those blood groups P and Yt^a which we had no available blood units or donors we successfuly faced the surgical problems of the patients with an autotransfusion programme. In the case of the third patient with anti-$\bar{c}$+Jk^b +unidentified to whom we didn't find any compatible unit, the necessary spleenectomy is going to be performed after erythropoetin treatment and autotransfusion. It is obvious that the big majority of the incompatible cases can be faced if there is available a panel of typed blood donors. In the rare blood group cases as well as the unidentified ones, growth factors and autotransfusion can solve the problems if they are not urgent. In another way, European and International blood bank of rare blood donors can be very helpful.

0620

THE MAXIMUM SURGICAL BLOOD ORDER SCHEDULE: IMPLEMENTATION IN A TERTIARY CARE FACILITY

D. Bervy, C. Chamberlain, A. Rauch, G.D. Wilner
Albany Medical Center Hospital, Albany, New York 12208 U.S.A.

The Maximum Surgical Blood Order Schedule (MSBOS) is a transfusion guideline designed to best optimize the blood inventory for elective surgical procedures. Following a review of the transfusion records of 778 elective surgical procedures, we undertook a study of the efficacy of a MSBOS implementation at a 675-bed tertiary care university hospital. A 6 month review and evaluation was done to determine physician compliance, cost savings, and impact on the crossmatch to transfusion ratio. Elective surgical procedures accounted for only 737 (23.7%) of the 3,105 packed red blood cells (PRBC) transfused during the 4 month review period. However, 40.4% of the total crossmatch procedures performed during this same period were used to provide these products. Implementation of the MSBOS resulted in a significant drop in the crossmatch to transfusion ratio (C/T), and has resulted in an estimated savings of $1,400/month in supplies and technologist time. Physician acceptance and compliance has been near 100%. We conclude that the MSBOS improves transfusion Service efficiency even in tertiary care settings where elective surgical procedures account for a minority of transfusion products.

0621

RELEVANCE STUDIES OF PRESCRIPTION OF TRANSFUSION OF RED BLOOD CELL CONCENTRATES.

D. Sondag, J.L. Houet - Immuno-Hématologie-CHU-
Blood Transfusion Centre-Liège-Belgium

Objectives : Despite selection of donors and the efficiency of screening tests for blood transmitted diseases, transfusion remains a therapeutic means embodying non-negligible secondary effects. Moreover, because blood and derivatives are collected from volunteer donors, these products should be used within their strict indications. The objective of this study is to evaluate the relevance of prescribing red blood cells concentrates, (RBC).
Material and methods : The study enrolled 451 cases and concerned 1273 RBC units. It was carried out in two general hospitals, one of which was a university hospital. Each case was examined in relation to an algorithm resulting in: acceptance of the prescription, further consultation with the clinician concerned, or, sometimes, in rejection.
Results :
- One third of RBC blood demands are not followed by any transfusion.
- On a global point of view, 50 % of blood units are not transfused at all.
- The mean number of blood units transfused per patient is 2.8.
  The major prescriptions are :

Type of pathology	Distribution (%) of transfused RBC hosp.A	hosp.B
Medical	36	32
Surgical	63	55
Gynecological	0	8
Pediatric	1	6

Conclusion : 91 % of indications were in agreement with the decisional algorithm. 9% were not immediately acceptable and required a revision.The majority of these latter prescriptions concerned patients suffering from malignant pathologies at the terminal stage and for whom comfort and psychological factors even more than established clinical indications, determined the decision.

0622

FROM CROSS-MATCH AND RESERVATION OF BLOOD TO TYPE & SCREEN AND DELIVERY ON DEMAND

J. Georgsen, S.T. Lillevang, S.E.H. Jacobsen, T. Kristensen
Dept. of Clinical Immunology, University Hospital, DK-5000 Odense C

Aims: Reduction of: (1) serology workload, (2) stores of blood, and (3) time from order to delivery.
Methods: The following alterations were made during 1993:
February: (1) Screening for irregular red cell antibodies was changed from a tube to a column agglutination technique utilizing plasma to facilitate automation, (2) all samples received for crossmatching screened for irregular antibodies on a 24 hours basis, and (3) Type & Screen introduced for patients with minimal risk of transfusion. **April**: Crossmatching performed in saline, only, i.e. enzyme- and antiglobulin techniques abandoned. **November**: Type & Screen introduced for all patients without irregular antibodies, i.e. no reservation of blood, but saline crossmatching and delivery on demand. Children younger than 7 years were excepted.

Results:	Monthly 1992	December 1993
Delivered units	1.885	2.080
Crossmatches	5.012	3.210
Blood inventory (*optimal*)	1000	790
No. of units outdated	96	15
Age of units at delivery (*average*)	4 weeks	2 weeks
Time from order to first delivery	90 min	45 min
Time from order to second deliveries	90 min	15 min

Conclusions: Crossmatch/transfusion ratio has been reduced from 2.8 to 1.5, blood stores by 21%, and outdating from 4.2% to 0.7%. On average, transfused units have a significantly shorter shelf-life. Time from order to first delivery has been reduced by 50%, while the time for second deliveries was cut down by 80%.

0623

ABCD-TEST, A SAFE PRETRANSFUSION PROCEDURE IN USE SINCE MORE THAN 10 YEARS

J. Säfwenberg[1], C.F. Högman[1], B. Cassemar[2]
1Department of Clinical Immunology and Transfusion Medicine, Uppsala, 2The EDP Working Group for Blood Banking, Sweden.

Objections have been raised against the use of the Type and Screen (T&S) procedure, particularly if it is used alone without further measures such as a ´rapid spin´saline cross-match. We have combined the T&S with a computerized delivery control, used in regular routine since 10 years, the ABCD-test (**A**ntibody screening, **B**lood group check, **C**omputerized **D**elivery control).

The blood group and the antibody status of the patients are stored in the computer. Immunization to red cell antigens disqualifies for ABCD-testing requiring cross-match. Test cells from 4 carefully selected donors covering a sufficiently complete antigenic spectrum are used. The serological techniques have been changed 3 times; since 4 years IAT/LISS in gel is used. A delivery slip with the patient's and unit's identifications is printed and attached to the unit. No further testing is performed.

95% of the patients qualify for the ABCD-test. The procedure reduces work-load by 65%. In 0.8% of the ABCD-tests a previously unknown immunization is detected and the patient is switched to cross-matches. Over 230 000 red cell units have been successfully transfused without reported clinical reactions related to red cell incompatibility. The procedure is considered to be safe.

0624

METHOD INTENSIFYING THERAPEUTIC EFFECTIVENESS OF ERYTHROCYTE MASS TRANSFUSION IN ACUTE POSTHAEMORRHAGIC ANEMIA

Sh.I.Shelegia, A.I.Abesadze, L.I.Ataneli-shvili, L.B.Okudjava, M.M.Kutateladze
Institute of Haematology and Blood Transfusion, Tbilisi, Republic of Georgia

The method intensifying therapeutic effectiveness of erythrocyte mass transfusion in posthaemorrhagic anemia has been worked out in the present work. It has been established that 40-45% loss of circulating blood causes sharp disorders in hemodynamic, hemorheological, hemostatic and acid-base systems. The proposed method with use of resuspended in rheopolyglucin erythrocyte mass (in proportion 4:1) with preliminary injection of alphaadrenoblockator promotes quick correction of posthaemorrhagic disorders. Restoration of hemodynamics, hemorheology and acid-base balance was found to develop simultaneously with improvement of peripheral blood and bone marrow composition. Correction of rheological showing and acid-base state are of leading importance in the mechanism of the positive effect of erythrocyte mass transfusion in the proposed scheme. The latter on its part promotes improvement of microcirculation, redeponation of erythrocytes and their inclusion in the blood circulation.

0625

ADJURETIN IN PROPHYLAXIS OF POSTTRANSFUSION DIC SYNDROME

M.G.Mdivnishvili, G.G.Iosava, A.I.Abesadze
Institute of Haematology and Blood Transfusion, Tbilisi, Republic of Georgia

According to our clinical and experimental data decrease of hematocrit to 25-30% or hemoglobin index to 8-10 g/l after acute hemorrhage causes hypoxia and significant changes in hemostasis. In the present work we have studied the changes in vessel-platelet interaction, megakaryocyte-platelet system, plasma coagulation factors in the state of acute hypoxia and attempted to correct these changes by means of intensive hemotherapy. Before the transfusion we have found stimulation in megakaryocyte-platelet system, in particular activation of daily thrombocytopoiesis and platelet aggregation Platelet count was elevated but generaly their life span decreased. Activity of plasma coagulation factors continued to be high whereas the effect of prostacyclin appeared to last only 15-20 min. The most interesting fact seems to be that transfusion of erythrocyte mass (10-15 ml/kg) causes hypercoagulation and DIC, while application of Adjuretin (1 mg/kg intranasaly) before transfusion promotes elevation of prostacyclin level and prevention of DIC in number of cases. Thus, Adjuretin stimulates endothelial cells antiaggregative activity and effective in prophylaxis of DIC syndrome.

0626

ERYTHROCYTE MASS TRANSFUSION IN COMPLEX THERAPY OF ONCOPROCTOLOGIC PATIENTS

J.G.Abesadze, I.Sh.Nadiradze, G.G.Nemsadze
Oncological Scientific Centre, Tbilisi, Republic of Georgia

It hasn't been yet established the importance of erythrocyte mass transfusion in complex therapy of oncoproctological patients, their doses and frequency are not known clearly. The aim of the present work was to investigate these issues. Patients witn cancer in various parts of large intestine including those with toxicoanemic forms were under our control. The complex therapy scheme included either a single erythrocyte mass transfusion in big doses(3oo-4oo ml) or 2-3 fold ones in small doses (13o-15o ml). Showings of peripheral blood and hemostatic system of the patient were studied in dynamics. It was shown that 2-3-fold transfusions of small doses of erythrocyte mass before a surgical operation do not cause any significant positive effect whereas a single transfusion of erythrocyte mass big doses was accompanied by increase of blood showing and correction of hemostatic system. More expressed positive effect was observed when a single transfusion of big doses of erythrocyte mass was made on the 3-4 day after a surgical operation. Thus the complex therapy of oncoproctological patients demonstrated the most favourable effect in cases with transfusion of erythrocyte mass big doses.

0627

BLOOD TRANSFUSION TREATMENT OF ANAEMIA IN CASE OF CHRONICAL RENAL DISEASES

BULGARIAN, HIGHER MEDICAL INSTITUTE-STARA ZAGORA
MANTOV, TODOROVA, PRODANOVA, PENCOVA

THE EFFICIENCY OF BLOOD TRANSFUSIANS TREATMENT OF MANIFESTED ANAEMIC SYNDROME HAS BEEN STUDIED IN 49PATIENTS WITH BILATERAL DIFFUSE RENAL DISEASES FOR A PERIOD OF FIVE YEARS. IN 43/87,7%/ OF THE CASES THE DISORDERS ARE COMPLICATED WITH CHRONICAL RENAL DEFFICIENS SYNDROME. ERYTHROCITE MASS OF 300 ML HAS BEEN TRANSFUSED TO PATIENS MAINLY BELONGING TO GROUP A /15-31%/ AND 0/18-37%/. THE EFFECT OF BLOOD TRANSFUSIONS AND THE FOLLOWING COMPLICATIONS IS BEING DESCUSSED.

0628

THE NECESSITY OF BLOOD TRANSFUSIONS IN CASES OF CHRONICAL HEPATIC DISEASES

BULGARIAN, HIGHER MEDICAL INSTITUTE-STARA ZAGORA
TODOROVA, MANTOV, PENCOVA, PRODANOVA

THE REASON FOR HOSPITALIZATION OF 33PATIENTS IS ANAEMIA, DUE TO CHRONICAL HAEMORRHAGES FROM VARICOSE VAINS OF OESOPHAGUS, HAEMORRHOIDES, EROSIVE GASTRITIS, HEPATIC DECOMPENSATIVE CIRRHOSIS/19-57,6%/, METASTASES IN THE LIVER/12-36,4%/ AND CHRONICAL ACTIVE HEPATITIS/2-6%/. THE PROLONGATION WITH THE TREATMENT BLOOD TRANSFUSION DEPENDS ON THE PRESENTATIONS AND REACTIONS OF THE OBSERVED ORGANISMUS. THE NECESSITY OF USING BLOOD TRANSFUSIONS, THEIR ZUSPICIONS EFFECTS ON THE COMMON STATUS AND THE LABORATORY RESULTS OF THE PATIENTS WITH HEPATIC DISEASES ARE DISCUSSED.

0629

IMMUNOMODULATIVE EFFECTS OF ULTRAVIOLET IRRADIATION (UV) IN PATIENTS WITH APLASTIC ANEMIA.

A. A. Ganapiev, S. I. Moiseev, O. E. Rosanova, T. V. Glasanova, K. M. Abdulkadirov.

Aplastic anemia (AA) is a serious disease characterizide by pancytopenia associated with a hypoplastic marrow. Response to immunosuppressive therapy would suggest a causative or perpetuating role for autoimmunity in development of this disease. We studied the influence of UV on lymphocyte subsets in peripheral blood in five patients with AA. In 4 patients initial data of lymphocyte subsets were: CD3+ 58,7; CD4+ 27,8; CD8+ 27,0; CD22+ 28,8; DR+ 28,8. UV was performed with germicidal lamp DRB8 (200-280 nm). The total dose of 1 UV treatment was 850 J/m². After the course of UV (4 procedures) observed decrease of CD3+ to 33,2% but the reduce of CD8+ were more decrease then CD4+: 10,0% and 21,8% respectivly. CD22+ lymphocyte subsets return to initial level but DR+ reduced not so significanly(29,9% and 18,2% respectivly). But in 1 patient was observed initial reduce of CD4+ 1,7% and CD8+ 3,7%, and the other data were CD3+ 45,5%, CD22+ 18,9%. After 4 UV were observed following results: CD3+ 46,2% CD4+ 32,4%; CD8+ 15,3% and CD22+ 4,4%. Thus, the use of UV in patients with AA have the immunomodulative properties.

0630

T CELL POPULATIONS IN MULTITRANSFUSED PATIENTS

M Amil, M Lima, C Gonçalves, E Coimbra[1], B Justiça
S Hematologia; [1]S Pediatria. Hosp S António -Porto, Portugal

It has been noted that transfused patients become more tolerant to transplant allograft and several studies have investigated the immunosuppressive effects of blood transfusion. This raised the issue of whether or how transfusion leads to non specific inhibition of immune function, increasing the risk of infection and cancer recurrence. In order to understand the immunological effects of blood transfusion we studied 24 patients (15 adults and 9 children) regarding to the number of previous transfusions, blood counts, and assessment of lymphocyte populations. Seven of the multitransfused children were followed-up for 6-10 months, and the study was repeated 1 year later. Lymphocyte phenotyping was performed by double staining with the following markers: CD19/CD3, CD8/CD4, CD45RA/CD4 and CD29/CD4. Results showed great intersubject variation but there was no correlation between the relative and absolute number of B and T cells and the number of transfusions. In the follow-up study, lymphocytes remained stable despite the increasing number of transfusions. These results suggest that 1) if non-specific immunosuppression occurs after blood transfusion it cannot be explained by an imbalance of T cell populations; 2) the relative proportion of lymphocytes is strictly regulated in each individual. Functional studies and further characterization of T cells concerning the expression of activation molecules are required.

0631

***IN-VITRO* INDUCTION OF PRIMARY CTL RESPONSE AGAINST PEPTIDES OF WILD TYPE OR MUTANT p53.**

Jos G.A. Houbiers[1,2], H.W. Nijman[1,3], S.H. van der Burg[2,1], A. Brand[1], W.M. Kast[1], C.J.M. Melief[1].
Depts of [1]Immunohaematology & Blood Bank and [2]Surgery, University Hospital, Leiden, The Netherlands

The p53 tumor-suppressor gene is mutated and/or overexpressed in many human malignancies and is therefore an attractive target for T lymphocyte immunotherapy of cancer. The HLA-A2.1 molecules gained above the background expression on T2 cells after incubation with a binding peptide probably all present that peptide, which makes T2 cells suitable antigen presenting cells Lymphocytes of an HLA-A2.1 donor were added to p53-peptide loaded T2 cells. On day 7 and 14 viable responding cells were restimulated. On day 21 the bulk responders were cloned by limiting dilution and expanded. The most efficient protocol resulted in highly specific CTL clones which lyse HLA-A2.1 target cells sensitized with the p53-peptide. The CTL lyse in loading peptide concentration and in an effector-to-target ratio dependent way down to 10-ng/ml and 0.3:1 respectively. The clones were HLA-A2.1 restricted, CD2, CD3, CD8, CD25, HLA-A2, HLA-DR and TCR-Óß positive and CD16 negative. Amino acid replacements showed the fine specificity and proved the importance of peptide position 5, (6, 7) and 8 for HLA-A2.1 restricted CTL recognition. Clones against mutant p53 peptides were also generated.

0632

IDENTIFICATION OF POTENTIAL CTL EPITOPES USING THE PROCESSING DEFECTIVE HUMAN CELL LINE T2

J.G.A. Houbiers[12], H.W. Nijman[13], S.H. vd Burg[12], J.W. Drijfhout[1], C.J.H. vd Velde[2], A. Brand[2], W.M. Kast[1], C.J.M. Melief[1].
Dept. of [1]Immunohaematology & Blood Bank and Dept. of [2]Surgery, University Hospital Leiden, the Netherlands

For identification of potential epitopes for cytotoxic T lymphocytes (CTL) we used an antigen processing defective human cell line 174CEM.T2 (T2). T2 expresses empty and unstable HLA-A2.1 molecules which are stabilized by peptide binding. This can be detected as an increase in HLA-A2.1 expression, measured by immunofluorescence using the mouse monoclonal antibody BB7.2. The synthetic peptides - e.g. of p53-protein - used for HLA-binding studies were selected using a dedicated computer algorithm which matches for the HLA-A2.1 specific motif. We succeeded in significantly upregulating the HLA-A2.1 cell surface expression after incubating the T2 line with synthetic p53-peptides. These identified HLA-A2.1 binding peptides are potential CTL epitopes of p53.

0633

EFFECTS OF SV-IV PROTEIN ON LEUCOCYTE SURFACE MARKERS

E.Cosentini *, V.Metafora°, S.Formisano * and S.Metafora°.
*Immunohematology - Medical School University "Federico II" Naples
°I.I.G.B. .C.N.R. Naples

SV-IV (seminal vesicle protein N°4, according to its mobility in SDS-PAGE) is a small protein produced in large amount by the epithelium of rat seminal vesicles, with interesting biological properties (immunosoppressive,antinflammatory,antiphagocytic,antithrombotic). Aim of this study was to investigate whether the expression of adhesion glycoproteins on leucocyte surface could be involved in the molecular mechanism underlying the immunosoppressive properties of SV-IV.

Materials and methods. a) SV-IV purification. The protein was purified to homogeneity from adult rat seminal vesicle secretion according to Ostrowski procedure. The purity of the protein was assessed by 15% PAGE in denaturing and non-denaturing conditions, by fingerprinting, aminoacid composition analysis, fast protein liquid cromatography (FPLC) and fast atom bombardment mass spectrometry. b) Flow cytometry analysis. Leucocyte markers determination was performed by direct immunofluorescence techniques on cells pre-treated or not with micromolar amounts of SV-IV, using the following FITC or PE monoclonal antibodies: anti-DR, -CD11a, -CD18, -CD54 purchased from B.D.. Fluorescence cells were analysed by flow citometer (FACScan Becton - Dickinson, California, USA.)

Results. The treatment of cells with SV-IV induced:
-a significant increase of CD54 and CD18 on lymphocytes and monocytes
-the absence of CD11a expression on lymphocytes
-a drastic reduction of DR and CD11a on monocytes

Conclusion. Micromolar amounts of SV-IV apparently change the expression of important molecules on the surface of immunocompetent cells. These data strongly support the hypothesis that SV-IV could inhibit the cell-mediated immune response by interfering with the cellular cooperation and/or antigen presentation.

0634

EXPERIENCE OF TRANSFUSIONS IN THE TREATMENT OF PATIENTS WITH TUBERCULOSIS AND HEREDITARY IMMUNODEFICIENT STATE

F.M.Abdullayev[I], A.A.Umnyashkin[2]
Institute of Pulmonary Diseases & TB, Baku, Azerbaijan.

We observed 49 patients with lung tuberculosis and concominant glucose-6-phosphate dehydrogenase deficiency in white cells. Because of low effect of antibacterial therapy component haemotransfusions (packed white cells and erythrocyte mass) were used in examined patients. The dose and frequency of haemotransfusions depended upon the patient's state. The donors were chosen according to antigene compability. The pronounced therapeutic effect was already detected during the first week after the beginning of transfusive therapy. Along with this the positive dynamics of immune indices sharply decreased before the treatment was noted. Thus, the increase of a number of CD5 lymphocytes was notified, CD4/CD8 index PHA and PPD-induced proliferation of lymphocytes levels, a number of CDI9, CD45R, CD23 lymphocytes normalized.

0635

INFLUENCE OF IMMUNOMODULATORS TO MONOCYTE FUNCTIONAL ACTIVITY IN PATIENTS WITH ACUTE MYELOID LEUKEMIA

I.A.Bagirov
Institute of Haematology & Blood Transfusion, Baku, Azerbaijan

Diusifon and levomisole were administered as immunomodulators to 26 patients with acute myeloid leukemia during induction in the period between cytostatic courses. We observed infectious complications in the 8 of ten patients (80%) used as controls, and only 12 of 26 patients (46%) that received immunomodulator demonstrated infectious complications. We achieved full clinical hematological remission in 5 controls (50%), and in 20 patients (76%) received immunomodulator. In patients who received immunomodulator, we noted the increase of monocyte count index and its functional activity (phagocytic activity and adhesive ability). We also observed lysozyme count increase in blood serum of these patients. In patients who received immunomodulator, we detected the correlation between phagocytizing monocyte absolute count recovery and acute myeloid leukemia course, e.g. remission - p^s=0.44 (p 0.05).

0636

USE OF IMMUNOMODULATORS IN ACUTE LYMPHOID LEUKEMIA PATIENTS

I.A.Bagirov
Institute of Haematology and Blood Transfusion, Baku, Azerbaijan

We administered thymus gland preparation (thymalin, T-activin) to 67 acute lymphoid leukemia (ALL) patients during induction in the period between the courses. The degree of immunomodulator efficiency was carried out by the study of clinical parameters and lymphocytic system cell functional activity. We observed infectious complications in 8 of 10 control patients (80%) while 12 of 25 patients (48%) who received thymalin (I) demonstrated different infectious complications. Only 17 of 42 patients (41%) who received T-activin showed infectious complications. We achieved remission only in 50% of patients used as controls, while in patients received immunomodulators, this index was equal to 89%. Immunomodulator use led to the lymphocytic system cell functional activity recovery in ALL patients. Administration of immunomodulators to ALL patients leads to the immune system normalization and helps to prepare optimal therapeutic regime in the hemoblastosis treatment.

0637

MONITORING OF IMMUNOLOGICAL PARAMETERS FOr THE BLOOD COMPONENT THERAPY.

V.N.Shabalin, N.B.Serebrjanaja, S.D.Volkova, L.D.Serova
1Research Institute of Clinical and Experimental Immunology, Moscow, 2Research Institute of Haematology and Blood Transfusion, St-Petersburg, Russia

34 patients with severe and mild hemophilia A were studied during massive blood component therapy consisted of antihemophilic plasma and criopreci-pitate.

Moreover 78 patients with septic diseases were also observed and treated with antibacterial therapy and leukocyte transfusion.

There were demonstrated the real decreasing of T-lymphocytes and NK-cells activity, increasing of immunoglobulin concentration and blast transfor-ming activity in the PHA presence in hemophilia patients with normal initial indexes of their immunity. Immune donor leukocyte transfusions activate the initial depressive immunity in sepsis patients.

The data showed that blood component therapy exerted modulate influence on different elements of immune system indicating the choice of the blood component administration associated with the type of basic disease and disorder degree of the immune system.

0638

BLOOD GROUP TYPE CARBOHYDRATE ANTIGENS AND HYPERACUTE REJECTION IN MOUSE TO RAT XENOTRANSPLANTATION

M. L. Gustavsson[1], G. Gannedahl[3], A. E. Bäcker[1], A. Olling[1], G. Tufvesson[2], B. E. Samuelsson[1]

[1]*Departments of Clinical Chemistry and Transfusion Medicine,*
[2]*Transplantation Surgery, Sahlgren's Hospital, Göteborg, Sweden,*
[3]*Department of Surgery, Uppsala University Hospital, Uppsala, Sweden*

There is a great clinical interest in the possibility of using animals as organ donors to humans. The greatest problem is that all donors, except anthropoid apes, give rise to a hyperacute rejection very similar to that after an AB0-incompatible organ transplantation when anti-A or anti-B antibodies are present in high titre.

To test possible approaches to avoid hyperacute rejection in the human situation we have a model where mouse heart is hetero-topically grafted to the neck vessels of the rat. The graft works for several days without rejection. Transplantation of a second mouse heart to the contralateral neck vessels gives rise to a hyperacute rejection of the graft within a minute.

Glycolipids from nine different organs have been prepared from the mouse donor and rat recipient strains. Sera from ungrafted rats show only weak and non-specific IgM and IgA antibody-binding to mouse glycolipids on a thin layer plate. Sera from grafted rats show clear IgG and IgM antibody binding to a neutral glycolipid migrating in the five-sugar region. The antibody pattern is similar to that after pig to human xenotransplantation.

The antigen has been identified by monoclonal antibodies, mass spectrometry and NMR to be the Forssman glycolipid and some of the induced antibodies can be adsorbed by the terminal Forssman disaccharide.

0639

MULTIPLE PLATELET TRANSFUSIONS INDUCE ANTI-MHC ANTIBODIES WHICH ARE DOWNREGULATED OVER TIME IN A MURINE TRANSFUSION MODEL.

John W. Semple[1], Edwin R. Speck[1], Victor Blanchette[2] and John Freedman[1].
1 Division of Hematology, St. Michael's Hospital, 2 Division of Hematology, Hospital for Sick Children, Toronto, Ontario, and the University of Toronto, Toronto, Ontario.

In humans, multiple platelet transfusions often lead to the development of anti-HLA (class I) antibodies (Abs) and a state of clinical refractoriness to subsequent transfusions. In order to study the immunology of platelet transfusions, a murine transfusion model was developed. BALB/c ($H\text{-}2^d$) recipient mice were transfused weekly (for 30 weeks) with 10^8 pooled platelets from CBA ($H\text{-}2^k$) and C57BL/6 ($H\text{-}2^b$) donor mice. Leukocyte contamination in the transfused platelets ranged from 1-4 $x10^3$/transfusion. Recipient mice were bled weekly via the tail vein (300 μl) and the sera were tested for the presence of anti-H-2 Abs by flow cytometry. Results show that in all mice, both anti-$H\text{-}2^k$ and -$H\text{-}2^b$ serum IgG Abs could be detected after five weeks of transfusions. Titres of anti-$H\text{-}2^b$ were found to be at least 3 fold higher than those of anti-$H\text{-}2^k$ at all times tested. The Ab titres steadily increased to maximum levels by 10 weeks and then, in 6/10 mice, declined to pre-transfusion levels by 15 weeks despite continued transfusions. In some mice, anti-MHC titres then reappeared to maximal levels. This apparent cycling of the anti-MHC Ab response generated by multiple platelet transfusions suggests that regulatory mechanisms are induced to downregulate the anti-MHC response. (Supported by the Canadian Red Cross Blood Transfusion Service).

0640

CYTOMEGALOVIRUS (CMV) INFECTION OF VERY LOW WEIGHT BIRTH (VLWB) NEONATAL PATIENTS.

C.R.Pallás, E.Gómez,C.Alba, M.C.Medina, F.Gilsanz[1], J.Otero[2]
Neonatology(Dr Belaústegui), and Haemotherapy[1] and Micro-biology[2] Departments. H. 12 Octubre. Madrid, SPAIN.

Objective:To analize leukocyte removed cellular blood products transfusion and breast milk feeding as vectors to CMV transmision in VLWB neonates. **Methods**:78 babies <1500g at birth were included and grouped as follows: group **I**, **CMV-** mother feeding or not the baby; **II**, **CMV+** mother not giving breast milk; **III**, **CMV+** mother giving breast milk **CMV-** in culture; **IV**, **CMV+** mother giving breast milk **CMV+** in culture. CMV detected by shell vial technique. PRC transfused through a RC50E filter and platelet concentrates were filtered with PLF1 (Pall Biomedical Ltd).WBC reduction >log3 and log4, respect. Adquired infection was diagnosed in average at 43 days when culture was negative for the first 2 weeks of life and 1 or more positive afterwards. **Results**: Average weight 1.180g. 83% of mothers were CMV+. Average number of transfusions in transfused patients was 2 and >80% of blood donors were CMV+. CMV infection rate in each group during treatment was:

	Group I	Group II	Group III	Group IV
%Transfu.	**62** (8/13)	**68** (15/22)	**39** (11/28)	**73** (11/15)
%Infected	**0** (0/13)	**0** (0/22)	**14** (4/28)	**53** (8/15)

Only babies feeded with breast milk from CMV+ mother were infected by CMV during treatment and infection frequency was significantly higher in group **IV**. 0% infected in groups **I** and **II**.**Conclusions**: High WBC reduction of PRC and platelets allowed to prevent CMV infection in newborns through their transfusion. Breast milk feeding from CMV+ mothers could however be considered as an important way of virus transmision, especially when CMV could be detected by culture.

0641

AUTOIMMUNE HEMOLYTIC ANEMIA AND WISKOTT-ALDRICH SYNDROME

Pinilla J, López R, Castañeda A, Cano I, Martín A, Rubio M, Santacreu M, Jiménez V, Martín MP, de la Cámara C. y Hdez Navarro F
Servicio de Hematología y Hemoterapia. Hospital "La Paz". Madrid (Spain).

The X-linked, recessive immunodeficiency, Wiskott-Aldrich syndrome, is characterised by thrombocytopenia with reduced platelet volume and impaired aggregation, immunological defects affecting both humoral and cellular responses, draining ears, eczematous dermatitis and bloody diarrhea. It has been described an increase in the IgM levels in this syndrome. Because that, there is an inability in the antipolysacharides antibody's production.

We describe an 8-month baby diagnosed of a Wiskott-Aldrich Syndrome who developed an autoimmune hemolytic anemia. This association has not been described before in bibliography. The patient was treated with prophylactic intravenous immunoglobulin (IVIg) (0,4 mg/Kg, three days a week) previously to the hemolytic anemia presentation. At this moment, the immunohematologic study was: DAT (polyspecific and anti-IgG) positive, score 10; antibody titre 128, score 63; haptoglobin (HPT) was normal. These findings were ascribed to the IVIg treatment, as it has been by several authors. A month later, an acute decrease in the hemoglobin (Hb) levels occurred with an increase in the lactic dehydrogenase (LDH) and bilirubin (BB) levels. The immunohematologic study was the same as it was above before except that the haptoglobin was extremely decreased. It not was started steroid therapy because of underlying disease. Then, a high dose IVIg treatment was begun (1 gr/kg). Hemolytic anemia improved with a progressive bioquimic parameters' normalisation (LDH, BB, HPT, Hb). There were no changes in the immunohematologic study because of the IVIg use. After that, the patient had an ear infection with a new hemolytic episode followed by sepsis and death.

0642

SIMULTANEOUS USE OF ANTITHROMBIN III AND PROTEINE C CONCENTRATES IN A CHILD WITH DISSEMINATED INTRAVASCULAR COAGULATION.

R. Favier[1], A. Deschamps[2], A. Tachet[1] and P. de Moerloose[3]. 1Hematological Laboratory, Hospital Trousseau, PARIS ; 2Hematological Laboratory, Hospital Rothschild, PARIS, France ; 3 University Hospital Geneva, Switzerland.

We report the difficulties of transfusion management in a child with DIC and venous thrombo-embolic disease. This 11 year old boy was admitted in our hospital for the diagnosis of deep venous thrombosis complicated by pulmonary embolism. These diagnosis were confirmed by venocavography and angiography. Laboratory investigations showed a platelet count at 100×10^9/l, APTT 39 sec (N<33 sec), fibrinogen 0.8g/dl, D-dimers>16mg/l, factorV 56%, ATIII 86%, ProtC 62%, ProtS 112%, plasminogen 88%. In spite of intravenous heparin, fresh frozen plasma, red blood cells DIC worsened biologically and clinically with bleeding. Therefore ATIII and ProtC concentrates were infused during 5 days. Bleeding stopped progressively and coagulation parameters returned to normal except platelets. However after stopping ATIII and ProtC concentrates DIC reappeared. ProtC concentrates alone were first reinfused and DIC was partially stabilized ; when ATIII was also added a complete normalization was obtained. Unluckily the patient developped ARDS and died, without autopsy performed. This atypical case points out the interest of the association of two coagulation inhibitor concentrates for the treatment of DIC, even if the basal levels of these inhibitors are in the lower part of the normal range.

0643

IMMUNOGLOBULIN'S CONSIDERATION IN THALASSEMIA-MAJOR PATIENTS

DOOSTDAR .S, ZANDIEH .T, NOOROZNIA .S, BEHNIA .S

Researching on 106 Thalassemia-major (2-18 years old) patients.
[The spleen of 54 of them had been taken.]
Comparing with 53 of checking group, from the statistics views, we came to this conclusion:

In 7-12 years old persons: The quantity of IgA didn'thave any considerable difference, but their IgM and IgG had.

Above 12 years old persons: The quantity of IgG didn't have any considerable difference, but their IgM and IgA had.

The conclusions show that IgG,IgM,IgA in this patients who are below 7 years old, it don't show any considerable difference, of course, we can see differance in above 7 years old patients.

In addition to the above conclusions, the test showed that the persons whose spleen were taken, had more natural Immunoglobulin's situation than the other patients.

0644

HOW SAFE IS BLOOD TRANSFUSION IN CHILDREN?

M Amil, T Fonseca[1], M Cunha, C Gonçalves, F Leite, L Vale[1], E Coimbra[1], B Justiça
S Hematologia, [1]S Pediatria, Hosp S António - Porto, Portugal

Transmission of infections to patients through blood products is a major risk in transfusion medicine. Children with leukaemia or congenital anemias are particularly at risk due to the large number of exposures. In order to evaluate the infectious risk at our Department concerning hepatitis B, C and HIV, we assessed 31 multitransfused children since 1981. All patients were immunized against hepatitis B. All blood donors are regular unpaid volunteers. It has been our standard practice to screen blood with ELISA for hepatitis B (since 1979), C (since 1990) and HIV (since 1984). Blood is also discarded whenever ALT is >80IU/l and anti-HBc positive. During the study period 876 blood exposures were carried out (mean 28, median 18).

Results showed that, before the first transfusion, one patient was anti-HBs, anti-HBc and anti-HBe positive and all others were negative. At the end of the study all patients are negative for hepatitis B antigens, hepatitis C and HIV antibodies. All children are anti-HBs positive following hepatitis B immunization.

Even with correct laboratory screening, the infectious risk still exists due the time gap between contact with the virus and positive serology. However the selection and characteristics of our donors as well as good laboratory practice gave a very low risk for patients after 876 transfusions.

0645

MONOCLONAL ANTI-D ANTIBODIES WITH BROAD SPECIFICITY FOR PARTIAL D

Anne Fletcher, Julie Watt
NSW Red Cross Blood Transfusion Service, Sydney, NSW Australia

Human monoclonal anti-D antibodies were produced from the B lymphocytes of immunised donors. Cell lines secreting anti-D were derived by Epstein Barr transformation and anti-D monoclonal antibody (Mab) secretion was stabilised by rosetting with D positive red blood cells. The cell lines were subsequently cloned. The antibodies were found to be specific for D positive red blood cells by conventional serological techniques and by flow cytometric analysis. The epitope specificity of Mab anti-D can be determined by reactivity with partial D red blood cells[1]. At least 8 D epitopes have been distinguished. By testing a variety of cells with partial D antigens (D^{III}, D^{IVa}, D^{Va}, D^{Vc}/D^{IVb}, D^{VI} and D^{VII}) we have determined the fine specificity of these anti-D Mabs. Several of the antibodies had the common specificity epD6/7; another two had epD4 specificity. Three antibodies had a broad specificity not previously defined. These antibodies reacted strongly with D^{III}, D^{IVa}, D^{Va}, D^{Vc}, D^{VI} and D^{VII} cells. They were also reactive with the recently described partial D phenotype, DFR, which is associated with FPTT[2]. Two Mabs reacted with all the partial D cells but were less stongly reactive with D^{VI} cells and thus resembled Workshop antibodies 103 (ESD-4) and 113 (BS221) which were previously described[3].

1. Tippett P (1990) J Immunogenet **17**: 247-257
2. Lomas C *et al* (1994) In preparation
3. Tippett P and Moore S (1990) J Immunogenet **17**: 309-319

0646

OBTENTION OF HUMAN ANTI-RHESUS FAB BY THE USE PHAGE DISPLAY LIBRARY

L. Edelman[1], P. Lafaille[1], E. Monchâtre[1], and J.C. Mazié[2]
[1]Institut Pasteur, Laboratoire d'ImmunoHématologie, Paris, [2]Institut Pasteur, Hybridolab, Paris, France.

Human monoclonal anti-Rhesus (D) clone D7C2 antibody of the IgM class was obtained by Epstein-barr virus immortalization of peripheral blood lymphocytes. Common positive erythrocytes and partial DIV Rhesus cells, were agglutinated whereas DVI cells were not recognized. 70% of Du were positive on opaline plates at room temperature. Immunoprecipitation of ^{125}I labeled R2/R2 red cells showed a protein of 30-32 kDa and was not obtained from in rr red blood cells.
mRNA was isolated from the clone D7C2 and used in order to obtain the Fab encoding cDNA. The cDNA was amplified by PCR and inserted inside the pComb 3 phagemide vector (kindly given to us by M. Lerner) as described by Barbas et al. (PNAS, 1991, 88,7978-7982). The Fab encoding gene was attached to the gene III of this f1 filamentous phage which allows the expression of the Fab at the surface of the filamentous phage. The phage Fab was isolated and used for in vitro studies. By cleavage of the gene III of the pComb 3 vector, a new plasmid was obtained which permits the expression inside the periplam of Escherichia coli the anti-Rhesus Fab without the phage. The biological activity of this Fab will be discussed.

0647

COMPARISON OF GEL ,COLUMN AGGLUTINATION TECHNOLOGY AND TUBE TEST IN ABO HAEMOLYTIC DISEASE OF NEWBORN

C.Mazzei,U.Gianatti,G.Imberciadori,
G.Barberis,F. Saccone,C.Durante
C.Trasfusionale,Osp.S.Corona,Pietra Ligure

The Gel-Test(DiaMed) and more recent Column Agglutination Technology (Ortho) can be easily used for detecting agglutinates.We tested cord cells of 640 infants and maternal sera by DAT and IAT,respectively, comparing reactivities observed in GT,CAT (according manufacturers) and conventional Tube Test, at 22 C.,at 37 C. and in IAT,using the same three cell pannel (Surgiscreen-Ortho). An ABO mother/infant incompatibility occurred in 90 cases (16%). 32 DAT+ (5%) were demonstrated by all methods and IgG anti-A were eluated from red cells;in 4 samples ,a DAT+ was detected by GT and CAT ;in other 3 cases a DAT weak positive was observed only by GT and we eluated (by ether and warm tre-atment of stroma) IgG anti-A,then reacting in IAT by all methods. Newborns showed a benign evolution of HDN with a little and transient increase in bilirubin level.The Gel-Test and CAT were more sensitive than conventional T.T. in diagnosis of ABO HDN particularly in those cases in which the amount of IgG anti-A on red cells is small (weak DAT+) and can be further reduced by washing, as required for performing DAT in Tube method.

0648

AutoAnalyzer Quantitation of Anti-c in Pregnancy

Fleetwood P J, Rowson DA, deSilva PM - North London Blood Transfusion Centre. Colindale Avenue, London NW9 5BG, UK.

Anti-c in maternal serum is commonly implicated as a cause of severe haemolytic disease of the newborn (hdn). AutoAnalyzer quantitation of anti-D using a bromelin - methyl cellulose technique and standard antibody preparations, is preferred in the UK for predicting the likelihood and severity of hdn. For anti-D, rising indirect antiglobulin test (IAT) titres correlate well with increasing quantitation. In a series of 72 antenatal patients with anti-c (309 samples), the antibody level was titred by IAT where appropriate and determined by AutoAnalyzer using the UK standard for anti-c. Some examples reactive only by manual polybrene or enzyme methods and not by IAT gave relatively high quantitation values (25 iu/ml), whereas others reacting strongly by IAT (titre 128) gave a low quantitation (0.9 iu/ml). Correlation between IAT titre and quantitation for this series was calculated to be 0.335. To date, no infants of patients in this study with anti-c levels <20 iu/ml, irrespective of the IAT titre, have required exchange or intrauterine transfusion, or suffered intrauterine death due to hdn.
Although correlating poorly with antibody titres, AutoAnalyzer quantitation was sensitive in detecting rising antibody levels. More cases will be studied to determine the clinical usefulness of this data.

0649

FUNCTIONAL DETECTION OF RBC- AND HLA-ANTI-BODIES IN HAEMOLYTIC DISEASE OF THE NEWBORN (HDN) BY A COMBINED PHOTOMETRIC BIOASSAY

U. Cassens[1], K. Gutensohn[1], H.P. Benn[1], H. Garritsen[2], W. Holzgreve[2], P. Kuehnl[1],
[1]Dept. of Transfusion Medicine, University Hosp. Hamburg, [2]Dept of Obstetrics and Gynecology, University Hosp. Muenster, FRG

The monocyte monolayer assay (MMA) is an useful functional test to detect the significance of RBC antibodies in HDN. Maternal HLA antibodies - which have possibly a protective effect in HDN - are detectable by an immune phagocytosis inhibition test (IPI).
We tested 18 maternal sera (multiparae with irregular RBC antibodies) in the MMA and IPI with panel monocytes. Furthermore, a combined photometric bioassay (MMA + IPI) was performed with paternal monocytes; they served as corresponding cells for potential maternal HLA antibodies.
MMA was positive in 10/18 sera and 5/10 MMA-positive sera were also positive in the IPI, indicating RBC- and HLA-antibodies. Three of these sera showed an markedly lower MMA-reactivity in the combined bioassay; the course of these pregnancies is uncomplicated so far. We conclude that this photometric bioassay might detect the discussed protective effect of HLA antibodies and could possibly improve the MMA to predict the severity of HDN.

0650

ANTIBODIES IN PREGNANCY

M.Djokic, N.Tijanic, D.Paunovic, R.Simonovic
Blood Transfusion Institute, Belgrade, Yugoslavia

We presented resultates of last five years (89-93) work in prenatal investigation. We investigated 34590 pregnant women with standard tests (ABO, Rh phenotype, screening antibodies, identification and titar). For the 14937 sera we performed microlymphocitotocsic test to HLA antibodies. We show resultates in the table:

antibodies (abs)	No of sampl. nvestigated	No positiv	%
all abs	34590	413	1,19
RhD abs	34590	290	0,84
other Rh	34590	64	0,18
other RBC systems	34590	59	0,17
HLA	14937	2376	15,9

Some higher % of senzitised RhD negative women (290 of 5534 or 5,24%) could means that Rh prevention wos insufficient.

0651

THE AMELIORATION OF HDN BY MATERNAL ALLOANTIBODIES WHICH INHIBIT THE CHEMILUMINESCENT (CL) RESPONSE OF HUMAN MONOCYTES TO ANTI-D SENSITIZED RED CELLS.

S.L. Shepard[1], A.G. Hadley[1], A.L. Noble[1], D. Filbey[2]
1IBGRL, Bristol, UK, 2Blodcentralen, Orebro, Sweden.

The severity of haemolytic disease of the newborn (HDN) may be predicted by measuring the CL response of human monocytes to red cells sensitized with maternal serum. Occasionally, women with biologically active anti-D (CL response above 20%) may deliver D-positive babies unaffected by HDN. In similar cases, Dooren *et al* [1], reported the presence of maternal antibodies, particularly anti-HLA DR52 and DR53, which inhibited the monocyte (FcγRI) -mediated lysis of anti-D sensitized red cells (iADCC); such antibodies may prevent the destruction of fetal red cells *in utero*. In the current study, sera were selected from women with anti-D who delivered babies with either severe HDN (group 1, n=12, anti-D level : 3-67i.u./ml, CL response : 29-196%), or who were unaffected (group 2, n=8, anti-D level : 4-945 i.u./ml, Cl response : 66-136%). Sera were tested for their ability to inhibit the CL response of monocytes pooled from 6 random donors, to red cells sensitized with monoclonal IgG3 anti-D. Sera from 4 of 12 (33%) group 1 cases, and from 6 of 8 (75%) group 2 cases, inhibited CL responses by over 30% (normal range = 0-20%, n=20). After platelet absorption of inhibitory sera, 1 of 3 sera (33%) from group 1, and 2 of 6 sera (33%) from group 2 remained inhibitory. These data suggest a role for HLA class I and class II FcγRI-blocking antibodies in the amelioration of HDN. Studies using paternal monocytes are necessary to elucidate the specificity of protective antibodies.

1. Dooren, M. C. *et al.* Lancet. 1992; 339:1067-1070

0652

KLEIHAUER TESTING AND ANTI-D IMMUNOGLOBULIN ADMINISTRATION

I.M. Bromilow J.K.M. Duguid
Mersey and North Wales Regional Transfusion Centre, Liverpool, U.K.

The Kleihauer test to detect foetal haemoglobin (HbF) is used to assess foeto maternal haemorrhage (FMH) in Rh(D) negative mothers. It is used antenatally following sensitising episodes (abortion, trauma, amniocentesis, etc) to assess if anti-D immunoglobulin (Ig) is needed. Postnatally in most European countries 1000-1500 i.u. of anti-D Ig is given and no Kleihauer test is performed. In the UK, 500 i.u. anti-D Ig is given, and a Kleihauer test is performed to assess the need for further anti-D Ig. There is currently no UK Quality Assurance Scheme for Kleihauer testing. A survey of Kleihauer testing in the Mersey region was undertaken using a simple questionnaire. All hospitals (n=24) replied. There was variation in technique used, method of assessing FMH and reporting. High and low power microscope fields were scanned in varying numbers from 3-50 fields. No hospital issued a report indicating the size of FMH nor with recommendation for anti-D Ig dosage. Kleihauer testing in this situation is intrinsically inaccurate measuring as it does HbF and not Rh(D) positive cells. If the dosage of anti-D Ig to be administered is to be assessed by measurement of FMH a more accurate and controlled technique (perhaps to specifically measure Rh(D) positive cells) should be used in order to decrease further the incidence of Rh(D) sensitisation occurring during pregnancy.

0653

RED CELL ALLOIMMUNIZED PREGNANCIES: PREDICTING THE NEED FOR INTRAUTERINE TRANSFUSION USING ULTRASONOGRAPHY AND DOPPLER

D.Oepkes, R.Meerman, F.Vandenbussche, R.Brand, H.H.Kanhai.
Dept. of Obstetrics, University Hospital Leiden, The Netherlands.

Objective To assess the value of ultrasonography and Doppler to predict the severity of fetal haemolytic anaemia.

Design Ultrasonographic measurements of the fetal liver, spleen, umbilical vein and placenta, and Doppler measurements of umbilical venous and fetal aorta flow velocities were performed before the first intrauterine blood transfusion. Multivariate regression models for the prediction of the fetal haemoglobin level were derived from the measurements.

Setting National referral centre for management of alloimmunized pregnancies

Subjects 40 fetuses in 39 red cell alloimmunized pregnancies

Results A logistic regression model incorporating the two Doppler parameters only, predicted the presence or absence of severe anaemia in nonhydropic fetuses with an accuracy of 90%. Positive predictive value was 89%, negative predictive value was 100%.

Conclusion In severe red cell alloimmunized pregnancies, Doppler blood flow velocity studies can be used to predict the severity of fetal anaemia. This may lead to a reduction of invasive diagnostic tests, to more accurate timing of intrauterine transfusions and thus to a higher survival rate.

0654

RED CELL ALLOIMMUNIZED PREGNANCIES: INTRAUTERINE INTRAVASCULAR TRANSFUSIONS IN THE NETHERLANDS

I.L.van Kamp, H.H.H.Kanhai, J. Bennebroek Gravenhorst.
Department of Obstetrics, University Hospital Leiden,
The Netherlands

Introduction Since the introduction of ultrasound-guided percutaneous fetal blood sampling in the early 1980's assesment of fetal anaemia and direct treatment by intravascular transfusions became feasible. We report the experience with this technique in our department, which is the national referral centre for management of severe alloimmunized pregnancies.

Subjects In a six-year period (1987-1992) 281 intrauterine transfusions were performed in 94 pregnancies (one twin pregnancy was included).

Results The mean gestational age at first transfusion was 26 weeks(18-34).The mean fetal haematocrit at first treatment was 17 L/L(5-35).Three intrauterine deaths occured obviously due to associated pathology, these pregnancies were excluded. Thirty-seven fetuses were hydropic and fourty-five had a gestational age of 26 weeks or less at first transfusion. Seventy-seven fetuses (84%) were liveborn after a mean of 3 (range 1-7) intrauterine transfusions.In the hydropic and low gestagional age groups the liveborn rate was 68% and 80% respectively.The mean gestational age of the liveborns at birth was 35 weeks.Four neonatal deaths occured resulting in an overall survival rate of 79%.

Conclusion Ultrasound-guided intravascular fetal transfusions are a wellcome addition to the management of red cell alloimmunized pregnancies.This method seems to be superior to the intraperitoneal approach especially in case of hydrops and when treatment is necessary in early pregnancy.

0655

INTRAUTERINE TRANSFUSION TO PREVENT FETAL DEMISE IN A CASE OF FETAL-MATERNAL HEMORRHAGE (FMH)

A.A. Konugres, D.M. Fountain, M-P. Thiet, G. Bowles-Johnson, O. Vincent
Brigham & Women's Hospital and Harvard Medical School, Boston, USA

The growing expertise of perinatologists has increased our capabilities of treating fetal patients with hydrops fetalis. The treatment by transfusion of hydrops fetalis due to FMH is reported.

A 28-year-old woman with unremarkable prenatal screen and normal fetal survey at 19 weeks gestation presented at 31.5 weeks with decreased fetal movement. Antibody screen, viral and bacterial cultures were negative. The Kleihauer Betke test was positive, 350 cc FMH was calculated (70 RBCs with fetal hemoglobin/1000 maternal RBCs). The patient underwent percutaneous blood sampling (PUBS). Fetal Hct was 5.6. The fetus was given a 40 cc intravascular blood transfusion (IVTR) resulting in improved fetal movement. Four days later, fetal movement was again decreased: ultrasound showed scalp edema, ascites; repeat PUBS Hct 9. The fetus was given a 70 cc IVTR. Daily biophysical profiles revealed resolving hydrops and improved fetal activity. Six days later, fetal activity was again sluggish. Patient opted for no further PUBS procedures and delivered at 32 weeks. The placenta was hydropic with no evidence of abruption. The infant's post-delivery Hct was 13.8, normal platelet count, and no evidence of coagulopathy. The newborn was transfused to a 48 Hct and on day 14 was discharged. The patient subsequently had a normal healthy infant after an uncomplicated pregnancy.

0656

INTRAUTERINE INTRAVASCULAR TRANSFUSIONS (IVT) IN RH HAEMOLYTIC DISEASE: INDIAN EXPERIENCE.

S.C. GUPTE, C.P. LULLA, S.S. KULKARNI, S. KORGAONKAR, R.H. MERCHANT, V.S. WALVEKAR
Institute of Immunohaematology, NWM Hospital, Parel, Bombay, INDIA

A total of 30 IVT, under USG guidence, were performed on 5 non-hydrophic and 4 hydropic fetuses between 25 to 34 weeks gestation. Fetal blood sampling was done if mother had fetal loss due to Rh-HDN, anti-D level was >20 IU/ml and/or amnitoic fluid showed Liley's zone II (end) or zone III. The IVT was performed when there was >2g/dl deficit in Hb level compared to normal value at that gestation and repeated upto 5 times at 1 to 3 weeks interval. The volume transfused was 20 to 130 ml based on fetal haematocrit (HCT), donor HCT, desired HCT and fetoplacental blood volume. The pre-transfusion HCT ranged between 9 and 28%. 5 nonhydropic cases received 2 to 5 IVT and all were liveborn. 3 infants did not require any treatment while the fourth received one exchange transfusion (ET). The fifth neonate who was born with rectal bleeding, was given platelet concentrate, fresh frozen plasma and simple blood transfusion. This child died on 3rd day due to bleeding from, multiple sites. Out of 4 hydropic fetuses 1 died within a week after 1st IVT and another after 4 IVT. Remaining 2 cases received 4 IVT each and delivered live child. One of them received ET while other did not need treatment. Thus our success rate was 80% in nonhydropic and 66% in hydropic series. There wase only one death (hydrops) related to procedure, hence the procedural mortality rate was 3.3 % (1/30).

0657

THE USE OF CRYOPRESERVED PACKED RED CELLS (PRCs) FOR FOETAL HAEMOLYTIC ANAEMIA.

S.Solinas[1], M.Masci[1], L.Piro[1], R.Paesano[2], V.Petrelli[2], G.C.Isacchi[1].
1 Dipartimento di Biopatologia Umana, Emato logia, Centro Trasfusionale. 2 II Clinica Ostetrica. Universita´ "La Sapienza", Roma, Italy.

OBJECTIVE:to report our experience with foe tal intravascular blood transfusion for the treatment of severe rhesus isoimmunisation using cryopreserved PRCs.METHODS:irradiated cryopreserved PRCs from Rh-negative (Rh-) and anti-Cytomegalovirus negative (CMV-) do nors were transfused into the foetal umbili cal vein. RESULTS:five intravenous transfus ions were performed in two pregnancies.Both foetuses showed hydrops.The pre-transfusion mean haemoglobin level was 6.15 g/dl, while the post-transfusion one was 11.9 gr/dl.Ces arian section was performed in both cases. Because of the haemolysis persistence, in one case two exchange transfusions were per formed still using the same kind of PRCs.At present time, the infants enjoy good health. CONCLUSIONS: foetal intravascular transfusi on is a highly effective treatment for foet al haemolytic anaemia.Since this particular kind of recipient needs the CMV- and Rh- blood,the cryopreserved PRCs supplies conti nually allow the Transfusional Service to dispose of such a rare type of blood.

0658

Induction of additional alloantibodies after intrauterine transfusions

H.E. Viëtor[1], H.H.H. Kanhai[2], A. Brand[1]
Dept [1]Immunohaematology and Blood Bank, and [2]Obstetrics, University of Leiden, The Netherlands.

Intrauterine transfusion (IUT) is the treatment of choice in severe haemolytic disease of the fetus. One possible complication of this procedure is the development of additional alloantibodies to red cell antigens. Between March 1987 and December 1992, 91 women with a blood group antagonism during pregnancy received a total of 280 ultrasound guided intrauterine transfusions. Additional red cell specific alloantibodies were detected in 24 women (26%). As the blood of unrelated donors had been used for the IUT, it was determined if these additional antibodies were directed against the donor or the fetal red blood cells. The immunizing source could be identified in 15 patients. In 11 cases, the additional alloantibodies were directed against fetal antigens and in 4 cases against donor antigens. The fetus and the donor shared the immunizing antigen in 4 cases and in 1 case the antibody occured naturally. There was only one case in which a primary sensitization against a donor antigen was proven. This study demonstrates that the use of maternal blood to prevent antibody formation after IUT is not indicated.

0659

IMUNIZATION AGAINST A LOW FRQUENCY ALLOANTIGEN, "IY" ON GP Ib/IX ASSOCIATED WITH FETAL/NEONATAL ALLOIMMUNE THROMBOCYTOPENIA

V. Kiefel[1], M. Vicariot[2], M. Böhringer[1], H. Kroll[1], A. Greinacher[1], C. Breitfeld[1], S. Santoso[1], C. Mueller-Eckhardt[1].

[1]Institute for Clinical Immunology and Transfusion Medicine, Justus-Liebig-University, Giessen, Germany,
[2]Centre Hospitalier et Universitaire de Brest, Unité d'Hémobiologie-Transfusion, France.

Recently, we observed a severe case of NAIT due to a platelet specific alloantibody against a low frequency antigen. After a normal first pregnancy, a 28 years old woman, Mrs I., gave birth to a thrombocytopenic child with large cerebral hemorrhage, who died on the 2nd day of life. Two years later, she became pregnant again and it was discovered by sonography that the male fetus had already a large hematoma. Maternal serum showed no reactivity in routine platelet antibody assays. Using the monoclonal antibody immobilization of platelet antigens (MAIPA) assay, an antibody against paternal platelet GP complex Ib/IX was identified. The corresponding antigen was detected in 1/233 German unrelated blood donors. Antibody binding assays with typsin-digested platelets (ELISA, immunoprecipitation with biotin labelled platelets) indicate tnat the antigen is not localized on the glycocalicin moiety of GP Ib_{α}, but may be situated on the remnant moiety of GP Ib_{α}, GP IX or $GPIb_{\beta}$.

0660

Maternal anti-HPA-1a levels and foetal platelet counts in FMAIT - a case report

B Dawkins. Red Cross Blood Bank, Brisbane, Australia.

The first child of a healthy female was diagnosed with ICH post-delivery. The infant's platelet count was $11x10^9/L$ at birth and subsequently rose to $462x10^9/L$ on day 5 after platelet transfusion. The mother was platelet type HPA-1b/1b while the father was heterozygous HPA-1a/1b. A second child was born without clinical abnormality and a platelet count of $218x10^9/L$. Maternal anti-HPA-1a levels were 1.284 on day 1 and 1.1184 on day 5 (MAIPA OD(T-B)). A third pregnancy commenced with maternal anti-HPA-1a levels of 0.801 at 7/40, 0.628 at 14/40, 0.389 at 20/40 - these lower levels persisted throughout the weekly sampling until delivery. Prednisone was given to the mother from 19/40 and IVGG (1g/kg/wk) from 24/40, until the day before delivery. At 22/40 PUBS revealed a foetal platelet count of $46x10^9/L$ (no platelet transfusion given) and the foetus to be HPA-1a/1b. The corresponding maternal anti-HPA-1a level was 0.443. At 29/40 PUBS was repeated and platelets were transfused after sampling. This time the foetal platelet count was $150x10^9/L$ and the maternal anti-HPA-1a 0.343. At the final PUBS (35/40) the foetal platelet count was $160x10^9/L$ and maternal anti-HPA-1a level 0.353. (Another foetal platelet transfusion was given.) This third infant was delivered by caesarean at 37/40 with a platelet count of $300x10^9/L$, no physical abnormalities evident (AGPAR score 9 and 10) and has continued to thrive.

In this case of FMAIT the MAIPA demonstrated falling levels of maternal anti-HPA-1a (at 14/40) before it was considered prudent to perform PUBS.

0661

A CASE OF NEONATAL ALLOIMMUNE THROMBOCYTOPENIA DUE TO ANTI-HLA-B44

K.S.Han[1], Y.J. Cha[2], S.I.Kim[3]
1Department of Clinical Pathology, Seoul National University College of Medicine, 2Department of Clinical Pathology, Joong-Ang University, 3Central Kil Hospital, Korea

We encountered a case of neonatal alloimmune thrombocytopenia(NAIT) due to anti-HLA-B44 and this is the first report of NAIT with the specificity of the causative antibody identified in Korea. Generalized petechia and purpura were the only abnormal findings at the time of birth. Platelet count was 31,000/uL. The mother's platelet count was 365,000/uL and she had no history of abnormal bleeding. Platelet antibody tests employing mixed passive hemagglutination and immunofluorescence revealed that the mother's serum was reactive against the platelets from the father, but was not reactive with her own platelets. The positive reaction was lost after chloroquine treatment of platelets. Antigen capture ELISA(ACE) and modified antigen capture ELISA employing monoclonal antibodies against platelet glycoproteins Ia, IIa, IIb, and IIIa were negative. Mother's serum was tested for lymphocytotoxicity against 49 donor lymphocytes and the specificity was found to be anti-HLA-B44.

0662

FREQUENCY AND CHARACTERISTICS OF POSTTRANSFUSION HEPATITIS (PTH) IN GREECE, WITH EMPHASIS IN HEPATITIS C.

K. Makris(1), A.Maniatis(2), V.Kouvelis(1), I.Drakopoulos(1), P.Petakou(1)
1 Blood Bank of KAT hospital, Athens, 2. University of Patra, Patra, Greece.

The purpose of this study was to determine: a) prospectively the frequency of PTH in Greece, b) the role of HCV in PTH and finally c) the efficacy of the screening of the blood donors.

During the period October 1989 - December 1991, a total of 143 surgical orthopaedic patients were examined and followed up with blood samples obtained, for a period of six months at 15 day intervals. PTH was diagnosed when ALT levels exceeded 2.5N. Anti-HCV screening was performed retrospectively in both the blood donors and the patients with a second generation ELISA and confirmation of seropositive samples with RIBA (2nd generation).

Patients were transfused with a total of 790 units of blood and blood products. For our retrospective screening 733 samples from these units were available. 16 samples (2,18%) were found with raised ALT levels (>1.5N) and 6 (0.81%) Anti-HCV positive. 18 (12.59%) of the transfused patients developed PTH. One (0.70%) developed hepatitis B and 17 (11.88%) non-A, non-B. In 8 (5.59%) patients seroconversion was observed in Anti-HCV screening and PTH was attributed to HCV infection while in 9 (6,29%) only an increase of ALT levels was observed. The patient that developed hepatitis B was transfused with four units one of which was positive for, Anti-HBc and Anti-HBe. From the 17 patients who developed NANBH, 5 (3.50%) were transfused with at least one unit with raised ALT levels and 7 (4.05%) with Anti-HCV positive blood.

We conclude that a) the frequency of PTH in our study was 12.59%, b) a proportion of PTH (40%) can be attributed to HCV, c) screening of all donations for Anti-HCV with a second generation ELISA test does not exclude infection of the recipient from HCV and d) we believe that we should screen all blood donations for raised ALT levels.

0663

HCV INFECTION IN FINNISH HAEMOPHILIACS

F.Ebeling, V.Rasi
FRC Blood Transfusion Service, Helsinki, Finland.

A national second-generation hepatitis C antibody (anti-HCV) assay survey was performed in 1993. Of the 282 patients, 204 (72%) were tested for anti-HCV (UBI HCV EIA, immunoblot as confirmation), anti-HBc and abnormal ALT (M >50 U/L, F >35 U/L).

Bleeding disorder	Anti-HCV+ n (%)	Anti-HBc+ n (%)	ALT abnorm. n (%)
Haemophilia A			
severe	74 (80)	41 (45)	33 (36)
moderate	9 (75)	6 (50)	4 (36)
mild	7 (21)	2 (6)	7 (22)
Haemophilia B			
severe	5 (100)	3 (60)	3 (60)
mild	17 (50)	13 (38)	10 (30)
FXIII deficiency	3 (30)	1 (10)	2 (20)
Von Willebrand's disease, severe	7 (41)	4 (24)	3 (18)
All	122/204 (60)	70/203 (34)	62/199 (31)

Anti-HCV was significantly associated with elevated ALT (p<0.0001). All patients were anti-HIV negative. Only two Finnish haemophiliacs have been found to be HIV-infected, owing to national self-sufficiency. This did not, however, prevent widespread infection with HCV. No anti-HCV seroconversions have been found in users of heat-treated (60°/72h) cryoprecipitate (8 pat.) after introduction of donor screening in 1990.

0664

PREVALENCE OF HCV-RNA POSITIVE PATIENTS IN A DIALYSIS UNIT IN GERMANY

M. da Silva Cardoso[1], K. Koerner[1], S. Epple[1], R. Krämer[2], D. Bundschu[2], B. Kubanek[1]
[1]German Red Cross Blood Bank and Dept. Transfusion Medicine, University of Ulm, and [2]Dialysis Unit of the Board of Dialysis and Transplantation Ulm e.V.

In order to establish the prevalence of HCV infections patients in the Dialysis Unit of the Board of Dialysis and Transplantations Ulm, we investigated a group of 195 patients by HCV RT/PCR. For the PCR we used at least two sets of nested primers for the most conserved region of the HCV genome. Serum samples were also tested for the presence of HCV antibodies with the ELISA second generation test from Ortho. The recombinant immunoblot assay RIBA-2 (Ortho) was applied to all ELISA reactive samples. One hundred sixty-five patients were found to be anti-HCV negative and 30 anti-HCV positive. Twenty-one out of 30 reactive samples could be confirmed positive by the RIBA-2. The other nine samples resulted either indeterminate (one) or negative (eight) by RIBA-2.

The HCV-RNA prevalence in our unit is though 15%, being not different from the anti-HCV prevalence, although not all the samples are simultaneously HCV-RNA^{+}/anti-HCV^{+}.

The data presented here suggest that in the hemodialysis population the antibody status of a patient has a very high prognostic value for viremia: we obtained over 95% correlation between PCR and RIBA in the antibody positive group.

0665

FREQUENCY AND CHARACTERISTICS OF ANTI-HCV POSITIVE BLOOD DONORS A RECOMMENDABLE ATTITUDE FOR BLOOD BANKS

SPANISH STUDY GRUOP OF DONORS WITH RISK OF TRANSMISSION OF HEPATITIS C
J. Montero, J.M. Echevarria, J.M. Hernández, E. Franco, D. Prados, J.M. García Bengoechea, C. Vigil, P. León, J.M. Barrera.
SPAIN.

Since the introduction of 2nd. or 3rd. generation enzyme immunoassays in blood donor screening, the frequency of HCV positive donors has dropped drastically, in direct relation to the greater or lesser prevalence of "habitual" donors at Blood Banks. The risk or PTH has subsequently dropped to values less than 1%.

In a prospective study carried out in 43 Blood Banks, representative of all the regions of Spain, a follow-up of the frequency of Anti-HCV reactive donations from 1990 to 1993 has been carried out.

Among the reactive donors found in the systematic sreening, 2900, as well as 700 who had been non-reactive but with high ALT, had been subjected to complementary confirmative tests. A broad and continually up-dated battery of assays, especially of the study of samples classified as "indeterminate", even with samples obtained in the follow-up of the donors 3 and 6 months after ther first study has been used for this purpose.

The comparison of the sociological, epidemiological, clinical and analytical data of the donors confirmed as Positive and Indeterminate, with regard to the Negative donors, with or without a rise in transaminases, as well as wilth a group of 900 non-selected donors as the Control Group, has made it possible to obtain a "profile" of the donors of each one of these groups, as well as to establish some criteria of attitude recommended to Blood Banks to follow the Anti-HCV reactive donors in the screening tests.

0666

PREVALENCE OF ANTIBODIES TO HEPATITIS C AND HCV-RNA IN BLOOD DONORS FROM SOUTHERN GERMANY

K. Koerner, M. da Silva Cardoso, S. Epple, B. Kubanek
German Red Cross Blood Bank Ulm and Dept. Transfusion Medicine, University of Ulm, FRG.

Since June 1990 the Red Cross Blood Service Baden-Wuerttemberg began to screen all blood donors with the Ortho anti-HCV ELISA. By performing the nested PCR with primers for the most conserved region of the viral genome, we could estimate that more than 80% (n = 301) of the second generation anti-HCV ELISA reactive donations with normal ALT are false positives. On the other hand in over 80% of the HCV-RNA positive donations, the presence of anti-HCV could also be confirmed by the second generation recombinant immunoblot assay (RIBA-2). Based on these data we began in 1993 to test all ELISA reactive donations with the RIBA-2. The blood donors with positive RIBA-2 results were informed by the blood bank and excluded from further donations. The total rate of anti-HCV RIBA-2 positive blood donors in the 2. and 3. quarter of 1993 was 55 per 100,000 blood donors; first time donors 133, repeat donors 47 per 100,000. Female blood donors had twice the rate of RIBA-2 positivity as male blood donors, 85 and 36 per 100,000, respectively. However, a high number of indeterminate anti-HCV RIBA-2 results (n = 122/293 anti-HCV ELISA positives, 42%) were attained. They will be analyzed by the RIBA 3. generation.

0667

MICROGEOGRAPHIC VARIATION OF HEPATITIS C VIRUS PREVALENCE DEPENDS ON THE IMMUNOGENETIC HETEROGENETEITY. STUDY ON A NARROW ITALIAN DISTRICT: THE PROVINCE OF PAVIA.

L.Salvaneschi, C.Daielli, F.Ambroselli, C.Pizzochero, A.Pastormerlo, R.Poma, C.Gatti, M.Martinetti.
Servizio di Immunoematologia e Trasfusione, IRCCS Policlinico S.Matteo,PAVIA-Italy

The motivation for presenting data on the microgeographic variation in the prevalence of the hepatitis C virus (HCV) is to recognize the possible adaptative nature of some genetic markers with respect to the cohabitation with certain pathogens.
Pavia is situated in Northern Italy, in South-West Lombardy. Pavia province is subdivided in three main areas: Pavese, Lomellina and Oltrepo'. These territorial distinctions have a different historical background and the distribution of HLA class I and II markers, performed on 928 healthy inhabitants, tight kept to this subdivision. Lomellina is genetically the most distant among the three geographical areas and it is characterized by the highest frequency of HLA-DR4. Pavese and Oltrepò are quite similar under the immunogenetic point of view, although with a peculiarity: HLA-DR3 is very frequent in the former while HLA-DR6 in the latter province.
The prevalence of carriers of anti-HCV antibodies, among 14,147 blood donors detected from May 1990 and February 1993, also revealed a geographical microvariation, being higher in Lomellina (3.9%) than in Oltrepò (3.5%) and in Pavese (2.4%). A peculiar distribution along the peripherical boundaries has been observed so that the in certain areas the level of HCV positivity was really high, raising a prevalence rate of 25.9% and 17.9 in villages of the extreme lands of Pavese territory. The immunogenetic profile of people living in these villages also revealed a characteristic behaviour, in term of a high frequency of HLA-DR3, the proper marker for autoimmune diseases. It would not be by chance if a high frequency of genomic exposure to HCV is located right where a favourable genetic background coexists.

0668

CHARACTERIZATION OF HEPATITIS C VIRUS ANTIBODIES POSITIVE BLOOD DONOR IN THAILAND AND JAPAN: A COMPARATIVE STUDY

T.Mazda[1], S.Tanprasert[2], C.Nuchprayoon[2], S.Nakahira[1], K.Nakata[1], T.Katayama[3], K.Fujisawa[1]
[1]Japanese Red Cross Tokyo Metropolitan Blood Centre, [2]National Blood Centre, Thai Red Cross Society, Bangkok, Thailand and [3]Tokyo National Chest Hospital, Tokyo, Japan

The assay of antibodies to hepatitis C virus (anti–HCV) was introduced for screening donated blood from November 1989 in Japan and January 1991 in Thailand. Anti–HCV positive rate evaluated by a commercial second generation kit on blood donor is similar in both countries, 0.6% in Thailand and 0.8% in Japan. The following dissimilarity in character was observed, however, in anti–HCV positive donors of both countries.

On HCV genotype: Genotypes of HCV were analyzed on 44 HCV RNA detected samples in Thai donors by PCR with type specific primers prepared by the method of Okamoto *et al.* 10 (22.7%) samples were showed type I; 32 (72.7%) were type II and 2 (4.5%) were mixed type (I+II). Type III and IV were not detected. While in 116 Japanese HCV RNA detected donors, type I was found in 1 (0.9%), type II 74 (63.8%), type III 32 (27.6%) and type IV 9 (7.8%). In both countries, prevalence of type II was the highest, and in Japanese type I was lowest while in Thai type I second highest.

On ALT value: Although 57% donor of anti–HCV positive in Thai were showed abnormal values (above 53 IU), in Japanese only 13% were showed abnormal values (above 35 Karmen Unit).

H.Okamoto *et al.* J Gen Virol 73: 673–679

0669

HEPATITIS C IN SOUTH AFRICAN BLOOD DONORS

T Tucker[1], A Bird[2], B Hinde[2], J Kannemeyer[3], B Gibbs[2], H Smuts[3], M Voigt[1]

1 UCT/MRC Liver Research Centre, Cape Town
2 Western Province BTS, Cape Town
3 Dept Virology, UCT Medical School, Cape Town

This study examines the prevalence of Hepatitis C Virus (HCV) antibodies in a cohort of South African donors and analyses the clinical characteristics of repeatedly reactive donors. All donors were screened using Abbot HCV EIA 2nd generation assay; if repeatedly reactive they were referred to Groote Schuur Hospital Liver Clinic for follow-up where serum was retested with Ortho HCV EIA 2nd generation assay. Selected donors were also tested using a polymerase-chain reaction (PCR) assay. From December '92 to September '93, 44906 donors were screened: 160 were repeatedly reactive with Abbott 2nd generation EIA giving a prevalence of 0,3%. 59 of these donors presented for clinical follow-up of which 38 were positive with Ortho EIA; $^{12}/57$ (20.3%) were PCR positive. In the PCR positive group, the majority (75%) had possible risk factors for HCV infection, whereas in the remainder of reactive donors <20% had possible risk factors. There were no signs of chronic liver disease although 8 donors had enlarged livers and the PCR positive group had a significantiy higher mean ALT level. It is concluded that HCV infection is of relatively low prevalence amongst South African donors. Discrepancies noted between two 2nd generation EIA kits may reflect differences in the local strains of HCV.

0670

A Preliminary study on the prevalence of anti-HCV amongst healthy blood donors in IRAN.

H.REZVAN,(PhD),I.AHMADI,(M.D),M.FARHADI,(M.D,PATH.) S.TAROYAN(B.SC.)

Objective:In order to obtain an insight on Prevalence of anti-HCV in IRAN,this pilot study was carried out on 15966 samples of voluntary donated at 21 selected centers with different geographical locations across the country.

Methods:Thesamples collected were first tested for anti-HCV using Elisa kits from UBI,USA,the reactive samples were double- checked by another Elisa, from Behring,Germany.Finally,the positive samples were confirmed using Lia.TEK.immunoblot strips from organon teknika.

Results:from the samples tested a total number of 114(0.7%)were reactive with first Elisa,on repeat of these samples 70(0.43%)were found to be double reactive and only 45(0.3%) of all the Elisa positive were confirmed by immunoblot.

Conclusion:the prevalance rate obtained in this study could be an indication for including the test in routine examination of blood donated.It is also important to have a correct algorithm for selection of true positive to avoid discrepancies in reported results.

0671

VIRAL SEROLOGY AND LIVER FUNCTION TESTS IN MULTITRANSFUSED PATIENTS IN WESTERN SIBERIA

Z.S.Barkagan,E.I.Buevich, A.Goncharova
Altai Medical Institute, Barnaul, Russia.

Serological examination was performed in 122 patients with severe forms of hemophilia A (101 cases) and hemophilia B (21 cases). The average age of the patients was 20.6. HIV-1 and HIV-2 were not registered. For the detection of hepatitis B determinations of HBsAg, HBeAg, and antibodies to HBs, HBc and HBe were used. On the basis of "two test criteria" it was concluded that 56.5% of patients were infected by HBV, and 67% by the HCV (EIA Abbott RIBA-2). About 42% of the investigated patients showed positive reactions both for hepatitis B and hepatitis C. Clinical manifestations of hepatitis was present only in 1/4 part of seropositive patients and one half of these patients had periodically abnormal liver function tests. The 2/3 of the investigated patients displayed also antibodies to CMV. All these data suggest that multivirus aggression is one of the main problems in reference to treatment of hemophilia. To reduce the risk of this complications we form the constant "donor-patient" pairs and resort to utilization of virus inactivated blood components, and leukocyte depletion from the transfused blood.

0672

DETECTION OF HEPATITIS C VIRUS (HCV) RNA IN ANTI-HCV POSITIVE VOLUNTEER BLOOD DONORS WITH NORMAL ALANINE AMINOTRANSFERASE (ALT) LEVELS

A. Rossini[1], G.B. Gazzola[3], A. Ravaggi[2], C. Mazza[2], E. Agostinelli[3], L. Biasi[1], E. Radaeli[1], E. Cariani[2]
1 3rd Dept. of Internal Medicine, General Hospital, Brescia, 2 Inst. of Chemistry, University of Brescia, 3 Blood Transfusion Service, Hospital of Chiari, Italy.

Since 1991 3795 blood donors were screened for anti-HCV with ELISA 2. Of 146 ELISA positive donors (3.8%), 75 (51.3%) were RIBA reactive (R), 25 (17.2%) RIBA indeterminate (I) and 46 (31.5%) RIBA non reactive (NR). All anti-HCV positive subjects were periodically tested for ALT levels. Serum HCVRNA was tested in 39 donors with normal ALT (determined every 3 months in the first year and monthly in the last 6 months of follow up). HCVRNA was positive in 16 subjects (14 RIBA R and 2 RIBA I) and negative in 23 (13 RIBA I and 10 RIBA NR). The 2 RIBA I subjects positive for serum HCVRNA were RIBA R on previous determinations. Liver biopsy was performed in 2 RIBA R and HCVRNA positive subjects, indicating chronic liver disease (1 chronic active hepatitis and 1 chronic persistent hepatitis). Conclusions: a)HCVRNA was detected in 41% of anti-HCV positive blood donors with persistently normal ALT b)RIBA 2 reactivity is associated with the presence of HCVRNA c)HCVRNA may be detected in subjects with RIBA I pattern d)all RIBA NR subjects were HCVRNA negative e)HCVRNA may be associated with chronic liver disease even in subjects with normal ALT levels.

0673

SIGNIFICANCE OF ANTIBODY TO PROTEIN ENCODED BY THE NONSTRUCTURAL 5 REGION OF THE HEPATITIS C VIRUS GENOME IN HEMOPHILIA PATIENTS

Takumi Kanesaki[1], Seiji Kinoshita [1], Giichi Tsujino [1], Keiichiro Yoshioka [1], Nobuko Ikegami [2], and Akihisa Takamizawa [3]
[1]Department of Pediatrics and [2]Clinical Research Institute, Osaka National Hospital, Chuo-ku, Osaka 540; and [3]Research Foundation for Microbial Diseases of Osaka University, Kannonji, Kagawa 768, Japan

[Purpose] We tried to determine which HCV antibody was correlated with disease activity. [Methods] Sequential serum samples were collected from 45 patients with hemophilia between 1986 and 1993. Three proteins (core, nonstructural[NS]3, and NS5) were expressed in recombinant E. coli that incorporated fragments of the putative core, NS3, and NS5 regions of the HCV genome, respectively. Antibodies to these proteins were detected by ELISA. HCV RNA was detected by the PCR assay. [Results] Antibodies to the core and NS3 proteins were repeatedly positive in all but one patient. The antibody to NS5 protein was repeatedly positive in 30 patients. Of these 30 patients, 28 showed an abnormal alanine aminotransferase (ALT) level and HCV RNA was detected in all 28 patients. Of the 15 patients negative for anitibody to the NS5 protein, 12 had a prolonged normal ALT level and HCV RNA was only detected in 4. [Conclusions] Antibody to the NS5 protein might be a useful serologic marker of disease activity in HCV infection.

0674

ANALYSING THE SEQUENCE DIVERSITY OF THE 5' NC-REGION OF HCV-ISOLATES FOUND IN SOUTHERN GERMANY

M. da Silva Cardoso, S. Epple, K, Koerner, B. Kubanek
German Red Cross Blood Bank Ulm and Department of Transfusion Medicine, University of Ulm, FRG

In this study we compared the nucleotide sequence of the 5' NC-region of HCV genome isolated from seven patients and two blood donors from Southern Germany. The two blood donors investigated showed reactivity in anti-HCV ELISA; one of them was RIBA-2 positive. RNA was extracted from the patient's serum, reverse transcribed and submitted to amplification (RT/PCR) with nested primers coding for sequences in the 5' NC region. The amplified fragments from six patients were cloned in the plasmid pBlue Script, while the fragments from the seventh patient and the two blood donors were directly sequenced after amplification. At the end we could identify two very distinct groups of isolates: the first very similar to the HCV prototype sequence (HCV1) with homology ranging from 99,5% to 98,7%; the second showing 91.7% homology to the HCV1. Group 1 isolates could be found in five patients and two blood donors. Group 2 isolates could be found in two other patients. Finally, we could observe neither nucleotide insertion nor deletion in the isolates described here.

0675

FOLLOW-UP STUDY ON ANTI-HCV POSITIVE BLOOD DONORS AFTER NOTIFICATION IN A REGIONAL BLOOD CENTER.

H.Kiyokawa,Y.Tsutsumi,K.Matsumoto,K.Tokunaga,K.Fukada,Y.Maeda.
Fukuoka Red Cross Blood Center, Fukuoka ,Japan.

Objective: Japanese Red Cross Blood Centers have been using 2nd generation anti HCV PHA screening test since February 1992.Notification has already been started for donors whose blood test results meet, the criteria. The purpose of this study was to know and analyze the clinical diagnosis of anti HCV positive donors.

Methods: Samples from donors were screened initially by 2nd generation anti-HCV PHA test, using an automated pretransfusion blood testing system (PK7200, Olympus) and all the positive samples were examined repeatedly using the usual microplate method by manual.According to the data of Japanese Red Cross HCV study group, it is known that if the titer of HCV positive sample shows more than 2,the probability of PCR positive almost 100%. Donors whose blood test, results meet the following criteria must be notified:

1) $>2^{12}$of titer on anti-HCV PHA test,or
2) $2^{11}>$anti HCV PHA $>2^{5}$and >36KUof ALT.

Anti-HCV test, results were mailed to donors to indicate counseling by local physicians from August through October 1993.

Results: 4050 of the 227,833 donors tested were positive for anti-HCV (1.77%). 1990 of the 4050 anti-HCV positive donors meet the criteria for notification. 839 of 1990 donors notified (42.2%) visited local physicians and diagnosed as follows:1) 229 asymptomatic carrier (27.3%) 2) 584 chronic hepatitis(69.6%) 3) 6 liver cirrhosis (0.7%) 4) 10 anti-HCV negative (1.2%).

Conclusions: The HCV intection in blood donors in Fukuoka seems to be associated with a high rate (69.6%) of chronic liver diseases. However, return rate of replies from consulting physicians to Fukuoka Red Cross Blood Center was rather low (42.2%).Still, we need further investigation to assess more precise incidence of the asymptomatic carriers and blood donors with definite liver diseases.

0676

THE INCIDENCE OF POST-TRANSFUSION HEPATITIS AFTER SCREENING OF DONOR BLOOD FOR ANTI-HCV ANTIBODY BY 2ND GENERATION OF PASSIVE HEMAGGLUTINATION

K.Osada[1],S.Takahashi[1],M.Shimizu[1],J.Watanabe[2]
1Department of Transfusion Medicine,Tokyo Women's Medical College
2The Japanese Red Cross Ohta Blood Center, Tokyo,Japan

Purpose. It is to know how more effective control of post-transfusion non-Anon-B hepatitis (NANBPTH) could be expected after introduction of the 2nd generation of anti-HCV antibody by PHA for screening since February 1992.

Methods. A prospective study to assess the effectiveness of this screening in Tokyo Women's Medical College had begun since May 1992. 292 patients with open heart surgery who were PHA negative before transfusions and received 5.5 units on average had been followed up for at least three months.

Results. The only one of these 11 patients who developed PTH and received 6.8 units on average showed seroconversion of anti-HCV antibody and detected HCV-RNA by PCR, although the other 10 patients were HCV-RNA negative by PCR.

One of the 7 blood donors who implicated to the patient with post-transfusion hepatitis C(PTHC) was HCV RNA positive by PCR.

Conclusion. Our present screening resulted rare incidence of PTHC. However, there remain some risk factors for PTHnon-C to be clarified.

0677

AN ANALYSIS OF THE EFFECTIVENESS OF BLOOD UNITS SCREENED FOR ANTI-HCV BY SECOND GENERATION ASSAY

S. Inaba[1], Y. Tsutsumi[2], T. Mori[2], K. Fukada[2], H. Kiyokawa[2], Y. Maeda[2], T. Katayama[3]
1 Blood Transfusion Service, Kyushu University Hospital, Fukuoka, Japan.
2 Fukuoka Red Cross Blood Center, Fukuoka, Japan.
3 Tokyo National Chest Hospital, Tokyo, Japan.

The Japan Red Cross Blood Center began screening blood for transfusion with the second generation anti-HCV assay in February of 1991. Serum samples of 551 anti-HCV negative patients who received homologous blood at Kyushu University Hospital between 1991 and July, 1993 were tested anti-HCV by passive hemagglutination test (PHA, DINABOT, the second generation assay) after a minimum followed up of 60 days to determine the effectiveness of the screening. Forty-seven (8.5%) patients were found to be anti-HCV positive by PHA. Of these three were found to be false negative because all other serial samples were PHA positive. Antibodies against core specific antigens were measured using the JCC-2 test (core specific, Ortho-Diagnostic) in the remaining 44 patients' samples, and 35 of them were found to be negative. Thus, nine of the 551 (1.6%) patients had seroconverted. In five anti-HCV cleared naturally, but remained positive for over 120 days after transfusion in four. ALT elevation indicating a clinical diagnosis of post-transfusion hepatitis (PTH) was found in only two patients (0.36%). Blood for transfusion to these two patients was from seven donor units, which we re-examined with all seven testing negative by both second generation assay and HCV RNA tests. We are in the process of collecting serum samples from the nine seroconverted patients for RNA analysis.

The incidence of PTH before the implementation of screening with c-100 ELISA (the first generation assay) was over 10% in Japan, and after the implementation of c-100 screening the incidence decreased to about 3%. In comparison, the effectiveness of anti-HCV screening with the second generation assay is excellent. Some questions, however, remain. The first is why we were unable to completely prevent HCV transmission, and the second is does seroconversion without ALT elevation indicate HCV infection or not.

0678

POST-TRANSFUSION HEPATITIS AND HCV SCREENING: A RETROSPECTIVE STUDY.

O.Giachino ,D. Lajolo ,M. Milan.
Centro Trasfusionale AVIS Torino. ITALY

22 cases of post-transfusion nAnB hepatitis (NANB PTH) in patients transfused in 1988,89,90 were studied. 8 patients had transfusion dependent ß-thalassemia and were included in this study because of no previously reported hepatitis, normal ALT values and no anti-HCV antibodies before hepatitis diagnosis. 14 patients were transfused after elective surgical procedures. The donors implicated in the 22 cases of hepatitis (108 for surgical patients and 45 that is the last 3 month donors for the multitransfused) were identified and a serum sample was obtained immediately after the reported hepatitis. The stored donor samples were later tested by both a 1st generation (ELISA 1) and a 2nd generation (ELISA 2) anti-HCV. 21 donors out of 153 (13.7%) were ELISA2 positive (0.7% in our population of first time donors p<0.01). Among the 21 HCV reactive, 9 were males and 12 females. The male-female ratio was .7 vs 2.2 in the whole implicated donor group. (p<0.05).12 donors were ELISA 1 reactive (57%). The other 9 were ELISA 1 negative, ELISA 2 positive. A seropositive donor was detected in 19 cases out of 22(86%).

The data show that 86% of NANBPTH could have been prevented by ELISA 2 screening (50% by ELISA 1).The sex of donors was statistically related to the risk of transmission. The female higher risk was likely to be a consequence of the ALT screening performed since 1983 with the same cut-off value in both sexes. A lower ALT cut-off for female donors is advisable, even after the implementation of HCV screening, in order to further decrease the residual risk of post-transfusion hepatitis.

0679

THE RECENT INCIDENSE OF POST-TRANSFUSION NON-A,NON-B HEPATITIS IN JAPAN SINCE THE IMPLEMENTATION OF THE ANTI-HCV SCREENING PROGRAM FOR BLOOD DONORS

T.Katayama, H.Baba, H.Fujii, Y.Hiyama, S.Inaba, S.Kawai, S.Kikuchi, K.Kiyosawa, K.Konishi, Z.Matsuura, K.Tadokoro, M.Takagi, M.Takimoto
Committee on Post-Transfusion infection. Ministry of Health and Welfare, Tokyo,Japan.

We report data on follow-up surveys of post-transfusion hepatitis at the 10 hospitals that participated in a study conducted by the Commettee on Post-Transfusion Infection of the Ministry of Health and Welfare.

There were 107 post-transfusion non-A, non-B hepatitis(PT-NANBH) cases(7.1%) among the 1507 patients who received blood in 1988 and 1989, when no anti-HCV screening was conducted.

Since November 1989, Japanese Blood Centers adopted the anti-C100 screening test (Ortho) to prevent hepatitis C. Among 1729, 42 patients developed PT-NANBH (2.4%) in 1990 and 1991. In spite of this screening procedure, we have witnessed 5 cases of post-transfusion hepatitis C(PT-HC).

In February 1992, the PHA test using the 2nd HCV-Ab(Abbott) was adopted for anti-HCV screening. The 18 cases of PT-NANBH were found among 1432 blood recipients(1.3%) from 1992 to July 1993. And 4 cases converted seropositive of anti-HCV.

0681

RISK FACTORS AND CLINICAL FEATURES OF BLOOD DONORS WITH ANTI-HCV

CK LIN[1], CL LAI[2], NK CHAN[1], JLP YOUNG[2], S LEONG[1]

[1] Hong Kong Red Cross Blood Transfusion Service
[2] Department of Medicine, Queen Mary Hospital, University of Hong Kong

The aim of this study was to determine the risk factors, physical and biochemical signs of blood donors with hepatitis C antibodies (anti-HCV).

Hong Kong Red Cross Blood Transfusion Service started mass screening of donated blood for anti-HCV since July 1992 using Abbott second generation anti-HCV EIA assay and Abbott MATRIX HCV for confirmation. HCV RNA detection by reverse transcription and polymerase chain reaction using nested primers was also performed. 123 Chinese voluntary non-remunerated blood donors with anti-HCV were interviewed and examined both physically and biochemically. Results were as followed:

Risk Factors	Accu-puncture	Tattoo	IV drug	Trans-fusion	Sex	Unknown
No. (%)	10 (8)	10 (8)	25 (20)	54 (44)	10 (8)	14 (12)

Physical signs	Spider angiomas	Palmer erythema	palpable liver	palpable spleen
No. (%)	59 (48)	29 (24)	54 (44)	2 (3)

Biochemical changes	ALAT > 53 U/L	ASAT > 34 U/L	GGT > 38 U/L	ALP > 118 U/L
No. (%)	39 (32)	68 (55)	20 (16)	10 (8)

Conclusions:

1. Blood transfusion was the most common risk factor.
2. Spider angiomas and palpable liver were detected in about 50% of subjects.
3. ALAT & ASAT were elevated in over 30 & 50% of subjects.

0682

IMMUNE RESPONSE AGAINST A SPECIFIC EPITOPE ON HCV NS-3 ANTIGEN IS CORRELATED WITH INFECTIVITY.

W. Habets[1], P. Boender[1], F. Jacobs[1], M Peeters[1], H. Peels[1], T. Cuypers[2], N. Lelie[2] and M. Mondelli[3].
[1]Organon Teknika, The Netherlands, [2] CLB Amsterdam The Netherlands,
[3] University Pavia, Italy

Infectivity of sera from patients with hepatitis C is best measured by nucleic acid amplification techniques such as PCR and NASBA. Such techniques however, are very costly, time-consuming and require expertise which is usually not found in routine hospital laboratories or bloodbanks. In a vast majority of cases, commercial anti-HCV antibody screening assays provide a good substitute, especially when the results are confirmed by supplementary assays like RIBA (Chiron Corp.) or LiaTek HCV (Organon Teknika). A problem arises however, when initial positive screening results cannot be confirmed unequivocally, in particular in those cases where the result of supplementary assays is "indeterminate".

We investigated a population of 75 donors and patients, positive in at least one commercially available HCV screening assay and indeterminate (C33c-only) in the RIBA assay. From this population 8 sera (11%) were found positive in a PCR assay using primers from the most conserved region of the HCV genome (5'UTR). This confirms previous observations that a small but significant percentage of RIBA-indeterminates should be considered carriers of the hepatitis C virus.

We further investigated whether a correlation would exist between PCR positivity and any serological finding. In our population no such correlation was observed with commercial assays from Abbott, Ortho or UBI, nor did the intensity of the RIBA pattern correlate with infectivity. However, when we employed an experimental HCV NS-3 inhibition assay in which antibodies in the patients serum compete with a human monoclonal antibody for binding to the HCV NS-3 antigen, we found that all 8 PCR-positive sera described above, effectively competed with the mAb, whereas only 1 of the 67 PCR-negative sera showed significant competition.

Our data show that the human monoclonal antibody defines an important epitope on the HCV NS-3 antigen which reacts with antibodies from viraemic patients, whereas PCR-negative sera react at different sites. The NS-3 inhibition assay might therefore provide an attractive alternative for PCR in those cases where RIBA results are (C33c) indeterminate.

0683

HCV GENOTYPES IN ANTI-HCV RIBA2 INDETERMINATE AND POSITIVE BLOOD DONORS

C. Capelli, D. Prati, P. Bosoni, F. Mozzi, A. Zanella, G. Sirchia. Centro Trasfusionale e di Immunologia dei Trapianti, Ospedale Maggiore, Milano, Italy.

Background: Biochemical and histologic findings of chronic liver damage are more common in viraemic RIBA2 positive than in viraemic RIBA2 indeterminate subjects. It is known that a different disease progression of HCV infection seems to be related to different HCV types. Aim: To evaluate HCV genotypes in RIBA2 positive and indeterminate blood donors. Methods: HCV genotypes were determined in 15 RIBA2 positive (group A, 13 with ALT > 40U/L) and 14 indeterminate (group B, 1 with ALT > 40U/L) blood donors by nested PCR (5'UTR region) and probe specific reverse hybridization assay (LiPA, Innogenetics); LiPA allows the determination of types 1 to 5 and subtypes. Results: Genotyping results of the two groups are given in the table.

	HCV subtypes			
group	1a	1b	2a	1a+1b
A	1(7%)	11(73%)	2(13%)	1(7%)
B	0	5(36%)	9(64%)	0

RIBA2 positive and indeterminate pattern was significantly associated with 1b and non-1b subtype respectively ($p < 0.05$ by Fisher's exact test). Comments: The finding of less aggressive HCV subtypes (non-1b) in most RIBA2 indeterminate subjects could account for their favourable clinical course.

0684

ISOTYPE SPECIFIC IMMUNE RESPONSE TO A B-CELL EPITOPE ON THE HEPATITIS C VIRUS CORE PROTEIN

K. Siemoneit, M. Cardoso, S. Epple, A. Wölpl, H. Wintersinger, K. Koerner, B. Kubanek
German Red Cross Blood Bank Ulm and Department of Transfusion Medicine, University of Ulm, Ulm, FRG

We have recently identified a 6-mer epitope (VYLLPR) within the N-terminus of the HCV core protein using a human monoclonal antibody (UL/F10). To evaluate the biological significance of this epitope we tested blood donors with a peptide ELISA. For this purpose we selected 223 anti-HCV ELISA (Ortho, 2nd generation) reactive sera. From these, 67 samples were reactive in the recombinant immunoblot RIBA-2 (Ortho, 2nd generation).

The RIBA reactive samples were divided into four groups: g1 c22 reactive, g2 c22/c33 reactive, g3 c22/c100 reactive, g4 c22/c100/c33/5-1-1 reactive. Additionally all these 67 reactive samples were tested by RT/PCR.

The analyses of the results showed that:

1. the epitope VYLLPR is highly immunoreactive (IgG1 restricted) in RIBA positive blood donors with a very low frequency of possibly false positive results, 2. PCR and anti-peptide assay correlated very well: more than 95% of the samples had coincident results in all subgroups, 3. correlation of anti-peptide and RIBA-2 varied from less than 10% in groups 1 and 3 to over 80% in groups 2 and 4.

In conclusion, if we consider the PCR as a standard method for detection of infectivity, screening of blood donors with the 6-mer peptide turns out to be more specific than the screening with the recombinant core protein (c22).

0685

PREVALENCE OF HEPATITIS A AND HEPATITIS C VIRUSES ANTIBODIES AND CHRONIC LIVER DISEASE IN RELATION TO HIV INFECTION IN ISRAELI HEMOPHILIACS.

A. Barzilai, E. Levin, P. Weiss, S. Schulman, D. Varon and U. Martinowitz.

The National Hemophilia Center, Sheba Medical Center, Tel-Hashomer, Israel.

One hundred thirty nine hemophiliacs were tested for human immunodeficiency virus (HIV), hepatitis A virus (HAV) and hepatitis C virus (HCV) antibodies. Forty three patients (30.9%) were HIV(+) and 96 (63.1%) were HIV(-). In the HIV(+) group 42 of 43 (97.7%) were seropositive to HCV in 2nd generation tests in comparison with 55 of 96 patients (51%), who were HIV(-), $p<0.001$. HAV antibodies were found in 28 of 43 patients (65%) in the HIV(+) group comparing with 33 of 74 patients (44%), $p<0.05$, in the HIV(-) group. Chronic liver disease was more common in patients with hemophilia who were HIV(+) and HCV(+): 19 of 43 (44%), in comparison with 23 of 96 (24%) of patients with hemophilia who were HIV(-) and HCV(+), $p<0.03$. These findings suggest that HCV and HAV infections are more common in HIV(+) hemophiliacs. Since the HIV(+) patients in Israel have been more heavily transfused with factor concentrates, it is likely that at least part of the HAV infections were mediated by transfusion of blood products. HIV infection seems to aggravate the course of chronic hepatitis caused by HCV.

0686

HCV: ANTIBODY PATTERN AND LIVER FUNCTIONALITY

S. Ciaffoni, G. Bovo, F. Schiesari, N. Pauletto, S. Migliozzi
Immunotransfusion Service,
Ospedale Civile, Bussolengo (VR), Italy.

The objective of our study was to value the relation between hepatic cytolytic parameters and the Hepatitis C Virus (HCV) antigens (C22, C33, C100 and 5-1-1). From Jan.'91 to Dec.'93 we studied 339 blood donors HCV-positive, using anti-HCV second generation ELISA assay. 8 determinations of Alanine transaminase and Aspartate transaminase, 6 anti-HCV ELISA assay and 3 anti-HCV second generation recombinant immunoblot assay (RIBA) were performed on each blood donor, at an opportune time. 100 of them were confirmed as positive, 56 indeterminate and 183 negative using RIBA assay. The results showed that there was an increase of transaminases more frequently and more marked from RIBA negative (5.5%) to RIBA positive subjects (79%) and proportional to the presence of one, two, three or four bands (16%, 62.5%, 84.2% and 100% respectively), indipendent of different associations between them. There was a nett predominance of anti-C22 reactivity when one band was present (73.2%) and of anti-C22 plus anti-C33 reactivities in the presence of two bands (89.6%).

0687

SUPPLEMENTARY HCV-ANTIBODY TESTING OF BLOOD DONORS

Mária Héjjas[1], G.A.Medgyesi[1], J.Szabó[1], P.Simmonds[2]
1Natl.Inst. of Haematol., Blood Transfusion and Immunol., Budapest, Hungary 2Dept of Med.Microbiol.Medical School,Univ.of Edinburg, Edinburgh, Scotland.

Rutin screening for anti-HCV was started in Hungary in 1992. In the first period of screening with Abbott EIA-2 a repeat reactivity rate of 0.98 % was observed. The system of supplementary testing was established on the basis of a previous pilot test comparing five different anti-HCV ELISA kits and two blotting tests. As a first step Wellcozyme anti-HCV ELISA was adapted. Donors strongly reactive ELISA ratio≥2.5) in both tests are permanently deferred. (ELISA ratio (E.R.)=optical density/cut off.) Those negative in the supplementary ELISA or weakly reactive (E.R.<2.5) in both tests are subjected to RIBA. RIBA positive donors are permanently deferred, indeterminates are excluded for one year and negatives are readmitted. 75 samples from donors permanently deffered were tested by PCR and 70 of them were found positive, whilst 3 out of 25 RIBA indeterminates (temporary deferral) were found PCR positive. Data of 16 months supplementary testing showed that RIBA testing included in the algorythm provided little useful information. In our proposed modified system any donor reactive in the screening ELISA and not deferred permanently will be deferred for one year and retested then. Those negative in the screening test will be readmitted when negative in both the supplementary ELISA and RIBA.

0688

HEPATITIS C VIRUS RNA DETECTION IN BLOOD DONORS WITH ANTI-HCV ANTIBODIES DETECTED WITH VARIOUS TESTS

E.Brojer, J.J.Stańczak, M.Radlińska, M.Sankowska, E.Kacperska, Z.Głoskowska - Moraczewska, H.Seyfried
Institute of Haematology and Blood Transfusion, Warsaw, Poland

Reverse transcription followed by two round PCR with primers complementary to the 5´ UTR was used for HCV RNA detection in sera of blood donors with anty-HCV antibodies. Sixty six HCV ELISA positive persons with different results in 4-RIBA test were investigated. In 48 of them HCV RNA was detected: in 30 out of 37 4-RIBA positive persons, in 11 out of 17 RIBA indeterminate and in 7 out of 12 RIBA negative sera.
In 15 persons with 4-RIBA positive results the HCV was detected in the first round of PCR. In all other cases two rounds of amplification were needed to obtain positive results.

0689

PARTIAL NUCLEOTIDE AND AMINO ACID SEQUENCE OF POLISH SUBTYPE OF HEPATITIS C VIRUS

J.J.Stańczak, E.Brojer, M.Radlińska, M.Gutowicz
Institute of Haematology and Blood Transfusion, Warsaw, Poland

Hepatitis C virus is a leading agent of posttransfusion hepatitis.About 40% of cases is an effect of infection with this virus. HCV is known a high genetic variability.Until now 16 genotypes,combined in 6 groups,have been described.They differ in virulency and pathogenicity.We have introduced modified RNA isolation and RT-PCR techniques for testing sera and tissue samples for the presence of genomic RNA of HCV. Nucleotide sequences of amplified fragments are sequenced with dideoxy chain termination method of Sanger et al.in order to determine a nucleotide sequences of Polish isolates.Partial nt sequence of highly conservative 5´UTR and hypervariable fragment of E/NS1 regions have been determined.Alignment of these sequences with previously described shows that sequence of 5´UTR is identical to HCV-US prototype,but significant differences were found in nt sequence,followed by predicted amino acid sequence,of E/NS1 region.
Here we report a partial nucleotide and predicted amino acid sequence of Polish subtype of HCV.

0690

COMMERCIAL HIV-1 IMMUNOFLUORESCENCE ASSAY (IFA) IN CONFIRMATORY ALGORITHMS FOR HIV-1/HIV-2 EIA.

Stramer, S.L.[1], Sapan, C.V.[2], Henderson, S.E.[3] and Tegtmeier, G.E.[3]
[1]Abbott Laboratories, Abbott Park, IL, [2]North American Biologicals, Miami, FL, and [3]Community Blood Center of Greater Kansas City, Kansas City, MO

Purpose: HIV-1 IFA and Western Blot (WB) were compared to HIV-1/HIV-2 "Third Generation" EIA (IgG and IgM detection) and an HIV-1 EIA (primarily IgG detection). Selected specimens were also tested for HIV-1 p24 antigen (Ag).
Methods: Specimens used in the evaluation included selected repository HIV EIA repeat reactives (83 WB IND and 15 suspect WB "false" POS), 10 HIV-1 seroconversion series (78 total specimens) and 12 HIV-2 samples (Cote d'Ivoire).
HIV-1 WB/IFA Results by Specimen Group:

		EIA Repeat Reactive		HIV-2		HIV-1 Seroconversion		
		WB POS	WB IND	WB POS	WB IND	WB POS	WB IND	WB NEG
IFA	POS	8	0	5	7	40(10)**	4(4)	0
	NEG	7*	83	0	0	2 (2)	9(4)	23(15)

*5 HIV-1 Ag EIA NEG **() No. HIV-1 Ag EIA
*2 QNS HIV-1 Ag EIA POS of 35 total Ag POS

Conclusion: In general, there is good agreement between the IFA, WB and HIV-1 EIA (HIV-1 EIA data not shown). However, all are less sensitive than newer generation (direct format) HIV-1/HIV-2 Ab EIAs. Therefore, for the confirmation of HIV-1 seroconversion, HIV-1 Ag should be assayed in addition to tests for HIV-1 Ab (IFA, WB or EIA). The IFA appears to have better specificity and better HIV-2 cross reactivity than does the WB; however, weak HIV-1 Ab reactivity that may be undetected by IFA and negative or indeterminate by WB would require additional testing for confirmation.

0691

A MICROPARTICLE ENZYME IMMUNOASSAY FOR THE DETECTION OF ANTIBODIES TO HIV-1 AND HIV-2 ON A RANDOM ACCESS AUTOMATED ANALYZER

W. Black, G. Hall-Steele, S. Stewart, S. Kramer, B. Sehgal, and D. Daghfal
Abbott Laboratories, Abbott Park, Illinois, USA.

Objective: To develop a combination HIV-1 and HIV-2 immunoassay for a random, continuous access analyzer with sensitivity equivalent to licensed assays. The clinical utility of this HIV-1/HIV-2 assay is for the qualitative determination of IgM and IgG antibodies against HIV-1 and HIV-2 in human serum or plasma samples as an aid in the diagnosis of HIV infection.
Method: Human serum or plasma sample reacts with microparticles coated with HIV-1 env, HIV-1 gag, and HIV-2 env proteins. Antibody captured on the solid phase reacts with biotinylated proteins to form an antigen-antibody-antigen complex. Bound antibody is measured by the addition of alkaline phosphatase anti-biotin conjugate and a fluorescent substrate. Sample handling, assay manipulations, and results reporting are continuously performed by the random access immunoassay analyzer. Assay performance is compared to that of other automated assay analyzers for HIV-1 and HIV-2 detectability.
Results: HIV-1 seroconversion sensitivity results are compared to other HIV assays on ten commercially available HIV-1 seroconversion panels. In all seroconversion panels tested, HIV-1 antibodies were detected with sensitivity equivalent to all other assays. Additionally, fifty HIV-1 and one hundred HIV-2 Western Blot confirmed positive samples are detected as positive. Specificity was evaluated on a totai of 2378 random diagnostic serum and plasma samples. Thirteen reactives were detected for an initial and repeat reactive rate of 0.54% . Ten samples confirmed positive. The confirming rate is 0.42%.
Conclusion: This study demonstrates the detectability of HIV-1 and HIV-2 antibodies in plasma and serum samples assayed in a continuous mode on a random access automated analyzer.

0692

EVALUATION OF AN AUTOMATED ASSAY FOR THE SIMULTANEOUS DETECTION OF ANTIBODY TO HIV-1 AND HIV-2 (IMx® HIV-1/HIV-2)

Webber, J. S.; Guckenberger, J.; Kewin, D.; Nordmark, K.; Minnert, G.; Spies, U;.and Bocher, M., et al.
Abbott Laboratories, North Chicago, Illinois, U.S.A.

A microparticle enzyme immunoassay (MEIA), capable of detecting antibody to both HIV-1 and HIV-2, has been developed using the Abbott IMx analyzer. Specimens from blood donors, diagnostic and hospital patients, individuals at risk for HIV infection, HIV-1 seroconversion panels, confirmed HIV-1 and HIV-2 positive specimens, and potential interfering specimens were tested in parallel with IMx HIV-1/HIV-2 and Abbott HIVAB HIV-1/HIV-2. Selected specimens were used to evaluate competitor combination tests. In this study, assays using a direct sandwich format (i.e. IMx and HIVAB) detect seroconversion approximately 1 week earlier than tests using indirect anti-human conjugates. The increased sensitivity is due, in part, to a demonstrated ability to detect early IgM response, as well as IgG antibody. The IMx assay detected all 300 HIV-1 and 200 HIV-2 reactive specimens. The IMx repeat reactive rate of 0.04% (1/2333) with donor serum and 0.52% (12/2296) with random diagnostic specimens was equivalent to HIVAB HIV-1/HIV-2. The IMx HIV-1/HIV-2 provides a useful tool for the simultaneous detection of HIV-1 and/or HIV-2 exposure in a fully automated instrument system.

0693

USE OF THE MULTISCREEN-TM TEST (ABBOTT) COMBINED SCREENING TEST FOR THE DETECTION OF HBs ANTIGENS AND HIV1+2 ANTIBODIES AMONG BLOOD DONORS.

B. Donéa, D. Sondag.
Blood Transfusion Centre, Liège, Belgium

The Multiscreen-TM HBs Ag - HIV1+2 (rDNA) EIA test from ABBOTT allows for the simultaneous detection of HBs Antigens and HIV1+2 Antibodies.
Results: 96.509 samples of blood from donors collected from 11/92 to 11/93 were tested with the Multiscreen-TM. As concerns 6.601 samples, the frequency distribution profile of Test Ratio (TR) shows that 91.86% of TR is lower or equal to 0.2, with a mean of 0.16 and a median of 0.10. From 96.509 samples tested, 95.857 are negative, 652 are initially reactive (0.67%), 191 are repeatedly reactive (0.19%). The 191 RR samples were tested with 2 supplemental tests, with a view to establish the etiological diagnosis of the reactivity.

HBsAg	EIA HIV1+2 - 3rd gen. Pos	Neg	Tot
IMX			
Pos	0	20(*)	20
Neg	83(**)	87	170
Tot	83	107	190

(*) 20/20 confirmed HBsAg positive.
(**) Western blot : positive (n=2); indeterminate (n=17); negative (n=64).

Conclusion: the Multiscreen-TM test and the automated equipment, FPC, PPC and VITAM from ABBOTT allow to safely and easily detect HBs antigens and HIV1+2 antibodies, with a single test. The partition of negative samples from positive is very clear-cut, the TR of negative sera are well-grouped in low values. The number of initially positive or repeatedly positive sera is not too high. The sensitivity for detection of HBs Antigens and HIV1+2 Antibodies is satisfactory.

0694

ADVANTAGES AND LIMITATIONS OF THE USE OF VARIOUS ANTIGENS IN AN IMMUNOASSAY FOR THE DETECTION OF EARLY HIV1 ANTIBODIES

S. GADELLE, B. EL MALIKI, C. LESAGER, C. CRABBE
SANOFI DIAGNOSTICS PASTEUR, 92430 Marnes (FRANCE)

OBJECTIVE :
• To determine the performance characteristics of an HIV1 Ab sandwich immunoassay using different HIV1 antigens, (the first ones being coated on the solid phase and the others labelled as conjugate), and
• to demonstrate their efficacy in detecting early seroconverters.

METHODS :
Well characterized panel samples (BBI, Serologicals, French National Society of Blood Transfusion/SNTS) were tested using different antigens : full lenght recombinant GP160, GP41 expressed in E. Coli, synthetic peptides mimicking the major GP160 epitope from various isolates (MN, LA1...) P25 expressed in E. Coli.

RESULTS :
Using different antigen (coated/labelled) combinations, variable sensitivities were obtained when detecting early antibodies. The coated GP160/ENV peptide LAI combination allowed the detection of the first Serologicals panel sample (n°2215) and did not permit the detection of SNTS panel sample n° 72. Opposite results were found using the coated GP41/labelled GP41 combination.

CONCLUSION :
The correct choice of epitopes involved in early Ab recognition as well as the genomic variability of the different known isolates must be carefuly considered in the development of new HIV Ab screening immunoassays.

0695

The use of a different assay for anti-HIV-1 repeatably reactive samples.

Rodríguez MA, Contreras C, Mattar MC. Banco de Sangre, Hospital Naval A. Nef, Viña del Mar, Chile.

Altough current reagents for anti-HIV testing have a high sensitivity and specificity, false reactivity still occurs and there is a need for complicate and expensive confirmatory testing.

As a search for an orientation, from 1992 we started performing a titration using a very sensitive modified gelatin particcle agglutination assay (Fujirebio INC, Japan) to every ELISA repeatably reactive sample (ELISA UNIFORM, Organon Teknika).

We have already tested over 7000 samples from patients and blood donors and found 34 to be repeatably reactive, of those only 8 were positive on titration with gelatin particles, and the remaining 26 were negative, although some of them showed some non-specific reactivity which cleared after absortion with unsensitised particles.

The results of confirmatory testing for the same samples were: 8 samples positives, the same that were positive on titration, 24 negative and 2 undeterminate (p24 only) none of those seroconverted later.

This approach gave us an orientation previous to the confirmatory results which of course will not allow the usage of the blood in the case of blood donations, but is helpful when patients are tested and comes to confirm again the high sensitivity and specificity of this simple and low cost technique extremelly useful in developing countries.

I would be of interest to repeat this experience with bigger figures.

0696

A novel one step HIV1/HIV2 antibody EIA utilizing magnetic microparticles and chemiluminescence on the fully automated Access® immunoassay system.

(N.Du Fou de Kerdaniel, A.Clément, C.Cucurou D.Riochet, JF.Delagneau; Sanofi Diagnostics Pasteur)

A one step, simultaneous EIA procedure has been developed for the detection of antibodies to the HIV1-2 viruses. The assay combines magnetic microparticles and chemiluminescence on the fully automated ACCESS®Immunoassay System instrument (Sanofi Diagnostics Pasteur). The format consists of the mixing of an instrument diluted sample, magnetic microparticles coated with protein A and conjugate reagent containing three HIV env peptides and a P24 full length recombinant coupled with alkaline phosphatase. Following the single 20 min. incubation at 37°C the particles and bound reactives are washed and the chemiluminescent substrate is added. Specific antibody is detected by measuring light (Relative Luminescence Units [RLU]) generated from the action of the bound conjugate on the substrate.

A total of 4799 normal blood donor samples (serum or plasma) were tested in the ACCESS instrument. The specificity was 99.73% including 7 Western Blot indeterminated (P24 reactive). No false positive results were found among 431 samples collected in pregnant women or in patients suffering from autoimmune, or infectious diseases.

The assay showed excellent sensitivity on several well known BBI (Boston Biomedica Inc) HIV seroconversion panels (initial reactive samples were K5+,Q5+,P5+,C3+,E10+,H6+,J3+). Sensitivity on fully converted sera or plasma is 100% [306/306] for HIV1 and for HIV2 [215/215]). A study of 4 sera (from negative to strong serum) showed a very good precision : intra assay < 6.57% and inter assay < 8.04%.

Conclusion : the ACCESS® immunoassay system HIV1-2 Ab EIA test provides rapid results with excellent sensitivity and specificity. The system instrument is fully automated and also allows random Access for testing each sample with multiple parameters.

0697

EVALUATION OF CHEMILUMINESCENT VS. EXISTING IMMUNOASSAY TECHNOLOGY B. Quint,* K. Mendel,* P. Buchaklian, R. Hu, J. Rogers, B. Peterson, G. Lindberg, R. Richerson, M. Hedblom and S. O'Brien. Abbott Laboratories, Abbott Park, Illinois, USA and *Abbott GmbH Diagnostika, Wiesbaden-Delkenheim, Germany.

There is an increasing focus in transfusion to automate laboratory testing while insuring the highest level of assay performance and process control. For this purpose, a system utilizing chemiluminescent immunoass ay (ChLIA) and microparticle capture technologies has been developed. The system fully automates all the steps of the assay procedure. Redundant checks and balances on critical system functions have been incorporated into the instrument design to insure that the entire assay process is in control.

In ChLIA technology, acridinium is used as the conjugate label with light energy being the final product. As little as a single photon emitted by the chemiluminescent reaction can be detected by the reader. In microparticle capture technology, particles as small as 0.2 microns in diameter are coated with the appropriate antibody or antigen and suspended in a liquid phase. The increased surface area of microparticles allows for more antigen/antibody bindings to take place. The improved kinetics allows the total assay process to be complete in less than one hour.

To assess the performance of the ChLIA assays, comparisons to commercially available ELISA and EIA methods have been performed. In these studies, the ChLIA technology showed enhanced sensitivity over traditional enzyme methods.

0698

THE USE OF MULTI MARKER RUN CONTROLS (ACCURUN 1, BBI) IN HIGHLY SENSITIVE THIRD GENERATION HIV-1 SCREENING ASSAYS.

W. Keur, J. Ariëns, H. Theunissen, J.A. Hellings
Organon Teknika B.V., P.O. Box 84, Boxtel, The Netherlands

Introduction
Improved intra-lab quality control procedures require the use of run controls, apart from the positive/negative control samples that are part of test kits from commercial companies. Multiple-marker run controls for several viral markers may be obtained from commercial sources. The availability of new, highly sensitive third generation assays necessitates evaluation of the use of run-controls, developed for earlier, less sensitive test systems.

Methods
Accurun I series 5000, 6000 and 7000 samples (positive and negative) were tested in two third generation ELISA tests for anti-HIV (Organon Teknika Vironostika HIV Uni-Form II and Murex Wellcozyme) and one second generation test (Ortho). These samples contain different levels of anti-HIV, in combination with (fixed) levels of, for instance, HBsAg, anti-HBc and anti-HTLV-I. The positive samples were tested 1:10 diluted as well. Further a dilution series of a strongly positive pool of human anti-HIV-1 positive sera was tested.

Results
The Accurun I series were all strongly positive (S/COV > 14) in the HIV Uni-Form II. In the Murex assay the values were 3.3; 6.9; 8.4 for the series 5000, 6000 and 7000 resp.. In the Ortho assay, however, we found S/COV 0.4; 0.7 and 4.9.
Accordingly, the detection limit of diluted samples in the third generation assays was much lower than that of the second generation assay (factor ≈ 100).
Dilution (1:10) of the Accurun I series 5000 (lowest titer) still gives S/COV of 4.1 in HIV Uni-Form II.

Conclusion
Run controls for intralab quality control need to be adjusted whenever new, more sensitive, generations of screening assays become available.

0699

EARLY DETECTION OF ANTI-HIV-1 IgM SEROCONVERSION USING A NEW THIRD GENERATION SCREENING ASSAY: VIRONOSTIKA HIV UNI-FORM II

W. Keur, A. Jacobs, J. v. Binsbergen, J.A. Hellings
Organon Teknika B.V., P.O. Box 84, Boxtel, The Netherlands

Introduction
Vironostika HIV Uni-Form II is a single step ELISA in a very user-friendly presentation form, with the enzyme-labeled antigen-conjugate presented as a freeze-dried sphere ready for use in the test well. The test concept: a double antigen sandwich, theoretically allows for extremely sensitive detection of antibodies of all classes (and species) including IgM, which is especially relevant for early detection of seroconversion.

Study design
Twenty commercially available anti-HIV-1 seroconversion series (181 samples) were tested by Vironostika HIV Uni-Form II, in comparison to a second generation ELISA (Ortho). An in-house IgM specific test was used to demonstrate the presence of anti-HIV-1 IgM.

Results
In 15 of 20 seroconversion series the third generation double antigen sandwich assay detects antibody earlier than second generation assays. This is clear from data of a direct comparison (Ortho) as well as from data on file with the providers of the samples.
Anti-HIV-1 IgM could be detected in all 20 series. In 16 of 20 series the earliest IgM positive sample coincided with the earliest positive sample in the Vironostika HIV Uni-Form II. In 2 cases the IgM-specific assay was positive earlier, in 2 cases later than the Uni-Form II assay.

Conclusion
Vironostika HIV-Uni-Form II provides a highly improved detection of early seroconversion to anti-HIV-1. The positivity coincides with the earliest detection of anti-HIV-1 IgM.

0701

SCREENING TEST OF HBsAg AND HIV ON BLOOD DONORS AND DIFFERENT HIGH RISK GROUPS IN THE NORTH OF VIETNAM

Nguyen Chi Tuyen, et al. National Institute of Haematology and Blood Transfusion, Bach Mai Hospital, Hanoi, Vietnam.

Hepatitis virus and HIV control are not routinely screened in blood transfusion centres (BTCs). So far only the BTC in Ho Chi Minh City and the National Blood Transfusion Centre in Hanoi are routinely screening hepatitis and HIV by ELISA blood tests.

Screening Test (HBsAg)	number	ELISA(+)	perc.
Blood donors	12,555	484	3.8
Hepatitis acute and chronic	1,481	661	44.6
Staffmember of hospital	103	12	11.6
Workers	189	36	19.0

Screening Test (HIV)	number	ELISA(+)	WB
Blood donors	17,384	2	0
Patients, suspect	1,343	0	0
Patients, polytransfusion	128	0	0
Drug addicts, I/V	260	7	0
Prostitutes	220	3	0
Prisoners	521	2	0
Matrons (W)	729	5	0
Repatriated refugees	5,328	2	0
Hotel staffmembers	150	0	0
Emigrants	777	2	0
Foreign workers	233	0	0
Total	27,073	23	0

0702

SIGNIFICANCE OF ANTI-HBc IN BLOOD DONORS. H. F. Polesky and M. Hanson. Memorial Blood Centers of Minnesota, Minneapolis, MN., U.S.A.

Routine screening of blood donors for antibody to hepatitis B core antigen (anti-HBc) was implemented in June, 1986. Since that time 5397 donations (over 10,000 components) have been discarded and more than 1500 donors permanently deferred due to reactivity in this test. More than 500 donors who were anti-HBc reactive have been non-reactive on a subsequent donation.

Of the anti-HBc reactive units 65 also were HBsAg positive, 90 were reactive by anti-HCV EIA, 5 had anti-HIV confirmed by western blot and 86 had elevated alanine aminotransferase levels.

From 1-1-90 through 12-31-93 of 254754 units drawn, 2111 (0.83%) were reactive for anti-HBc by EIA. Of these 1141 (54% were anti-HBs reactive by RIA with a ratio (sample/neg control) = >5. The presence of both anti-HBc and anti-HBs usually indicates prior infection with and recovery from HBV infection. Donors who have both antibodies are unlikely to transmit HBV to recipients.

Screening of blood donors for anti-HBc results in the loss of a significant number of components that present minimal risk to blood recipients. With the availability of sensitive screening tests to identify carriers of hepatitis C virus it may be appropriate to revise current recommendations on the use of anti-HBc in donor screening or to allow re-entry of donors who have only anti-HBc and are anti-HBs positive.

0703

HBV VACCINATION AMONG STREET DRUG ADDICTS. A SUCCESSFUL EXPERIENCE IN NORTH-EAST ITALY

S. Ciaffoni[1], N. Pauletto[1], S. Migliozzi[1], G.L. Bovo[2], F. Lugoboni[2], P. Mezzelani[3].
1 Blood Transfusion Service, Bussolengo(Verona)
2 Center for Drug Addicts, Bussolengo (Verona)
3 Institute of Clinica Medica, Verona.ITALY

Objective.Since 1985 all Intravenous Drug Users (IVDUs) attending the Centre for Drug Addicts of Bussolengo (Verona) have been tested for hepatitis B virus (HBV). 234/568 (41,2%) were seronegative.
The authors decided to carry out a campaign of vaccination. Aim of this study is to analyze the compliance with the vaccination program.
Methods. From December 1988 the seronegative IVDUs were recruited for vaccination with a recombinant vaccine requiring an initial injection followed by 1 and 6 months boosters. No favourable condition (i.e. methadone or naltrexone manteinance program, admission to hospital or therapeutic community) was given to any of the IVDUs who decided to undergo the vaccination. We only stressed the azard of HBV infection.
Results. Compliance with the vaccination program has been very high: 179 IVDUs (76,5% of HBV seronegatives)have been recruited into the vaccination program and only 12 (7%) have dropped out. Among 179 IVDUs who started the vaccination program six or more months ago, 162 (93%) have completed all 3 injections. Antibody response was measured in 105 patients, of whom 97 (92%) developed anti-HBV.
Conclusions. These data prove that a HBV vaccination program among IVDUs is feasible with a large compliance. This original experience is encouraging. We would suggest that additional HBV vaccination programs be undertaken and planning started for possible testing of hepatitis C virus and HIV vaccines with IVDUs.

0704

COMPARATIVE SENSITIVITY EVALUATION BETWEEN THE ORTHO NEW HBsAg ELISA AND LICENSED HBsAg ELISAs.

G.Green, T.Maiore, L.A.Shablesky, B.Healey, D.Achord and A.V.Le[1], J.A.Jarricot[2], G.Pizzocolo[3], P.Morel[4] and C.Janot[5].
1 Ortho Diagnostic Systems Inc., Raritan, NJ, USA, 2 J&J International France, 3 Uni. of Brescia, Italy, 4 CRTS Besancon, France, 5 CRTS Nancy , France.

ORTHO new HBsAg ELISA is an improvement of the current ORTHO Antibody to HBsAg ELISA Test System 2. Eight HBsAg licensed EIA tests were evaluated, each of which was tested separately against the ORTHO new HBsAg ELISA at ODS-Raritan. The sensitivity panels used were BBI PHA803, PEI panel, ORTHO dilutional sensitivity panel and the LNS panel. The ORTHO new HBsAg ELISA was tested in both the stationary format and agitation format. The sensitivity of the ORTHO new assay in the stationary format was equivalent to one licensed test which was used with agitation. No test kit used in the stationary format had sensitivity equivalent to ORTHO new HBsAg ELISA. All the 9 subtypes in the LNS panel were easily detected. It was clearly the best test kit when the incubation was carried out with agitation. The limit of detection was 0.2 ng/mL HBsAg/ad (ad) and 0.1 ng/mL HBsAg/ay (ay) for the BBI PHA803, 0.05 ng/mL ad and ay with the ORTHO dilutional sensitivity panel, 0.03 IU/mL ad and ay with the PEI panel and 0.12 ng/mL ad+ay with the LNS panel. The limit of detection without agitation was 0.3 ng/mL ad and ay with BBI PHA803, 0.1 ng/mL ad and ay with the ORTHO panel, 0.06 IU/mL with the PEI panel and 0.22 ng/mL ad+ay with the LNS panel. These results are consistent with the comparative field trials in which the ORTHO new HBsAg assay demonstrated sensitivity superior to the licensed test kits. When tested against 10 BBI seroconversion panels, the ORTHO new HBsAg assay detected HBsAg earlier than the 2 licensed HBsAg test kits in 50% of the cases. Consequently, the modifications made to the current ORTHO Antibody to HBsAg ELISA Test System 2 have resulted in a superior ability to detect weakly reactive HBsAg containing specimens over the licensed test kits. Comparative field trials indicated that specificity was not compromised. Specificity was greater than 99.90% (N=4125).

0705

EVALUATION OF A USER-FRIENDLY HIGH PERFORMANCE MICROELISA SYSTEM FOR DETECTION OF HBsAg

I. de Boer, P. v.d. Wiel, J.A. Hellings

Organon Teknika BV, Boxtel, The Netherlands

Objective
A new microelisa system was developed for detection of HBsAg in serum or plasma. The system is based on highly purified, fully characterized bioreagents and has a novel presentation of HRP-labeled anti-HBs in the form of a freeze dried sphere, already present in the microwell. This test, the Hepanostika HBsAg Uni-Form II, has been evaluated in-house as well as in a routine bloodbank setting to establish performance characteristics, in comparison to other commercial assays.

Methods
Sensitivity panels were based on WHO and PEI standards, as well as commercially available low-titer panels. Specificity was tested using panels of RF+ sera and sera with high levels of Hb, bilirubin, lipid and protein, respectively. Sera with up to 240.000 PEI U/ml of HBsAg were tested to study a possible high dose hook effect. In bloodbank studies over 2000 samples of fresh plasma and serum were tested. Behring Enzygnost and Abbott Auszyme tests were used as a comparison.

Results
Detection limit of the assay was found to be less than 0.06 PEI U/ml (ad) and 0.03 PEI U/ml (ay) or less than 0.14 IU/ml WHO (ad). Normalized responses found with the ACCURUN 1 multi-marker run controls series 5000, 6000 and 7000 from BBI are 2.3; 2.1 and 2.2, respectively. No reactivity was found with any of the possibly interfering samples. No high dose hook effect was found. Specificity in blooddonors was found to be better than 99.8%. All these data compare favourably to the other commercial assays. Total assay time is less than 2 hours and when the MicroPlate Processor 3000 is used lab tech time has been reduced to 3 min per plate/run.

Conclusion
Hepanostika HBsAg Uni-Form II is a highly sensitive and specific test system with an extremely user-friendly test procedure.

0706

IMMUNOASSAYS FOR HBsAg, ANTI-HBs, AND ANTI-HBc ON ABBOTT AxSYM™.

AM Spronk, LS Schmidt, BM Edwards, S Taskar. Abbott Laboratories, Abbott Park, IL, USA

A clinical study for the qualitative determination of HBsAg and anti-HBc, and the quantitation of anti-HBs on the Abbott AxSYM, a high volume, random/continuous access fully automated immunoassay analyzer, is described. Samples (in barcode labeled primary tubes or sample cups) and reagents were placed into the instrument which completes all the assay steps.

Reactivity for HBsAg and anti-HBc was based on a cutoff calculated from the signal of the negative Index Calibrator.
HBsAg Confirmatory testing was fully automated. Anti-HBs concentrations were calculated from a standard curve. The AxSYM made automated dilutions for anti-HBs samples at >1000 mIU/mL to bring them into the range of the standards.

Sensitivity on AxSYM was 0.24 ng/mL for HBsAg and 0.3 PEI Units/mL for anti-HBc. Between run reproducibility (CV) of samples near the cutoff ranged from 4 to 5.5% depending on the assay. Samples from blood donors, hospital patients, and individuals reactive (R) for HBsAg, anti-HBc or anti-HBs and with other diseases were assayed by the AxSYM and IMx® analyzers. Agreement between analyzers of the HBsAg and anti-HBc results are below. Correlation (r) of anti-HBs concentrations was 0.976 with a slope of 1.018 (N=304 reactives among 1845 specimens).

Results by AxSYM for these HBV markers have acceptable reproducibility, sensitivity and specificity with the benefits of high throughput, minimum sample handling, and test results for multiple markers from a single sample within minutes.

	HBsAg			anti-HBc		
Test Population	N	R	Agree	N	R	Agree
Blood Donors	2052	4	99.95%	1370	45	99.85%
Hospital patients	835	7	99.76%	674	71	100.00%
HBV+ & Serial bleed	277	236	98.91%*	145	136	97.24%
Anti-HBc+	NT	NT	NT	122	122	100.00%
Diseases & others	97	0	100.00%	100	34	100.00%
Total tests	3261	247	99.82%	2411	408	99.79%

*Discordant samples were confirmed by AxSYM Confirmatory.

0707

PERFORMANCE OF QUALITY CONTROL PROCEDURES FOR HBsAg ASSAYS: CONTROL CONCENTRATION VS SENSITIVITY TO ERRORS

G.Green, T.Maiore, L.A.Shablesky, D.Achord, E.Page and A.V.Le[1], R.N.Carey[2]
1 Ortho Diagnostic Systems Inc., Raritan, NJ, USA, 2 Peninsula Regional Medical Center, Salisbury, MD, USA.

Historically, positive control (PC's) for HBsAg ELISAs have been designed as reagent controls to indicate that all critical reagents have been added and are functioning properly. With minimal emphasis on demonstrating the analytical sensitivity of the assay in each run, PC's have been targeted with ODs substantially above assay cutoff. There is currently interest in providing PC's with ODs close to cutoff for the purpose of gaining information about the analytical sensitivity of this assay. Studies were conducted using the ORTHO new HBsAg ELISA. Experiments were designed to test the effectiveness of controls having various concentrations of HBsAg ranging from near cutoff to fairly strongly positive in predicting assay problems. The conjugate concentration, primary incubation time, primary incubation temperature, sample volume, substrate concentration and substrate incubation time were varied over a wide range from the prescribed conditions of the assay. Assay failure was defined as the inability to detect a specimen at the threshold sensitivity of the assay (0.1 ng/ml). These data show that, with this assay, there is a linear relationship in response to changing assay conditions between the ODs of all PC's studied (target OD 0.06 to 1.2) and the signal to cutoff ratio of the threshold standard (0.1 ng/mL). High OD PC's detected a loss in sensitivity due to reduced sample volume better than low OD PC's. In all other cases, the linear relationship was slightly stronger for the PC's with ODs substantially higher than cutoff. The within run precision was better for the high OD PCs than the low OD PC's. The results demonstrate that PC's with ODs substantially above cutoff could be at least equally effective, and may be superior to controls with OD's at or near cutoff in their ability to verify that assay performance has not been compromised, when statistically-derived control limits are used.

0708

USE OF EXTERNAL CONTROLS IN INFECTIOUS DISEASE TESTING.

M. Hanson and H.F. Polesky. Memorial Blood Centers of Minnesota, Minneapolis, MN. U.S.A.

Borderline controls prepared from "confirmed" positive units are run with each batch of donor viral marker screening assays to monitor test performance. An HBsAg control with an expected RIA ratio of 2.5 is used. Controls for EIA methods (HCV-2, HBc and HIV-1,2) have an expected sample/negative cutoff (S/CO) of 1.5-3.0.

Results from multiple lots of Abbott HBsAg (RIA), Ortho anti-HCV and anti-HBc and Genetic Systems anti-HIV-1,2 were analyzed. To determine within and between lot variation the lot mean sample/negative control (S/N) was determined for HBsAg. The lot mean S/N for the HBsAg control ranged from 2.2-3.4 for runs tested on 2 hour initial incubation and 2.3-3.8 with overnight incubation. For EIA tests the lot mean cutoff OD and the mean S/CO for in-house controls were calculated. Lot mean cutoff OD ranges for anti-HCV, anti-HBc and anti-HIV-1,2 were .695-.932, .489-.585 and .273-.290 respectively. On control samples the lot mean S/CO for anti-HCV ranged from 1.54-2.25, anti-HBc from 2.0-2.84 and anti-HIV-1,2 from 2.57 to 4.35. Less than 1% of runs had control values outside the acceptable range.

All reagents evaluated except HBsAg showed consistent reactivity within and between lots. While these controls are not used to determine the validity of test runs they are useful for monitoring variations in sensitivity and evaluating cutoff values from run to run and between reagent lots.

0709

EVALUATION OF CYTOMEGALOVIRUS INFECTION IN INFANTS FOLLOWING EXCHANGE-TRANSFUSION

T. Zandieh, S. Cavyani, M. Rakhshan, L. Hamidpour; Iraian Blood Transfusion Service, Ostad, Nejatollahy Ave, Tehran, Iran

The prevalence of IgG as well as IgM antibodies against CMV was determinded by ELISA method in 100 exchange-transfused (E-T) neonates, the mothers and the donors whose blood was used. The studies were repeated on the infants 2 months after the E-T.
A significantly higher prevalence of anti-CMV was observed in infant sera 2 months after E-T (48 %) compaired with infant sera before exchange (14 %) and with sera from mothers during feeding of infant or before that (1 %). It is concluded that newborns are at high risk for transfusion-transmitted CMV infections. It is determined that the volume of perfused blood to the infant is directly proportional to rate of transmittance of infection to infant (P 0.05), but other variables such as age, sex, blood group, and weight are independent on the basis of these results. It is suggested that: 1 - If possible, one should try to use blood that has shown anti-CMV Negative for infants being sero-negative and are born from CMV Ab-negative mothers.
2 - If it is not possible, it should be tried to use W.B.C. free-blood or blood with the least amount W.B.C. e.g. washed red blood cells.

0710

ROLE OF LEUKOCYTE DEPLETION IN THE PREVENTION OF TRANSFUSION INDUCED CYTOMEGALOVIRUS INFECTION IN THALASSEMIC PATIENTS.

T.Lombardo[1], V.Frontini[1], G.Ferro[1], P.Sergi[1], F.Di Vincenzo[2]

1Serv. Talassemia, 2Lab. Analisi Osp. Ferrarotto USL 35 Catania Italy

Blood from donors with latent human Cytomegalovirus (CMV) infection is capable of transmitting the virus to susceptible recipients. Thalassemic patients with impaired immune response and receiving transfusion therapy are at risk for transfusion transmitted CMV infection. The putative source of virus is the leukocyte and this infection can be prevented by sierological screening of blood donors or by leucocytes depletion by filtration.In order to verify the role which plays red cells (RBC) filtration to prevent CMV infection, we carried out a study on the group of the transfusion dependent thalassemic patients CMV seronegative. Since january 1987, 17 patients(9 male 8 female, ranging in age from 8 to 35 years) with thalassemia major and thalassemia intermedia(TI), were observed for serological evidence of viral infection, by the collection of serial serum samples. All the patients were regulary transfused: from 15 to 50 units/years. Two patients are undergoing at bone marrow transplantation (BMT) and 2 patients with TI had pregnancy. Every unit before transfusion was wasched on saline, centrifuged at 3000 x g for 20'. Saline and buffycoat were discarded and then RBC filtered with 3log.lab filter (Leucostop LDSS-Miramed-Mirandola-Italy). WBC residual was counted still to november 1990 in Burker chambre and then in Nageotte. Howewer residual WBC was always fewer <5 x 10 E6. Transmission of CMV was evaluated clinically and by measuring the levels of IgG anti-CMV antibodies with a specific ELISA (Sorin-Italy). None of the patients had clinical symptom or evidence of seroconversion. The data in this preliminary study indicates that filtration of blood products with 3log filters prevents the development of transfusion associated CMV infection in CMV sero negative patients undergoing transfusion therapy. In our opinion in thalassemic patients to reduce the risk is of interest for different motives: the infection is associated with substantial morbidity and mortality; some of them may be candidates for BMT. Howewer because the detection of infectious donors is not readily adaptable to the blood bank setting, WBC reduction of blood components, through filtration is a convenient and effective way to markedly reduce or eliminate the occurence of CMV infection in high-risk patients populations.

0711

ANTI-CMV SCREENING: COMPARISON OF 3 METHODS IN A SELECTED DONOR POPULATION

B de Vries, A Hoekstra, L de Boer, RL McShine, PC Das, CTh Smit Sibinga
RC Blood Bank Groningen-Drenthe, Groningen, NL

Previous anti-CMV negative (90%) and first time donor samples (10%) were comparatively tested in Abbott MEIA IMx IgG (IMx); IgG+M Behring ELISA (B) and CMV Scan Latex IgG+M anti-CMV tests. Discordant repeated results from routine work load were arbitrary subjected to an IgG and IgM anti-CMV ELISA test (University Hospital Groningen).
RESULTS:

n=260		IMx neg	B neg	IMx pos	B pos
L					
A	neg	215	217	4	2
T					
E	pos	12	12	29	29
X					

Discordant to LATEX		Positive EIA IgM	Positive EIA IgG
pos/neg	n=12	0	1
neg/pos	n= 4	0	2

Specificities: Latex 95% B 100% and IMx 99%. Sensitivities respectively: Latex 94%, B 97% and IMx 97%.
CONCLUSION: IMx and B anti-CMV tests demonstrated satisfactory, specificity and sensitivity for effective clinical use of CMV-negative blood products.

0712

MICROTITRE PLATE METHOD (MTP) FOR ROUTINE ALT SCREENING OF BLOOD DONORS : PERFORMANCE OF AN ALGORITHM TO ELIMINATE FALSE NEGATIVE RESULTS DUE TO HIGH ALT LEVEL.

M.PERNELLE[1],M.MUSSON-GENON[1],M.C.GUIMONT[2],J.M.JEGO[1]
1 SANOFI DIAGNOSTICS PASTEUR, Marnes (FRANCE)
2 Hôpital BEAUJON, Clichy (FRANCE)

Samples with high ALT level cause rapid substrate depletion resulting in absorbance values with a bad linear correlation coefficient. With very high ALT level, the substrate depletion is extremely rapid and completed in the first minute of the kinetic. These samples could display near zero enzyme units and therefore be founded false negative.In order to identify these samples without dilution, we have compared the ALT enzymatic kinetic of 41 patient sera with ALT values between 100 and 5000 UI/l with normal sera.
For this study, we used the MTP for routine ALT screening that we have developed with the ALT/GPT kit from SANOFI DIAGNOSTICS PASTEUR. Absorbance changes were monitored using a programmable rate reading photometer.
The results showed that under the assay conditions, the highest determinable value of ALT without sample dilution is between 200 and 250 UI/l. The rapid substrate depletion, which caused bad linear correlation coefficient below the accepted threshold in calculation or which caused false negative samples, was readily identifiable by the very low level of absorbance at the first minute of the kinetic.
Conclusion of this study was that we could use a cuf off value for both linear correlation coefficient and first minute absorbance. In that case we detected 100 % of samples with high ALT level (> 200 UI/l) without false negative result.

0713

EVALUATION OF A MICROPLATE METHOD FOR BLOOD DONOR ALT SCREENING

F Schmitt[1], JM Jégo[2], M Pernelle[2]
1 Laboratoire de Biochimie A, Hopital Necker, Paris, France, 2 Sanofi Diagnostics Pasteur, Marnes la Coquette, France

Introduction:

The aim of this study was to evaluate the microplate adaptation of the "ALT/GPT" kit from "Sanofi Diagnostics Pasteur".

For this, the microplate and "Cobas Fara*" adaptations of the "SDP ALT/GPT kit" and "Biotrol bireagent kit" were studied

390 donnor samples from the hospital blood bank, one sample with 300 IU/L ALT activity and two control sera with 16.4 IU/L and 8 IU/L ALT activity were simultaneously tested.

Résults:

Corrélation coefficients:

	ALT/GPT Cobas Fara	Biotrol microplate	Biotrol Cobas fara
ALT/GPT microplate	0,9488	0,9257	0,9393

Intra and interassay variability: no significative difference was shown

The quantification range of "ALT/GPT kit" analysed with dilutions of a sample with 300 IU/L of ALT activity was from 0 IU/L to 200 IU/L

Conclusion:

The microplate adaptation of the ALT/GPT kit from SDP is an efficient method for the blood donor screening with equivalent performances than the classical biochemical method.

*Cobas Fara is an automate from Roche)

0714

ALT MICROTITERPLATE QUANTIFICATION FOR BLOOD DONOR SCREENING

A Blanchard de Vaucouleurs[1], J Roger[1], JM Jégo[2], M Pernelle[2]
1 Centre de Transfusion Sanguine des Armées, Clamart, France, 2 Sanofi Diagnostics Pasteur, Marnes la Coquette, France

Introduction:

The aim of this study was to evaluate a microplate method for ALT quantification developped by "Sanofi Diagnostics Pasteur".
994 non selected samples (from male subjects) were simultaneously tested with the "Abbott method on VP" and the SDP microplate adaptation of the "SDP ALT/GPT kit" and the "Biotrol bireagent kit".
5 control samples (with 20 IU/L and 145 IU/L ALT activity) were also tested.

Résults:

Correlation coefficients:

"ALT/GPT from SDP" versus "Abbott VP": 0.8496 (y=0.88183+3.08657)
"ALT/GPT from SDP" versus "Biotrol": 0.9151 (y=0.90009+1.94493)

Inter assay variability:

	Abbott	Biotrol	SDP
20.5 IU/L control	14.76%	13.59%	10.34%
82 IU/L control	3.06%	4.38%	3.41%

Intra assay variability:

	56 IU/L control	82 IU/L control
SDP	6.46%	8.06%

Concordance levels between the three methods were greater than 99%

Conclusion:

With reproducibility equivalent to the Abbott method especially at the cut off, with a quantification range from 0 IU/L to 200 IU/L), the SDP microplate method is an efficient solution for blood donor ALT screening.

0715

EVALUATION OF THE HAMILTON MICROLAB F.A.M.E. FOR HBsAg AND ANTI-HIV 1+2

P. Bachmann, A. Rudolf, J.J. Burckhardt
ZLB Central Laboratory, Blood Transfusion Service SRC, Berne, Switzerland

The **F**ully **A**utomated **M**icroplate **E**LISA processor (Hamilton Microlab F.A.M.E.) for viral marker serology works with EIA technology. We evaluated HBsAg (Sanofi Pasteur, **routine condition** (RC) **vs F.A.M.E.**) and Anti-HIV 1+2 (Enzygnost Anti-HIV 1/-HIV 2, OWRP 20/21, Behring, RC on **BEP II vs** Wellcome Anti-HIV, VK 54/55, Murex on **F.A.M.E.**) and obtained the following results:

Result/ Marker	Sample Size	Routine Condition				Microlab F.A.M.E.			
		IR	%	RR	%	IR	%	RR	%
HBsAg	4'202	**46**	**1.09**	4	0.10	5	**0.12**	3	0.07
Anti-HIV 1+2	28'825	161	0.56	26	0.09	123	0.43	77	0.27

IR = initially reactive RR = repeat reactive

For HBsAg, the automated processing with the F.A.M.E. results in an almost tenfold reduction of IR samples!

For Anti-HIV 1+2, all of the RR samples tested under RC were negative upon confirmation. However 11/77 samples RR with the F.A.M.E. showed one or more bands in Western blot (WB); none of these was a true positive. The enhanced sensitivity of the Anti-HIV 1+2 with the F.A.M.E. most likely caused the higher rate of RR results compared to the other test under RC.

0716

EVALUATION OF A DRB 1,3,4,5 TYPING SYSTEM (INNO-LIPA) AND COMPARISON WITH PCR-SSP AND NESTED PCR-SSP

H.R. Lang, H. Beeser
Dept. of Transfusion Medicine, University Hospital Freiburg, Germany

We compared a newly developed, commercially available DRB 1,3,4,5 (rSSO) typing system with described PCR-SSP and nested PCR-SSP typing protocols.
The DRB 1,3,4,5 (rSSO) typing system is a reverse dot blot which is modified to use stripes instead of dots. All DNAs used for this study were of patient origin and were pretyped by PCR-oligotyping. The overall goal of this study was:

1. to compare the resolution of the 3 tests employed,
2. to determine the sensitivity and specificity of these tests,
3. to compare the handling of the different tests in daily routine work (acceptance by technicians).

The overall result of the study demonstrates that identical typing results are obtained with the different methods, but that in terms of reliability the rSSO test system performs much better than the other tests and obtains higher acceptance by technicians.

0717

HEMOVIGILANCE : FROM BLOOD TRANSFUSION SAFETY TO PUBLIC HEALTH. SEROLOGICAL RESULTS BEFORE SURGERY

JP. Aufeuvre[1], C.Fretz[1], A.Boudifa[1], B.Riou[2], P.Viars[2], P.Opolon[3], JJ.Fournel[1].
1-Transfusion Center, 2-Dept. of Anesthesiology, 3-Dept. of Hepatology, Hôpital Pitié-Salpêtrière, 75651 Paris cedex 13, France.

Objectives : to evaluate the serological status of every patient admitted to hospital prior to surgery as the first step of an hemovigilance program for transfused patients.
Methods : routine testing was proposed to 5216 hospitalised patients before surgery, from July 1992 to March 1993. HBs Ag, HBc Ab, HCV Ab, HIV1+2 Ab and HTLVI/II Ab were screened with ELISA tests. Retrovirus were confirmed with Western Blot and HCV Ab with Immuno Blot.
Results : 928 (17,8%) subjects were positive for at least one marker. 298 (5,7%) had a marker of an active infection of whom 21 patients were positive for 2 or more markers. Positive patients had a transfusion history more often than negative patients (p=0,0001).The prevalence of HCV infection, patients' age and chronic evolution make HCV infection a public health concern.
Conclusions :
1) prevalence of viral markers in hospitalised patients is high,
2) other routes of contamination than transfusion exist,
3) diagnosis of infection before surgery will enable counselling and early treatment. Follow up of transfused patients is in progress and will help to determine the actual incidence of transfusion transmitted viral infections.

	tested	HIV Ab	HTLV Ab	HBs Ag	HBc Ab	HCV Ab
Nber	5216	47	30	69	798	169
%		0,9	0,25	1,3	15,3	3,2

0718

RETROVIRUSES AND HEPATITIS B (HBV) AND C VIRUSES (HCV) MARKERS AMONG BREAST MILK AND BLOOD DONORS

MONCHARMONT P., VOISIN A. AND DEGOTTEX J.
C.R.T.S. LYON - BP 7015 - 69342 LYON CEDEX 07 - FRANCE

Purpose : Since 24.11.1992, anti-HIV 1+2 antibodies, anti "Human T Lymphotropic Virus I/II "(HTLV I/II) antibodies, anti-HCV antibodies and HBV surface antigen (HBs Ag), are screened in all breast milk donations in France. We have compared the prevalence of these markers in breast milk and female blood donors.
Methods : Serum samples collected in breast milk and blood donors were tested for anti-HIV 1+2, anti-HTLV I/II and anti-HCV antibodies and HBs Ag by using screening tests and if necessary by confirmation testing. Statistical analysis was performed with the X^2 test.
Results : From 1.01.1993 to 30.09.1993, 16,900 female blood donors and 559 breast milk donors were screened. Age range is from 18 up to 43 years. None blood or breast milk donors are found anti-HIV 1+2 or anti-HTLV I/II seropositive. Twenty five out of the 16,900 blood donors (0.15 %) and 3 out of the 559 breast milk donors (0.54 %) have positive or indeterminate profil in HCV RIBA 3.0 (ORTHO DIAGNOSTICS SYSTEM) (X^2 = 5.06; $p < 0.05$). None breast milk donors are HBs Ag positive but 10 are found in blood donors (0.06 %) (X^2 = 0.31; non significant).
Conclusion
Female blood donors and breast milk donors have low prevalence of retroviral markers. In the other hand, anti-HCV antibodies are more frequently observed in breast milk donors and HBs Ag remained only observed in female blood donors.

0719

PREVALENCE OF VIRAL INFECTIONS TRANSMISSIBLE THROUGH TRANSPLANTATION IN FRENCH ORGAN DONORS OVER A 48 MONTH PERIOD

Sellami F, Claquin J*, Girard M, Lefrère JJ
Hôpital Saint-Antoine, Paris *France-Transplant

Objectives: To determine the prevalence of viral infections in organ and tissue donors through serologies performed before transplantation.
Methods: From 1990 to 1993, serums from organ donors collected in Parisian intensive care units were sent to our laboratory to be virus-screened.
Results: The results per year (with percentage) over a 48 month period are given in the table:

	1990	1991	1992	1993
N°samples	424	481	424	358
anti-HIV+	8 (1.8)	7 (1.4)	10(2.3)	5 (1.3)
p24 ag+	ND	1 (0.2)	3 (0.7)	ND
HTLV-I+	1 (0.2)	0 (0)	0 (0)	1 (0.2)
HBs+	12 (2.8)	9 (1.8)	5 (1.1)	3 (0.8)
anti-HCV+	10 (2.3)	19(3.9)	14(3.3)	13 (3.6)
anti-HBc+	ND	ND	58(13.6)	43 (12.0)

Conclusions: The frequency of viral infections among organ donors from the Paris area emphasizes to reinforce policies of excluding donors at risk of viral infection, in order to increase safety with respect to organ or tissue transplantation.

0720

PREVALENCE OF HEPATITIS E VIRUS (HEV) ANTIBODIES IN BLOOD DONORS IN SPAIN

D.Castellà, M.Urrecho, M.Claparols, L.Massuet, E.Argelagués.
Banc de Sang de l'ICS. Barcelona. Spain.

Hepatitis E has been defined as enterically transmited hepatitis which causes epidemics and sporadic outbreaks in tropical and subtropical developing countries and which is associated with the ingestion of contaminated water. However, cases have occasionally been reported in Europe and USA, frequently linked to trips to endemics areas.
Material and methods. At the ICS Blood Bank in Barcelona a study was set up to determine the frequency of HEV in BD. The study included 775 samples.
An EIA test(Abbott) was used for the detection of IgG HEV antibodies in which two recombinant antigens, derived from the Burma strain and expressed in E.Coli, were used as solid phase antigens: SG-3 and 8-5.
All positive repeated samples were sent to Abbott laboratories (Illinois USA) for confirmation by supplementary analysis which included an EIA test with recombinant proteins, for the detection of specific IgM antibodies, another EIA test employing two sinthetic peptides of the Burma strain, and a Western Blot test using recombinant proteins.
Results.Of the 775 samples studied 2.8% were positives at the first determination with 2.2% being later confirmed as positive for HEV antibodies.
No samples proved specific IgM antibody positive.
Conclusion.With these results we have demostrated that sporadic cases of, HEV antibodies do exist in our country although clinically they go undetected.

0721

PHARMACOLOGY OF 8-METHOXYPSORALEN (8-MOP) AFTER INFUSION TO NORMAL HUMAN SUBJECTS. J. Stickney[1], V. Billiard[2], P. Gambus[2], J. Barr[2], L. Corash[1], J. Tessman[1], and S. Shafer[2]. [1]Steritech, Inc., Concord CA; [2]Palo Alto VA Hosp., Palo Alto CA. U.S.A.

The 2 objectives of this study were: 1. to assess the effects of escalating doses of 8-MOP (5, 10, and 15 mg infused for 60 min; N=6, each dose) on selected vital signs, and general well-being; 2. to determine the pharmacokinetics (PK) of 8-MOP administered IV. Data were collected over a 10 hr. period. The drug did not alter heart rate (HR), mean arterial blood pressure (MAP), or respiratory rate (RR). For the 15 mg dose (mean ±S.D.):

	HR beats/min	MAP mmHg	RR resp./min
Baseline	61±12	89±6	19±6
60 min	62±10	88±3	20±5
120 min	62±13	86±7	19±5
240 min	67±9	92±6	20±3

PK parameters for the 15 mg dose were: peak plasma concentration, 186±71 ng/ml; plasma elimination half time, 67 min. The volume of distribution was 0.77 l/kg and the clearance 10.1 ml/min/kg. No adverse reactions were reported. Thus, at doses greater than those required for bacterial inactivation in random donor platelets (Lin, et al. Blood **82** (Suppl.1):205a,1993), 8-MOP produced no adverse reactions, and peak plasma concentrations were comparable to those routinely observed following oral administration for treatment of psoriasis and mycosis fungoides (cutaneous T-cell lymphoma).

0722

STORAGE OF PLATELETS IN SYNTHETIC MEDIA: PRESERVATION OF *IN VITRO* PLATELET FUNCTION FOLLOWING PHOTOCHEMICAL DECONTAMINATION

L. Lin, M. Rheinschmidt, K. Metchette, L. Corten, B. Behrman, & L. Corash. Steritech Inc., Concord, CA, U.S.A.

The objective of this study was to develop a cost-effective synthetic medium: (1) to store platelets for transfusion, and (2) to prevent platelet injury during photochemical bacterial inactivation. This photochemical decontamination (PCD) technique is based on activation of 8-methoxypsoralen (8-MOP) by long wavelength ultraviolet light (UVA, 320-400 nm). Since 8-MOP binds non-specifically to serum albumin, the use of a synthetic resuspension medium with reduced plasma concentration increases the concentration of free 8-MOP in platelet concentrates (PC) and enhances PCD efficiency. In this study we evaluated three new physiological solutions: S2.22, S3.0, and S4.0. The *in vitro* function of platelets resuspended in these media with 15% residual plasma after 5 days of storage at 22°C was the same as control standard PC in 100% plasma. Following PCD treatment in S2.22, S3.0, or S4.0 under bactericidal conditions (25 ug/ml of 8-MOP and 3 Joules/cm² of UVA) in 15% plasma (**Blood** 82: 205a, 1993) and 5-day storage, *in vitro* platelet function was preserved. In contrast, when three other experimental synthetic media, PASII (**Transfu. Sci.** 11:353, 1990), AS-18 (gift from C.Y. Chong, Miles), and PSM (**Blood** 80: 260a, 1992), as well as a commercial product, Plasmalyte-A (Baxter), were similarly evaluated, *in vitro* platelet function was compromised. These results indicate that S2.22, S3.0, and S4.0 are superior storage media, and are able to protect platelets from UVA-induced damage.

0723

EVALUATION OF STANDARD PLATELET STORAGE CONTAINERS FOR USE OF PHOTOINACTIVATION OF VIRUSES USING ULTRAVIOLET-A (UVA) RADIATION

N.Yerram, S.Sowemimo-Coker, S.C.Park, T.Goodrich, P.Forster, S.Crandall. M.S.Platz* and R.Goodrich. Cryopharm Corporation, Pasadena, CA,
*Department of Chemistry, The Ohio State University, Columbus, OH, USA

Photodynamic inactivation of viral contaminants using a combination of photosensitizer and UVA light for platelet concentrates is being developed by several investigators. Since platelets do not absorb in UVA radiation (320-400 nm) spectrum, the photosensitizer present in platelet concentrate can be selectively activated with UVA radiation. In order to activate the sensitizer in platelet storage containers, the plastic material should be transparent to UVA light. Therefore, in the present study we have evaluated UVA transmission characteristics and photoinactivation efficiencies of model bacteriophage φ6 for various blood containers. We measured the UVA transmittance of seven different plastics using a UVA radiometer and spectrophotometer at a wavelength of 365 nm. The results indicate that there is a significant difference between radiometer and spectrophotometer readings. The significantly lower transmission values observed with the spectrophotometer are due to the light scattering effect. Despite this difference, 6-7 logs inactivation of model virus was obtained (300 µg/mL of CP-38, 1.2 J/cm^2) regardless of the plastic used, indicating that viral reduction levels correlated more closely with the radiometer values. Contrary to previous suggestions in studies based on spectrophotometer readings, the results in the present studies suggest that most of the plastic containers that are currently being used by most blood banks for storage of blood components can be used for photoinactivation procedures using UVA radiation.

0724

INACTIVATION OF PATHOGENIC VIRUSES IN HUMAN PLATELET CONCENTRATES WITH A NOVEL PSORALEN. S. Wollowitz, D. Cook, H. Londe, C.V. Hanson, L. Corash, L. Lin, and S. Isaacs. Steritech Inc, Concord, CA, USA.

Efficient photochemical inactivation (PCD) of viruses in platelet concentrates (PC) using UVA light requires psoralens(Ps) with enhanced nucleic acid binding and reduced dark mutagenicity. We synthesized and screened over 100 new Ps to optimize the PCD process. S-59(100 uM + 5J/cm^2 UVA), a primary amino functionalized Ps, inactivated 10 $^{5.3-5.7}$/ml cell-free and cell-associated HIV in PC, as determined by plaque assay followed by blind passage. 150 uM S-59 (3 J/cm^2 UVA), inactivated > 10 $^{6.7}$ cell-associated HIV. PCD utilizing 0.1-100 uM S-59 + 5 J/cm^2 UVA inhibited expression of p24 by latent HIV infected cells(OM 10.1). Duck hepatitis B virus(>10 ^{6}/ml), a model for HBV, was completely inactivated by S-59 (100 uM, 5 J/cm^2 UVA). Hepatitis C virus (molecular titer = 2.5 x 10 ^{5}/ml) was inactivated as demonstrated by RT-PCR inhibition assay. Stored platelets (5 days post-PCD treatment) retained in vitro function within allowable limits for transfusion. Genotoxicity of S-59 was examined in mammalian and bacterial systems. Murine micronucleus formation, Chinese hamster ovary (CHO) cell gene mutation, and CHO chromsomal aberration were acceptable. Native S-59 was weakly mutagenic in one Ames test strain (TA1537) without metabolic activation; but after PCD, S-59 was non-mutagenic in all strains. These results demonstrate that S-59 is a promising Ps for effective decontamination of PC.

0725

CLINICAL EXPERIENCE WITH OCTAGAM-A SOLVENT DETERGENT (SD) VIRUS INACTIVATED IV GAMMAGLOBULIN.
B. Brenner, Institute of Hematology, Rambam Medical Center and Bruce Rappaport Faculty of Medicine, Haifa, Israel.

Safety and efficacy of Octagam® (Octapharma), a solvent detergent (SD) virus inactivated IV gammaglobulin was evaluated in 61 patients who received 185 infusions with a total amount of 5415 grams. Half-life evaluated in 12 primary hypogammaglobulinemia patients was 28±3 days. In 25 chronic lymphatic leukemia patients and 3 multiple myeloma patients, monthly infusion of 0.4 gr/kg Octagam was safe and effective in increasing IgG levels. In 12 patients with ITP, infusion of 1-2 gr/kg of Octagam was safe and effective in increasing platelet count and in arrest of bleeding. In 6 patients with antiphospholipid syndrome monthly infusions of Octagam were found to be safe. Adverse reactions following Octagam infusion were uncommon, mostly mild and all were transient. Viral safety assays for HIV, HBV and HCV were all negative.

0726

VIRUS VALIDATION OF A NEW POLYVALENT INTRA-VENOUS IMMUNOGLOBULIN (OCTAGAM)

L. Biesert[1], A. Goudeau[2], H. Suhartono[1], L. Wang[1], H.D. Brede[1], H. Rübsamen-Waigmann[1]

1Georg-Speyer-Haus, Frankfurt/Main, Germany,
2CRTS, Montpellier, France

In-process samples of Octagam, an intravenous IgG preparation (IVIG), were spiked with both transfusion-relevant viruses and a large number of model viruses. The following steps were analysed: Cohn precipitation, solvent/detergent treatment, pH 4-step, storage at low pH in the liquid state. Aliquots collected at different times in order to obtain inactivation kinetics were titred on susceptible cells. Infectivity was determined by endpoint dilution. The virus titres were calculated according to Spearman-Kaerber. The inactivation and removal of viruses has been studied following established guidelines from the EU CPMP Ad Hoc Working Party on Biotechnology/Pharmacy.

Virus	Genome	Envelope	Step	RF*
HIV-1	RNA	yes	Cohn	≥5.5
			SD	≥5.3
			pH 4	≥7.1
PRV	DNA	yes	Cohn	≥7.3
			pH 4	≥5.4
Polio-1	RNA	no	Cohn	≥3.8
Cox-B6	RNA	no	pH 4	2.7
			storage	3.1

* RF: reduction factor (log TCID50)
The results of these representative studies demonstrated the high viral safety of Octagam.

0727

CHROMATOGRAPHICALLY MANUFACTURED INTRAVENOUS IMMUNOGLOBULIN G

VIJAYLAXMI RAY, MAYA PARIHAR, S.JOBANPUTRA & M.B.AGARWAL.

NATIONAL PLASMA FRACTIONATION CENTRE
K.E.M.HOSPITAL, BOMBAY-12 (INDIA)

Intravenous Immunoglobulin G (IV IgG) is being imported in India at enormous cost. Hence it was decided to manufacture this product at our centre. The centre is engaged in manufacture of blood products using screened starting plasma & virus sterilisation of final product.

The average yeild of IgG is about 5 gms/lt of plasma. It is found to be 90% monomeric and meets all other standards. The IgG is formulated to 5% ready to use solution & stored at 4°C.

To study the efficacy of product a clinical trial on 23 patients of ITP was carried out. 62% of the patient showed good response,17% showed partial response & about 21% showed poor response. Pre & post blood samples were tested for HBsAg & anti HIV. No viral transmission was seen in any of the patients after receiving IV IgG.

Thus IV IgG manufactured in India is found to be equally safe & effective compared to imported product. The IV IgG is also being tried in other autoimmune diseases.

0728

VIRUS FILTRATION OF FACTOR IX INCREASES PRODUCT SAFETY AND PURITY

L. Hoffer, D. Josic, H. Schwinn
OCTAPHARMA Pharmazeutika ProduktionsGmbH,
Vienna, Austria.

Applying combinations of different virus inactivation or virus removal principles the suppliers of blood products intend to reach the highest possible degree of product safety.
The efficacy of a new virus removal system (Viresolve ®) based on a tangential flow membrane filtration which was introduced in our standard Factor IX (F IX) production protocol was evaluated. At present Viresolve 70 and Viresolve 180 membranes are available having exclusion limits of 70 and 180 kD respectively. Virus retention potency was measured with different model viruses (Polio, SV-40, Sindbis, Reovirus-3). Log reduction values were between 3.5 and 7.2 and are strongly dependent on virus diameter.
While performing filtration additional purification of the product occured. So far 3 trial batches starting from 1000 kg plasma were run. The routine F IX production process includes solid phase extraction, chromatography and the solvent/detergent virus inactivation. At the stage of virus filtration 15 kg of F IX-solution with an average contents of 30 IU/ml and 80-120 U/mg protein specific activity are to be processed. After filtration an increased specific activity of F IX close to theoretical values was found. High molecular weight impurities were retained by the membrane, wich could be demonstrated clearly by SDS-Polyacrylamide-electrophoresis.

0729

A Double Virus-Inactivated, Highly Purified Factor VIII-Concentrate

H. Schwinn, M. Stadler, Dj. Josic, F. Bal, W. Gehringer, I. Nur and R. Schütz
Octapharma AG, Haus im Park, CH-8866 Ziegelbrücke, Switzerland

In an assessment of the risks of virus transmission by clotting concentrates it is clear that the currently practised procedures for virus inactivation are not equally effective against all types of viruses; neither a pasteurisation nor the Solvent Detergent (S/D) process alone are adequate enough to inactivate viruses that are strongly resistant to heat and organic solvents. In this connection, human parvo virus B19 and hepatitis A virus (HAV) are of particular concern. In order to improve this situation which still poses a risk to the haemophiliac patients, we have developed a more effective pasteurisation process that could be easily applied to our factor VIII (FVIII)-process in addition to the S/D-treatment already well-established. We were prompted to initiate experiments using temperatures above 60°C by two recent publications, which demonstrate that HAV becomes instable at temperatures exceeding 62°C. It is the purpose of this paper to present our progress in:

- achieving a pasteurisation procedure for FVIII at 63°C for 10 hours with no discernible change in the structure of the factor VIII/von Willebrand factor (FVIII/VWF)-complex owing to a newly developed composition of stabilizers
- applying this pasteurisation procedure to a purified FVIII fraction, that has already been submitted to a S/D-treatment: Doing so, we are able to perform two independent virus inactivation steps, as has been recommended (IABS-Meeting in Cannes, France, November 1992).
- introducing a second purification step on an anion exchange resin, achieving an additional virus reduction over our presently manufactured FVIII preparation.

Numerous animal studies proved the double virus-inactivated FVIII concentrate to be well-tolerated and without side-reactions. The effectivity of the 63°C heating step against different types of non enveloped and enveloped viruses is published elsewhere.

0730

Extraction of Triton X 100 and its Analysis in Human Plasma, Virus Inactivated by the Solvent / Detergent Method

Ales Strancar
BIA d.o.o., Adamiceva 4, 61000 Ljubljana, Slovenia
Horst Schwinn and Djuro Josic
Octapharma Produktionsges.m.b.H., Oberlaaer Str. 235, A-1100 Wien, Austria

For the inactivation of lipid-enveloped viruses during the production of fresh frozen and lyophylized human plasma the solvent/detergent method developed by Horowitz at al. was applied (Horowitz, B.; Bonomo, R., Prince, A.M. Chin, S.N., Brotman, B. 8 Shulman, R.W. Blood 79 (1992), 826). In this process, the solvent tri-n-butylphosphate is removed by extraction with castor oil. The removal of non-ionic detergent Triton X 100 is performed by solid-phase extraction using reversed-phase. Different polymer- and silica based supports were tested. The highest capacity for Triton X 100 was achieved with C_{18} silica gels. These supports bound more than 0.1 ml Triton X 100 per one ml support. In practice, none of the proteins, e.g. clotting factors, bound to the support and therefore, flow through the column. Their biological activity was hardly affected.

Another main application of such sugars is far quantitative: detergent analysis during the production process. The use of special columns allowing direct sample injection could be introduced. It is a simple method for very fast in-process analysis of Triton X 100 in human plasma by reversed-phase chromatography under isocratic conditons.

0731

PRACTICAL INTEGRITY TEST METHOD FOR VIRUS REMOVAL FILTER FROM THE VIEWPOINT OF PROCESS VALIDATION

H. Nakano[1], T. Sato[1], T. Noda[1], S. Manabe[1],
1. Asahi Chemical Industry Co., Ltd., Tokyo, Japan

It is necessary for the each production lot of plasma fractionation products to make sure that all the process worked well.

In this meaning, integrity test is necessary for each production lot to make sure that filtration process for virus removal worked well.

Integrity test should be considered to detect any kind of pore size change which affects the virus removability.

Two typical pore size changes are conceivable during filtration as follows;

(case 1) Extremely large pores formed by the breakage of membrane

(case 2) Pore size distribution shifts to the larger mean pore size

Case 1 is the supposed worst case for the correlation between virus removal and integrity test value.

Taking both case 1 and case 2 into consideration, novel integrity test method was developed.

Which is composed of the combination of the leakage test and the gold particle removability test or the leakage test and the liquid forward flow test.

0732

SMALL SIZE VIRUS REMOVAL MECHANISM AND ITS REMOVABILITY BY THE FINTRATION OF "PLANOVA15"

T. Sato[1], H. Nakano[1], S. Manabe[1], A. M. Losokoff[2],
1. Asahi Chemical Industry Co., Ltd., Tokyo, Japan
2. BRFF, Ijamsville, MD, USA

Recently, several problems were reported for the plasma derived products contaminated with small size viruses, such as Hepatitis A virus and Parvo virus.

Newly developed filter "PLANOVA15" is very effective for the removal of small size viruses possible in the plasma derived products.

This filter was validated using polio virus as the model virus, and therefore it can remove, for example, polio virus, Parvo virus and Hepatitis A virus effectively.

In this presentation, the removal mechanism of small size viruses using "PLANOVA15" filters and the actual removability were introduced.

For example, logarithmic rejection coefficient of polio virus is more than 4.5 (average is more than 6.0), Parvo virus is about 4.3 and Hepatitis A virus is also more than 4.0.

"PLANOVA15" is already used for the commercial plasma derived Factor-IX product in Japan, and also for the plasma derived Factor-VIII product in USA in the near future.

0733

EFFECT OF VARIOUS FACTORS ON THE RATE OF INACTIVATION OF THE MODEL VIRUS, SINDBIS, DURING LOW pH INCUBATION OF INTRAVENOUS IMMUNOGLOBULIN

Andrew MacGregor, I.F. Young, R.W. Herrington
Bioplasma, CSL Limited, Melbourne, Australia

In order to assess the tolerance of the low pH virus inactivation step used in the Intragam® process at CSL (process licensed from Pharmaceutical Division, Miles Inc. - identical to their process for Gamimune-N®) to deviations from the specified conditions, the effects of varying pH, immunoglobulin concentration, protein concentration and temperature on the rate of inactivation of the lipid-enveloped model virus Sindbis were studied.

At a temperature of 27°C and at pH 4.25, more than 6 logs ($TCID_{50}$) of virus were inactivated in 3 days. Rate of inactivation slowed significantly at pH 5 or above.

When the temperature was held at 0°C and the pH at 4.25, there was no detectable inactivation of virus over a three week period. Furthermore, at 35°C the rate of inactivation was significantly greater than that observed at 27°C.

When protein concentration was increased, the rate of virus inactivation also increased, but this was not related to the presence of specific antibodies to Sindbis in the immunoglobulin preparation.

These results support the efficacy with respect to the destruction of lipid-enveloped viruses of the conditions of incubation which are employed for the virus inactivation step in the manufacture of Intragam®.

Intragam® is a registered trademark of CSL Limited.
Gamimune-N® is a registered trademark of Miles Inc.

0734

VIRUS INACTIVATION AND REMOVAL DURING THE PURIFICATION OF HIGH PURITY FACTOR IX 9MC/REPLENINE

P.L. Roberts, C.P. Walker
Bio-Products Laboratory, Elstree, Herts., UK.

Treatment of prothrombin complex concentrate, an intermediate in the 9MC/Replenine high purity factor IX process, with solvent/detergent (0.3% Tri-n-butyl phosphate/1% Tween 80) was evaluated in laboratory 'spiking' studies and shown to be effective in inactivating a range of enveloped viruses. In addition, the subsequent copper chelate affinity chromatography step was also shown, using a small-scale model, to contribute to virus reduction. Significantly, this step was effective against non-enveloped viruses such as the hepatitis-A-like picornavirus polio, as well as enveloped viruses. Virus reduction values for the two process steps are given below.

Virus	Virus Reduction (log) Solvent/ Detergent	Affinity Column	Total
Sindbis	≥7.1	6.9	≥14.0
VSV	>5.5	-	>5.5
HSV-1	>5.6	-	>5.6
Vaccinia	2.4	≥5.9	≥8.3
HIV-1	≥6.3	-	≥6.3
Polio-1	0.0	4.6	4.6

0735

COMPARISON OF HAEMOGLOBIN TESTS BY HAEMOCUE[R] AND SYSMEX K1000 IN 211 DONORS

J.de Wildt-Eggen, M. Bins
Bloodbank Zwolle, the Netherlands

During two months Hb-test of 162 donors, who did not meet the Hb-criterium (m<8.4, f<7.8 mmol/l) as determined by Haemocue (fingerprick; method A) were compared with the Hb-tests from the Sysmex K1000 (venous blood, EDTA; method B). As a control Hb-tests were also compared in 49 donors with Hb-values passing this criterium.

Results:	Method A	Method B	(A-B)
mean duplo	0.18±0.12	0.02±0.04	0.32±0.29
range duplo	0-0.8	0-0.2	0-1.85
mean low Hb	7.5±0.4	7.5±0.5	
mean norm Hb	8.8±0.7	8.8±0.6	

Conclusion: The mean values of the Hb-values were the same for methods A and B, although the mean difference between both was 0.32 mmol/L. The difference between duplo-determinations was much smaller in method B. Of the donors (n=162) who were rejected for low Hb by method A 24 would have passed the Hb-test by method B. Of the donors who met the criteria (n=49) in method A one would have been rejected by method B.

0736

HIV EDUCATION : AN UNUSUAL TRANSFUSION RESPONSE

J M Pearce, C Sims, A van Zyl

Western Province Blood Transfusion Service

Our participation in a gay-associated voluntary HIV study in 1984 gave us experience and insight into counselling. Subsequent voluntary work and continuous exchange of information has further maintained our credibility with this association and decrease Pattern I type transmission to our recipients. When testing was introduced to our Service in 1985, we continued counselling our own positive donors, sexual partners and families. Until alternative test sites were available we offered counselling and testing to 300 "high risk" individuals to minimise the misuse of the donation process for this purpose. Due to our experience and knowledge, we have advised many developing AIDS intervention organisations and now have a wide network of medical, legal, psychosocial contacts and services which can be used to the ultimate benefit of our HIV positive donors. Our counselling staff are also responsible for the Autologous Unit, Transfusion Transmitted Disease investigations and HIV look back programme. The senior member supervises Public Relations, Donor Promotions, Records and Clinic procedures. This integrated system ensures rapid feedback of changing epidemiological data which can be implemented in new screening procedures, as well as current statistical information for potential recipients, medical practitioners and press. Our screening techniques and teaching programmes have been adopted by other organisations and disseminated elsewhere in the continent. The open and responsive attitude to the risks involved in transfusion has improved public perception and resulted in responsible press reporting.

0738

AVIS AND ITALIAN TRANSFUSIONAL SERVICE.

V. Saturni, G. Marescotti, G. Callegari, Bosello, G. Dian.
Area Sanitaria AVIS Nazionale.

The blood voluntary association AVIS was born in Italy in 1927, among the first European nations and since it acts to divulge the blood donation's culture in all over national territory. It results divided in: municipal, provincial and 22 regional structures. Our targets: - scolastic and universitary popolation; - organized group; - family medical doctors; - mass-media and blood donors.Our instruments: - audiovisival material; - newspapers (Es. "TUTTINSIEME"); - scientific meetings. Our aims: - to mantein informed the AVIS members; - to give the instruments for a coscience of the donation to the non members; - to make sanitary culture about the donation-transfusion themas. These activities have permited us to reach very important results. At 31/12/92 infact the AVIS members, all periodic, anonimous, voluntary and non remunerated donors, were 777.241, with 1.356.632 blood donations and with a donation index of 1,74. Of particular interest is the increment of donors/population ratio (1,292 in 1987 and 1,403 in 1991). Furthermore we have sensitized our blood donors to apheresis, with good results. The AVIS (regulated by its own "Statuto") and all transfusional activity are governated in Italy by Law 107/90. Therefore AVIS is a propositive strenght of great impact into the social , sanitary and solidaristic Italian substrate, with great benefits for our transfusional system.

0739

DONOR RECRUITMENT PROBLEMS IN THE CZECH REPUBLIC

V. Veselý

Blood Transfusion Center, Medical Faculty Hospital, Praha 2, Czech Republic

Rather simple altruistic model of blood donation was expected after political changes in the year 1989 in Czechoslovakia, now Czech Republic.

Underestimated blood donor recruitment policy lasting for years, necessary changes in blood production and supply, and general attitudes of the public makes not only the substantional changes impossible but substantional measures must be taken to prevent further deterioration of the recruitment policy.

The scientific Society Blood of Transfusion Medicine plays an important role in the task not to deteriorate the voluntary non-remunarated universal blood donation and mantaining the blood supply and national self-sufficiency.

0740

DONOR MANAGEMENT INFORMATION SYSTEM: AN INVESTMENT IN THE FUTURE.

Los APM, Smit Sibinga CTh.
R.C. Blood Bank Groningen-Drenthe, NL

Adequate evaluation of policy on motivation, recruitment and retention of blood donors forms an essential aspect of donor management. Registration of relevant donor characteristics in an Extended Donor Data Base (EDDB) provides opportunities for systematic evaluation of donor policies.
APPROACH: Existing donor database is extended with new variables: reason & location registration, donation in labour-hours y/n, average donation time, way of traveling to donor-site (time & distance), reason of resignation (deferral). These data are obtained from the donors through interviews / questionnaires, coded, and entered in the EDDB.
PROSPECTIVE: Continuous entry in the EDDB of data obtained, provides a dynamic and growing data pool for continuous consultation. In the EDDB donors can be 'followed' anonimously. Example: first-time donors are flagged according to reason / location of registration (action A or B). The long term effect of action A and B can be evaluated in terms of donor career (registration period) of newly registered donors, and donor retention (% deferrals + reasons). Lapse of donors can be related to circumstances (donation in labour-hours, necessary donation time, reasons / location of registration, etc.).
CONCLUSION: New registrations and lapse can now be followed systematically. Choices can be made for policy measures which are most effective (long term) in relation to efforts and costs, and which guarantee a stabile and consequently safe donorbase.

0741

BLOOD TRANSFUSION AND AIDS: RESULTS OF SELF-EXCLUSION PROGRAM AND ANTI-HIV TESTING IN THE NORTH OF THE NETHERLANDS 1983-1993.

Los APM[1], de Vries AH[1], de Wit HJC[2], Smit Sibinga CTh[1].
1R.C. Blood Bank Groningen-Drenthe, 2R.C. Blood Bank Friesland, the Netherlands

Since April 1983, blood donors are informed on risk factors for HIV infection and asked to refrain from donation if a risk factor is apparent (self-exclusion program). Since May 1985 each donation is screened for anti-HIV. Results of both policy measures are compared and presented in terms of safety of blood transfusion practice.
RESULTS: Donorbase extended from 60,000 (1983) to 75,000 donors (1993). Yearly deferral because of an indicated risk factor is around 60 donors (total 662). Total number of tested donations: 765,000 since 1985. HIV positive donations: 12 (0.0016%) of which 5 (0.0006%) seroconversions. All HIV positive donors had a risk factor which was denied and/or not mentioned at donor interview. Look back of previous donations (seroconversions only) revealed no contamination. Total amount of blood products from screened donations, distributed to regional hospitals: > 1.1 million, from which there was no clinical report of HIV transmission.
CONCLUSION: Adequate information to donors on risk factors and continuous evaluation on efficacy of information, combined with anti-HIV screening are the best guarantee to prevent transfusion associated HIV infection. The policy of self-exclusion and anti-HIV screening has resulted in safe blood products and therefor a safe blood transfusion practice in the North of the Netherlands over the past ten years.

0742

EPIDEMIOLOGICAL CHARACTERISTICS OF PATIENTS RECEIVING RED CELL TRANSFUSIONS

Mahes de Silva[1], D S Wijayatilake[2]
[1]North London Blood Transfusion Centre, [2]Charing Cross Hospital Medical School, London UK.

A knowledge of the characteristics of patients requiring blood transfusion is valuable for planning blood collections. The blood groups of the patients, their ages and the diseases for which transfusions are given all provide useful information. This information may also be helpful in making decisions regarding tests that are done on blood donations.

A retrospective study was carried out on patients who received blood transfusions during a three month period at 7 large hospitals in London.

2591 patients received red cell transfusions, an average of 370 patients at each hospital. A total of 8132 red cell units were transfused.

1205 patients were male and 1386 were female.

The blood group distribution of patients receiving red cell transfusions was as follows:

Blood group	O	A	B	AB	RhD+	RhD-
% of patients	44	41	12	3	83	17

The age distribution of patients receiving red cells was as follows:

Age (years)	0 to 12	13 to 60	>60
% of patients	7	37	56

Surgical patients accounted for 48% of patients who were transfused, 24% had haematological diseases and 16% of patients were treated for other medical conditions. The reason for transfusion was not available for 12% of patients.

0743

A PESSIMIST'S SCENARIO: BLOOD SUPPLY PROBLEMS IMMINENT IN U.S.

Leslie H. Vogt, Virginia Blood Services, Richmond, Virginia, USA.

While the collection of allogeneic whole blood in the United States declined only slightly (-0.2%) from 1988-1992, blood donations will decline dramatically in the next two years causing the blood delivery system to become dysfunctional. Hospitals have formed or joined consortia that negotiate contracts with low-cost blood providers regardless of geographic relationships. Blood shortages now occurring because of business downsizing, seasonal variations, and ineffective recruitment techniques will be exacerbated by the new procurement methods. The blood "substitutes" now being developed for specialized uses will further confuse donors, who may erroneously assume their blood is no longer needed. Blood, viewed as a commodity by consortia, will become harder to obtain from donors who have always thought they were giving blood for use in their own communities. Donors and businesses will stop contributing blood and time to their local blood center. Blood will become a high-cost, rationed drug. Unable to affect donor behavior to counteract negative effects of this environment, blood centers will issue repeated emergency pleas that will be ignored, forcing centers to seek blood from other countries, where quality and safety procedures may differ. The system, burdened by blood shortages and ineffective management techniques, will collapse.

0744

COMMUNICATING EFFECTIVELY WITH DONORS

P.J. Miscall, A.M. Rose, American Institutes for Research, Washington D.C., USA.

Effective communication with blood donors can help to reduce the chances of transmission of HIV and other infectious diseases via transfusion. In many countries, high levels of HIV incidence is causing concern for the safety of the blood supply. Current blood tests are good, but the "window period" between infection with HIV and detection of HIV antibodies is an obstacle for all transfusion services. With this in mind, we must focus on effective communication techniques to improve the safety and adequacy of the blood supply.

To address these issues, the World Health Organization/Global Programme on AIDS supported a research effort by the American Institutes for Research (AIR). The purpose of this effort was to develop practical recommendations to improve blood donation systems in developing and economically restricted countries. The focus of this effort was on improving methods to more effectively recruit, educate, and retain voluntary, non-remunerated donors.

Communication materials used to recruit and retain blood donors were examined from many countries. Three transfusion programmes in developing countries were examined through in-depth investigation on site. Workshops were conducted with staff from several sites in each country. Working with these transfusion programs, recommendations for recruiting, educating, and retaining safe donors were developed.

The recommendations demonstrate that improvements in communication can be made with limited resources. Increasing staff involvement in a donor communication program, increasing the involvement of key local and national leaders, and monitoring and evaluating the impact and effects of the program will lead to a strategy which will be appropriate for each country.

0745

Blood Service Restructuring in New Zealand

D G Woodfield
Department of Transfusion Medicine, Auckland, NZ.

Internationally, health costs are increasing and this is a problem in Western countries. Because of this, health restructuring in NZ has taken place. The new format is based on contestability and competition between health providers. The public health service is to remain substantially funded by the taxpayer. It is postulated that the changes will stabilise costs of health care.

Blood Services are to have policies consistent with overall health directions. All voluntarily collected blood is now placed under the stewardship of a Blood Transfusion Trust, that controls permits required for blood collection, and approves Contracts for blood processing and its supply to health providers. Six regional blood services are replaced by 23 Hospital based Crown Health Enterprises (CHE), each with responsibility for their own blood services. Competition between CHE for the collection, processing and supply of blood is envisaged. Blood services are to have zero budgets and will retrieve all costs from a CHE, which is funded by one of four Regional Health Authorities, in turn funded from Government. No direct charges will be made to patients in private or public hospitals for the supply of blood and blood products.

The objective is to control blood transfusion expenditure, and retain the voluntary donation system without any charges being passed on directly to patients. Current policies of national self sufficiency in blood are to be maintained. These policies are a new method to ensure that competition and contestability are part of the future policies of Blood Services in New Zealand.

0746

HOW TO PROMOTE THE BLOOD DONATION IN THE UNIVERSITARY COLLECTIVE.

Flores, J.A.; Roig, R.J.; Rey, E.; Puente, V. y García - Villaescusa, R.

GALICIA REGIONAL BLOOD TRANSFUSION CENTER. SANTIAGO DE COMPOSTELA (SPAIN)

In this paper we present our experience and results in the first campaing to promote blood donation in the Santiago de Compostela University (SCU).

MATERIAL.- The SCU is divided in two different campus (north and south) and has about 29.500 students registered. They are distribuied in 15 Faculties and 6 Universitary Schools.

METHODS.- The work to promote blood donation in this field was divided in the next items: (1) The blood promotion team had a meeting with all Deans, School Directors and Students Representatives to show our intentions and ask for their collaboration. (2) Distribution of publicitary supports (videotape, posters, brochures, information and quotation letters to blood donors), and (3) Small talks, course by course, and room by room, in each and everyone Faculties and Scools of this universitary district.

CONCLUDING REMARKS.- In this first campaign we have reached 1.704 blood donations. The 99 % of these are new blood donors. The percentage between men / woman there was about 32 % for men and 68 % for women. The age was since 18 to 37 in the 77 % of these new blood donors.

0747

MOTIVATION OF DONORSHIP IN AZERBAIJAN

Ch.D.Asadov
Institute of Haematology and Blood Transfusion, Baku, Azerbaijan

There are two donor types in Azerbaijan: active and voluntary donors. Active donors are those who donate blood (plasma, blood cells) on regular basis with certain intervals. They do it for the financial inducement and represent about 10% of all donors. About 40% of voluntary donors are donors-relatives. The research was carried out using the method of anonymous questionnaires and was aimed at the study of various characteristics of donorship motivation in Azerbaijan. The main tasks of the research were: to examine sexual, age, educational, employment aspects in motivation of donorship; to reveal drawbacks in practical work of stationary and mobile blood supply service as viewed by donors; to find out the administration's reaction to the participation of its employee in donor activity. The analysis shows that 30% of donors give their blood voluntarily "to help a sick man"; 20% do it for money or extra free days; the rest indicate a number of various reasons, either connected with the privileges that are given to donors, or with moral standards. Having analysed the attitude of different social and age groups to donorship, we shall be able to approach the donorship propaganda in different ways.

0748

VARIATIONS IN BLOOD COLLECTION IN GREECE

C. Politis, J. Yfantopoulos
Hellenic Red Cross Blood Transfusion Centre, Athens, Greece.

The regionalization of health services has been a prime objective of the health care system worldwide. However, in Greece, despite the legislative intentions of various governments a comprehensive regionalization of health services has not yet been achieved. In the blood sector, from the analysis of data at na'tional level, we note 24.46 patients discharged per hospital bed, 9.45 blood donations per bed and 0.38 donations per patient discharged. These figures fit in the world bank category of the industrial market countries as calculated by Leikola in WHO/ISBT regions (the corresponding figures are 7-9 donations per acute hospital bed and 0.41 donations per hospital admissions). However, the analysis of data at regional level yields significant discrepancies in the blood collection and distribution per population, hospital bed and patient discharged from hospital. At a prefecture level there is also variation in the blood donation from the patients' environment and volunteers, which is partly explained by differences in the GDP per capita. Further analysis is required to assess the relative needs of the population in conjunction with the medical and socio-economic establishment. We would also approximate the medical aspects by using a crude indicator of hospital beds per population. These indices suffice to provide a general picture of the factors that influence the supply of health services at a county and regional level.

0749

BLOOD DONORS DEFERRAL. COMPARISON BETWEEN VOLUNTARY AND DIRECTED DONORS.

K. Maragos, J. Spiliotopoulou, N. Sevastos, L. Dadiotis, N. Vgontza, G. Theodossiadis, A. Lagiandreou, E. Digenopoulou, J. Georgopoulos, Ir. Kontopoulou
1st R.T.C. Hippokration Hospital, Athens, Greece.

A safe blood supply can be established through intensive selection of donors and blood screening. In Greece, a country of 10 million inhabitants, 500.000 units of blood are donated yearly. Despite the effort to establish a voluntarily donated blood supply, till now, the major source of blood (60%) comes form the non renumerated directed donors from patient's families. In an effort to clarify the deferral rate and the reasons for it, between non renumerated voluntary and directed donors we prospectively analyzed the causes of deferral of 15.593 donors, 4.082 were voluntary and 11.510 directed. The overall deferral was 2.490 (15,96%), 292 (7,15%) for the voluntary and 2.198 (19,09%) for the directed.

analysis of the reasons for deferral

reasons	total	voluntary	directed
medical history: a) permanent	3,18%	0,85%	4,01%
b) temporary	5,14%	1,88%	6,29%
clinical evaluation	7,62%	4,38%	8,77%

The most common causes of deferral were anemia and abnormal blood pressure. From our findings it becomes obvious that voluntary blood donors are aware about the restrictions and rules for blood donation that have introduced to protect donors and recipient. A safe blood supply can be established through voluntary donation and not directed one. A vigorous effort has to be applied towards this direction through education-motivation of the general population.

0750

TRANSFUSION MEDICINE IN BULGARIA - PRESENT STATUS AND FUTURE PERSPECTIVES

M.Kirova, D. Shinkov
National Centre of Clinical and Transfusion Haematology
Sofia 1756 , Bulgaria

The present status of transfusion medicine in Bulgaria does not meet the requirements of hospital practice. The grave decrease of the number of voluntary blood donors from 44 per 1000 in 1988 to 24 per 1000 in 1992, the outdated equipment (blood collecting in glass bottles), the improper use of blood (33% of the donated blood transfused as whole) brought a serious shortage of blood components and particularly of plasma products (in 1993 was produced 194000 I.E. cryoprecipitate and 24 kg albumin per 1 mln population.

The deep crisis imposed a revision of the global strategy in transfusion medicine. Three main programs were developed: for blood donor recruitment, for the reconstruction and reorganisation of the transfusion network and program for its technological renewal. This includes the fast possible introduction of plastic bags in the blood banks, a measure which is expected to increase the amounts of donated blood by 12000 l, and those of plasma by 8000 l (donated by the same number of donors).

Another measures is the renovation of the system for post graduate specialist training and the establishment of a program for undergraduate medical training in transfusion medicine.

0751

SELF-EXCLUSSION IN BLOOD DONORS

MARIN-LOPEZ A.+*; LOPEZ-PARRA S. * ; BRAVO-HERNANDEZ G; HERNANDEZ-DE-LOJO JM.*

* MEDICINA TRANSFUSIONAL Y HEMATOLOGIA DE PUEBLA.
+ HOSPITAL GENERAL DE PUEBLA

INTRODUCTION.- TRANSFUSIONAL MEDICINE SERVICES INCLUDE PROCEDURES SUCH AS THE SELF-EXCLUSION METHOD TO DRECREASE THE FREQUENCY OF TRANSMISSIBLE DISEASES FOUND IN BLOOD DONORS BY THE USE OF A QUESTIONAIRE WHICH EACH DONOR MUST COMPLETE PRIOR TO THEIR DONATION.

MATERIALS AND METHODS.- FROM JANUARY 1992 TO OCTOBER 1993, 2096 BLOOD DONORS WERE INCLUDED IN THIS STUDY. EACH APPLICANT WAS TO FILL OUT A QUESTIONAIRE CONCERNING THE SELF-EXCLUSION METHOD.

RESULTS.- 154 (7.34%) OF 2096 BLOOD DONORS WERE EXCLUDED FOR THE FOLLOWING REASONS: 26 (1.24%) FOR ANEMIA, 10 (0.48%) FOR MEDICINAL THERAPY PRIOR DONOR, 11 (0.52%) HIGH RISK PATIENTS, 7 (0.33%) FOR TATOOS. ONLY 20 (0.95%) OF THE 2096 BLOOD DONORS ANSWERED THE QUESTIONAIRE STATING THAT THEIR BLOOD WAS SAFE WITHOUT THE RESULTS OF SEROLOGICAL TESTING, WHICH GAVE NEGATIVE RESULTS. 1922 BLOOD DONORS ANSWERED THE SAME QUESTIONAIRE STATING THAT THEY ALSO HAD SAFE BLOOD YET THEIR SEROLOGICAL RESULTS CAME BACK POSITIVE FOR THE FOLLOWING: 2 (0.10%) FOR HIV, 8 (0.41%) FOR HVC, 3 (0.15%) FOR VBH AND 12 (0.62%) FOR Hbc.

DISCUSSION.- THE DATA RECEIVED REVEALS THAT THE NUMBER OF DONORS WHICH HAD POSITIVE SEROLOGICAL TESTING WAS NOT ANY LESS THAN THE NUMBER OF DONORS WHICH PARTICIPATED IN THE SELF-EXCLUSION METHOD.

0752

HIV INCIDENCE IN WESTERN CAPE DONORS

J M Pearce, B Gibbs, C Sims, B Hinde

Western Province Blood Transfusion Service, Cape Town

This study outlines the incidence of HIV positivity amongst Western Cape donors. Initially our confirmed positive donations were from predominantly male homosexuals (Pattern 1 infection) changing quite abruptly in 1991 to heterosexual males and females (Pattern 2 infection). 75% were new donors with 25% being repeat donors. 3 donors had seroconverted between donations. Look back was instituted in all recipients of repeat donors. With the exception of 4 donors identified in 1985 at the start of testing, no transfusion transmitted disease infections have been found amongst recipients from known donor seroconversions. A total of 1020396 donations have been tested with only 91 positive donations, an incidence of 0,008%. This compares favourably with the national donation incidence of 0,05%.

Significant changes in donor screening questionnaires were instituted in 1991 to accommodate behaviour risks apparent in our Pattern 2 donors. Personal interviews were initiated for certain clinic venues and will be phased in throughout the region in early 1994. Demographically and geographically the Western Cape has an overall low incidence of HIV in comparison to South Africa as a whole, as evidenced by prevalence surveys in regional antenatal clinics, and those reported to the South African Institute for Medical Research.

0753

THREE DONOR GROUPS TESTING FOR ANTI HCV-ANTIBODIES.

M-K. Sultsmann

Tartu Univercity Maarjamõisa Hospital Laboratory of Immunoanalysis, Tartu, Estonia

One of the problems of Estonian blood transfusion service is the diagnostic of hepatitis C. We screened blood sera of donors of Tartu and South-Estonia. The screening was performed by Helsinki Red Cross Blood Transfusion Service and Maarjamõisa Hospital Laboratory of Immunoanalysis. We used ELISA-method for detecting HCV antibodies: Behring, Organon-Teknika, Wellcozyme/Murex, ORTHO.

We tested 900+1570+654 donors. The prevalence of anti HCV-ab was 0,7 %. The results need to be controlled by confirmatory tests (e.g. ORTHO RIBA 2). The group of 654 donors was studied in addition as for fermentative function of liver (ALT; AST; γ-GT) and comparatively anti HBc total and HBsAg.

Analysing the results of group diagnostic and comparing the prevalence of different indicators it proves true that estimating of surrogate marker anti HBc total and the activity of ALT is not sufficient to guarantee safe transfusion. Specific tests are most reliable for detecting anti HCV. We must find opportunity for virus diagnostic according to the experience of developed countries.

0754

INCIDENCE OF HEPATITIS B SURFACE ANTIGEN AND ANTI-HIV IN BLOOD DONORS IN BOMBAY

DR. MAYA PARIHAR, DR. V.RAY

Department of Transfusion Medicine,
K.E.M.Hospital, Parel, Bombay, India

In India, screening of blood for HBsAg & anti-HIV 1 & 2 is mandatory. At our centre, from 1989-1993, screening results of 1,15,009 donors were compiled to know the incidence of these viruses. Our is a public hospital based Blood Bank with 40% relative replacements from the lower socio-economic strata and 60% voluntary donations.

% POSITIVITY OF UNITS COLLECTED

YEAR	HBsAg	Anti-HIV	
1989	3.6#	0.8	Method : **ELISA**
1990	3.3	0.6	# RPHA + ELISA
1991	2.7	1.6	* Anti-HIV 1&2
1992	2.7	2.0	introduced
1993	2.2	1.9*	

Relative donors showed a higher positivity for both HBsAg and Anti-HIV than the voluntary donors. Similarly, males had a higher positivity as compared to female donors.

Though the incidence of HBsAg is higher in our part of the world, a recent study on Anti-HCV among 1000 donors showed an incidence of 1.16% which is similar to that reported in the Western population. This test is not yet mandatory.

0755

POSSIBLE ACQUISITION OF HIV DURING INITIATION INTO STUDENT OCCULT CLUBS. A. ADEGBOYE, E.E.EZE. OA UNIVERSITY, ILE-IFE, NIGERIA.

Purpose: To report a scenario of possible HIV spread through exposure to infected blood during 'initiation' into occultism.
Methods: R.A., a male teenage law student of OAU, Nigeria was brought into the Emergency room of OAU Teaching Hospital following matchet cuts on face, inflicted by hooded students. He proved HIV+ve(double reactive ELISA). Epidemiologic investigations were done.
Result: Medical history showed no drug use nor sexual contact with persons at risk for HIV infection. He has never been transfused with blood/blood products, never been operated(including all surgical and dental) on. Serotests for Syphillis and HBV were negativ However, he was exposed to other persons' blood during 'club initiation' 6 months ago. He did not know the HIV serostatus of these newly initiated members he 'mixed blood' with
Conclusion: Since no other risk factor for HIV infection could be established in this patient, HIV transmission might have occured during the initiation ceremonies he participated in which occasioned exposure to other persons' blood.

0756

HBV, HDV, HCV MARKERS AMONG HEALTH CARE PROFESSIONALS IN REPUBLICAN CENTER OF HAEMATOLOGY AND BLOOD TRANSFUSION, SOFIA

V.Magaeva[1], A.Gushterova[2]
1National Drug Institute, Sofia Bulgaria, 2Blood Bank, Military Hospital, Sofia Bulgaria

Bulgaria belongs to the countries with intermediate HBsAg carrier rate 2-7% in general population. Risk of contracting hepatitis B infection in medical occupation is about 10 fold higher that in general population.

We investigated health care professionals in Republican center of haematology and blood transfusion for HBV, HCV, HDV infection in connection with vaccination against hepatitis B. The aim of this study was to evaluate the prevalence of serum HBV, HCV, HDV markers in health care professionals, whose work in blood bank according their function and place of activity.

The results of that study are shown below:

markers function	HBsAg	anti HBs	anti HBcIgG	anti HCV
doctors	0/25	8/25	5/25	1/25
lab. techn.	2/50	14/48	16/50	2/50
technicians	1/24	5/18	10/24	2/24
	3/99	27/91	31/99	5/99

*Conclusion:*There is strong correlation between duration of work in blood bank and infection with hepatitis viruses. We recommend HBV vaccination according results, for employers all health care professionals and students before starting medical activities.

0757

INFECTIOUS WASTE HANDLING IN BLOOD TRANSFUSION CENTERS IN INDONESIA AS COMPARED WITH BELGIUM

D.Van Caekenberghe (1), W.Gardjito (2)
1 Military Hospital, Brussels, Belgium,
2 Dr. Soetomo Teaching Hospital, Surabaya, Indonesia.

Blood bank infectious waste is peculiar in that wet infectious waste prevails.

In Belgium infectious waste has to be declared to a special state agency, it has to be collected in specially designed single use containers, it has to be stored cooled or frozen, and has to be picked up regularly for incineration at an authorized incineration plant. Incineration is preferred for hygienic and aesthetic reasons. The cost for incineration is one to several US $ per kg.

In Indonesia environment protection regulations do exist, but a comprehensive body of regulations regarding infectious hospital waste has not yet been issued. Should the example of the industrialized countries be followed? The economic reality in developing countries is different. Whereas public funding is scant, cheap labour is abundant.

Small scale steam pressure sterilization of wet infectious waste could offer a low-budget, labour-intensive alternative, yielding sterilized liquids (that could be passed to the sewers or used as a soil fertilizer),and sterilized packing material (that could be tipped with domestic waste).

0759

PROGRESS IN THE STRUTURING OF THE INFORMATIONAL SYSTEM OF THE CENTER FOR BLOOD TRANSFUSION

I. Maslovaric (1), V. Libek (2), P. Kusljevic (1), N. Nedeljkovic (1)
1. Blod Transfusion Institе of Serbia - Beograd
2. KBC Zemun , Zemun Yugoslavia

A well-adapted informational system in great degree facilitates and increases the reliableness of the operation of the Center for Blood Transfusion.

The Clinical Center "KCB Zemun" has an advanced informational system which functions very successfully. The entire set of computer programs, procedures and related documentation associated with the system comes from the fourth generation of software (Progress). The system monitors all the phases of the operation from the time a unit of blood is taken to the time it is given to a patient. A data-base is established in which the history file of a patient, protocol of the taken units of blood, results of the completed blood analyses, products in the unit of blood, results of the interreactions, and issuing of the unit of blood - are all given.

The system automatically runs a data-check to make certain that all the data are complete, and then prints the corresponding labels (blood type, phenotype, HBsAg, anti - HIV, TPHA, name of product, date when it was taken, expire date, identification no.bar code). Since the system is able to run a complete data-check in a very short period, we can acquire all the desired data without any delay.

We will take this opportunity to mention that our informational system is very flexible in terms of its enhancement, and thus allowing improvement in the operation of the Centers for Blood Transfusion.

In conclusion, only a highly organized informational system can provide prosperity in research undertakings such as those conducted at our Center, as well as at others.

0761

PLASMA FRACTIONATION IN INDIA

VIJAYLAXMI RAY & MAYA PARIHAR
NATIONAL PLASMA FRACTIONATION CENTRE
K.E.M.HOSPITAL, BOMBAY-12 (INDIA)

Prior to 1987 plasma fractionation in India was with private organisation who obtained plasma from professional donors by plasmapheresis. The Government of India undertook to set up the first plasma fractionation centre using voluntary donor blood. The centre was started at K.E.M.Hospital where in 1988 component therapy was initiated to save plasma for fractionation. Thus centre not only introduced optimal use of voluntary donor blood but also the better patient management became evident.

At present there are about six blood banks (1993) which are making blood components. The plasma input to centre was only from K.E.M.Hospital in 1989, now supplies only 40% of the plasma, while 60% of the plasma is coming from other blood banks in Bombay. The products made in this centre, like Albumin 5% & 20% are meeting the demand of the city and is not imported into the country.

Thus introduction of plasma fractionation has been an impetus to improve the transfusion practice and awareness in component therapy in Bombay city which is the largest medical centre in India.

0762

NEEDS FOR SAFE BLOOD IN DEVELOPING COUNTRIES

E.J.Watson-Williams.E.C.Technical Assistant, Blood Transfusion Service, MOH, Lusaka, Zambia.

Introduction. Blood transfusion practices in the developing world have changed little since 1960. Provision of assistance to screen for HIV has revealed many deficiencies compared with standards demanded in developed countries.
Problems. 1. There is no organised voluntary donor base, due to lack of public education, donor recognition, transport and facilities and trained staff. 2. Fear of HIV testing (lack of confidentiality, possible erroneous result and inadequate quality of counselling and care). 3. Constant blood shortage leading to inappropriate selection of recipients. 4. Outdated laboratory equipment and procedures that threaten safety to staff and patients. 5. Large numbers of life threatening anaemias in childhood and pregnancy and haemorraghic complications of parturition. 6. Many small, remote and understaffed hospitals. 7. Lack of funds.
Solutions. Provide financial assistance (not more than 10c per head per annum) and training for. 1. Physician specialists in B.T. medicine. 2. Donor recruiters and counsellors. 3. Donor facilities and transport. 4. Re-equip laboratories and introduce safer methods. 5. Screen blood for all detectable transmissible diseases (not only HIV). 6. Improve nutrition and primary health care. 7. Educate hospital staff to reduce demand for isologous blood.

0763

DONORS AND DONATIONS IN YUGOSLAVIA NOWDAYS

Gradimir Dimitrijević, G.Dimitrijević
Department for blood transfusion, Novi Sad, Yugoslavia

What can we say?A country where 90% of the population is poor(according to UN a poor person is one with less then 1 dollar per day),where the health system is collapsed and where we still have blood donors.Old ones,but new ones are coming.Motivation--altruistic or idea to help to a member of a close family or close friend,(directed donations).Dependent on nationality of a donor and are we collecting blood in rural or urban area.From apound 30000 donations per year in our dept.we finished 1993.year with around 16000 donations.Some of the benefits donors had,thay all lost.Despite all this,they are still coming but the scale is slowly going towards directed donations, rather than altruistic.We are convinced that they will all come again if overall situation becomes as it was some few years ago.Donations are still not payed and are volunteer bases,even if they are directed donations.Donors on any pf the apheresis procedures are extremly rare,due to the equipment shortage.All together:"Eppur si muove".

0764

BLOOD BANKING STAFFS IN DEVELOPING COUNTRIES

Melani Wikanta, Indonesian Red Cross Central Blood Transfusion Service

Since 1969 Blood Transfusion Service in Indonesia have been coordinated by Central to combat the high paid donors and incoordinated management.

To meet the need of blood bank staffs throughout the country, a regular six month course of trainees had been taken without officially regulation from the government, and yet it ccould have been running the Blood Transfusion Service year by year.

Up to now there are 27th course with 1.068 Blood Transfusion assistants throughout the 138 Blood Transfusion Chapters.

To improve the carrier and financial status of Blood Transfusion Assistants, many efforts have been tried with struggle and at least this year there will be an approval by Department of Health, and the improvement from six month course to 1 year Diploma I has been taken.

0765

BLOOD TRANSFUSION SERVICE IN AZERBAIJAN

Ch.D.Asadov, G.B.Abbasova
Institute of Haematology and Blood Transfusion, Baku, Azerbaijan

The blood donor and supply service is an integral part of Azerbaijan care system. The service includes the network of Haematology and Blood Transfusion Institute, Blood Transfusion Stations and Departments (Blood Banks). Nearly 150 physicians and 300 paramedical personnel are involved in Azerbaijan Blood Transfusion Service. The financing of Blood Transfusion Service is based on direct state support. Usually blood is collected from nearly 160.000 donors per annum. About 198.000 whole blood units, 66.000 (41.2%) of which are used for transfusion, are collected annually. All blood units are tested for anti-HIV-1, HbsAg. Plasma is collected from 2300 donors by single or double plasmapheresis (number of plasma donations - 15.000). The production department exists in Haematology and Blood Transfusion Institute and in Baku, Ganja and Guba Blood Transfusion Stations. Near 3700 l of plasma is fractionated there per annum. Computer system is worked out for Blood Transfusion Stations. It is intended for: a) centralised registration and efficient donor research; b) improvement of blood, its component and preparation calculation organization; c) carrying out of statistical works.

0766

ABOUT HAEMOPHILIA PROBLEM IN ESTONIA

K.A.Orgulas,M.A.Veske,J.R.Tamme '
Children Hospital,Tallinn,Estonian Blood Centre,Tallinn,Estonia.

7;46 Haemophilia is a very important problem and needs support and help from goverment as it is actual in ESTONIA but all difficulties encountered can`t be explained by economic situation. There are 45 haemophilia patients in Estonia. Today we are seeking for optimal organization of care in our country. Haemophilia assotiation was organized in november 1992. It´s purpose is to take care of patients and integrate with similar assotiations in other countries (Finland, Latvia, Lithuonia) Self-sufficiency is a most important condition for reducing transmission of infectious diseases. For replacement therapy of haemophilia A we use fresh frozen plasma separated from an individual unit of whole plasma and frozen within 6 hours after collection and single-donor cryoprecipitate. The main problem is to provide an adequate supply of plasma. In order to avoid disruption of needed therapy for haemophilia patients our Blood Centre has taken steps to increase the supplay of fresh plasma for factor VIII and to improve quality of cryoprecipitate production. We do not have imported blood products. Haemophilia patients are treated-cured with fresh frozen plasma or cryoprecipitate, that are produced from Estonian donors blood.

0767

SELF-SUFFICIENCY IN BLOOD AND BLOOD PRODUCTS - IS A REAL THING IN BULGARIA?

T. Lissitchkov[1], P. Vatkovsky[2]
1National Center of Clinical and Transfusional Haematology, 2Republican Center of Haematology and Blood Transfusion, Sofia, Bulgaria

Self-sufficiency in blood and blood products must be a goal of a national transfusional policy of every country. The whole transfusional system in Bulgaria has to be modernized according new contemporary knowledge and practice. The number of the blood donations are reduced to the half than in 1988, the production of Factor VIII in Sofia in 1988 was 1030000 U but in 1993 - only 240000 U. The blood preservation is old fashioned one. Plasma fractionation is a smallscale, plasma preparations are not virusinactivated. The use of blood and blood products in clinical practice is unsuitable (42.8% of blood and 17.1% of fresh frozen plasma in Sofia are in clinical practice).

There is in Bulgaria a new long term donor recruitment programme, a project for modernisation and restructuring of the of the transfusional system, plan for new plasma fractionation.

But in spite of all these activities the self-sufficiency in blood and blood products will be a real fact no sooner that five years.

0768

STRATEGIES FOR THE REVIEW OF TRANSFUSION PRACTICES IN YUGOSLAVIA

N. Nedeljkovic[1], S. Mitrovic[1], M. Antic[1], V. Gligorovic[1], N. Tijanic[1], N. Suvajdzic[2], M. Petrovic[2], M. Colovic[2], M. Pajevic[3], Lj. Lovric[4], S. Gruden[5], M. Jelic[6], Lj. Nikolic[6], G. Bunjevacki[7], D. Veljkovic[7], D. Mitrovic[8]

1 Blood Transfusion Institute of Serbia, 2 UCC Institute of Hematology, 3 Clinical Center Zvezdara, 4 Clinical Center „Dr D. Misovic„, 5 Clinical Center Zemun, 6 Institute of Oncology, 7 Institute of Maternity and Child Care, 8 Institute of Pathology University School of Medecine, Belgrade Yugoslavia

In our practise modern transfusion principles were successfuly applied. They covered blood collection, serological processing of blood units, technological preparations of blood products and rational utilization of whole blood, blood components and blood derivatives. In the last three years (1991, 1992 and 1993) aberrations from these principles have taken place.

A referential team of transfusiologists monitor doctrines of good production and clinical practise using retrospective, comparative and prospective surveilance methods. The obtained data suggest fall of the number of voluntary blood donors by 29% with rise of special (targeted) donors from 10% to 60% of the total number of donors. The level of blood products production has been generally lowered with the steepest fall of Standard Platelet Concentrate production were the correlation coefficient of the negative trend was 0.959 ($p<0.05$). The number of plasmapheresis and cytapheresis procedures has also fallen (-1.000, $p<0.05$) as well as plastic systems for blood transfusion (-0.999, $p<0.05$). The total consupton of Whole Blood has increased from 20% to 65% of the total number of transfusions due to the respective decrease of blood products production.

Shortages of medical supplies (trifold and fourfold plastic bags), discontinued maintenance of equipment due to lack of spare parts, fall of number of voluntary blood donors have led to irrational consumption of Whole Blood and endagered a large number of acute and chronic patients whose survival and quality of life depend on blood product transfusion.

0769

THE ROMANIAN BLOOD TRANSFUSION SYSTEM, FOUR YEARS AFTER THE REVOLUTION

Marcu, I., Nat. Inst. Health Services & Management, Bucharest, ROMANIA

The Romanian BTS, outdated, overstaffed and centralized, had to be reformed. Financial and technical support from the European Union was offered but little was used. A National Program was introduced in 1990 but the progress was very slow. The little progress towards decentralization of the BTS, achieved in 1991-1992, was reversed in 1993, in part due to lack of adequate legislation and insufficient internal financing, but also because of a limited outlook of the Administration. Lack of support from the policy makers in the field of healthcare for recruitment of voluntary, non-paid blood donors has postponed, maybe for several years, the development of this type of donation. Teaching of Transfusion Medicine is currently marginal. An additional problem is the persistent attempts of private foreign companies to establish for-profit plasmapheresis in the country. Training of staff in modern techniques, introduction of bags, efforts to develop voluntary non-paid blood donation should be encouraged. Analysis by experts will hopefully redirect the evolution of the BTS, provided that suggestions for change are accepted by the Administration. International organizations should support the change.

0770

USE OF PROSTAGLANDIN E_1 DURING PREPARATION OF PLATELET CONCENTRATES.

SG.Mitchell, RJ.Hawker, VS.Turner.
West Midlands Blood Transfusion Service, Birmingham, U.K.

Prostaglandin E_1 (PGE_1) has been shown to be an inhibitor of platelet activity. It may therefore have a role in inhibiting activation and then maintaining platelets in a resting state during storage.

Ten volunteer donors took part in a paired study to investigate the benefits of adding *in vitro* PGE_1 during preparation of platelet concentrates (PCs) by routine techniques. PGE_1 (560μM final concentration) or a control solution was added to the platelet rich plasma prior to a 18.5×10^3 g min centrifugation to pellet the platelets. The resulting platelet concentrates were stored in a volume of 65ml for 5 days at 22°C with agitation in PL1240 units. A sample of the PC was then labelled with ^{111}Indium and autologously reinfused. The remaining platelets were assayed for *in vitro* function and biochemistry. Blood samples were taken from the volunteers over the next 5 days for determination of *in vivo* platelet recovery and survival and some donors had gamma camera images taken to determine organ distribution.

No significant *in vitro* differences were found after the storage period apart from LDH content and large particles. 7 out of 10 of the PCs had better aggregation responses to ADP following 5 days storage with PGE_1 and 3 out of 4 had lower ß-TG release.

(n=10)		$+PGE_1$	$-PGE_1$
HSR(%)		38.4	32.0
Aggregation(%)	ADP 3.2μM	22.8	18.1
	ADP 32μM	69.1	55.4
LDH Release(%)		10.0	11.3
LDH Content (IU/10^{11}plts)		122	155
ß-TG Release (μg/10^9plts)		11.7	20.9
Aggregates $>45\mu m^3$ (10^7/L)		141	338

In vivo recoveries were similar: 41.4%($+PGE_1$) v. 44.4%($-PGE_1$) with no difference in organ distribution at 24hrs, but survivals were reduced ($p<0.05$) in the presence of PGE_1: 5.8 days v. 6.9 days.

Although PGE_1 did not improve platelet characteristics after 5 days storage, it did facilitate easier and faster platelet resuspension following centrifugation obviating the need for "resting".

SUBJECT-INDEX

ORAL PRESENTATIONS

Virus inactivation of plasma products
0149 0150 0151 0152 0202 0203 0204 0205 0206 0207

QA of blood component preparation
0160 0161 0162 0163

Cryopreservation of blood cells and stem cells
0165 0166 0167 0168

Monitoring hemolytic disease of the Newborn
0170 0171 0172 0173

Virus inactivation of cell concentrates
0183 0184 0185 0186

R-DNA plasma products and convential clotting factor concentrates
0189 0190

Collection and transplantation of stem cells
0193 0194 0195 0196 0227 0228 0229 0230 0231 0232

Pediatric transfusions
0210 0211

Hepatitis B virus
0213 0214 0215 0216

Storage and preservation of red cells
0218 0219 0220 0221

Transfusion in developing countries
0222 0223 0224 0225 0226 0244 0245

Hüfner Memorial Symposium
0232

New plasma products
0234 0235 0236 0237

Storage and preservation of platelets
0249 0250 0251 0252

POSTER PRESENTATIONS

Blood Groups
0259 0260 0261 0262 0263 0264 0265 0266 0267 0268 0269 0270 0271 0272 0273 0274 0275 0276 0277 0278 0279 0280 0281 0282 0283 0284 0285 0286 0287 0288 0289 0290 0291 0292 0293 0294 0295 0296 0297 0298 0299 0301 0523 0524 0525 0526 0527 0528 0529 0530 0531 0532 0533 0534 0535 0536 0537 0538 0539 0540 0541 0542 0543 0544 0545 0546

Antibody Detection (including Anti-HLA)
0302 0303 0304 0305 0306 0307 0308 0309 0310 0311 0312 0313 0314 0315 0316 0317 0318 0319 0320 0321 0322 0323 0324 0325 0326 0547 0548 0549 0550 0551 0552 0553 0554 0555 0556 0557 0558 0559 0560 0561 0562 0563 0564 0565

Leukocyte Removal and Filtration
0327 0328 0329 0331 0332 0333 0334 0335 0336 0337 0338 0339 0340 0342 0343 0344 0345 0346 0347 0348 0349 0350 0351 0352

Quality Assurance
0353 0354 0355 0356 0357 0358 0359 0360 0361 0362 0363 0364 0365 0366 0367 0368 0372

Clinical Aspects of Blood Transfusion
0373 0374 0375 0376 0377 0378 0379 0380 0381 0382 0383 0384 0385 0386 0387 0388 0389 0390 0391 0392 0393 0394 0395 0396 0397 0398 0399 0400 0401 0402 0403 0404 0405 0406 0408 0409 0410 0412 0413 0414 0415 0416 0417 0418 0419 0420 0421 0422 0424 0425 0426 0427 0428 0429 0430 0431 0617 0618 0619 0620 0621 0622 0623 0624 0625 0626 0627 0628 0629 0630 0631 0632 0633 0634 0635 0636 0637 0638 0639

Apheresis
0432 0433 0434 0435 0436 0437 0438 0439 0440 0441 0442 0443 0444 0446 0447 0448 0449 0450 0451 0452 0453 0454 0455

Transfusion Transmitted Diseases
0456 0457 0458 0459 0460 0461 0462 0463 0464 0465 0466 0467 0468 0469 0470
0471 0472 0473 0474 0475 0476 0477 0478 0479 0480 0481 0482 0483 0484 0485
0486 0487 0488 0489 0490 0491 0492 0493 0494 0495 0496 0497 0498 0499 0500
0501 0502 0503 0504 0505 0506 0507 0508 0509 0510 0662 0663 0664 0665 0666
0667 0668 0669 0670 0671 0672 0673 0674 0675 0676 0677 0678 0679 0681 0682
0683 0684 0685 0686 0687 0688 0689 0690 0691 0692 0693 0694 0695 0696 0697
0698 0699 0701 0702 0703 0704 0705 0706 0707 0708 0709 0710 0711 0712 0713
0714 0715 0716 0717 0718 0719 0720

Alternatives and New Products
0511 0512 0513 0514 0515 0516 0517 0518 0519 0520 0521 0522

Quality Assurance of Component Preparation
0566 0567 0568 0569 0570 0571 0572 0573 0574 0575 0576 0577 0578 0579 0580
0581 0582 0583

Storage and Preservation of Blood Cells and Bone Marrow
0586 0587 0588 0589 0590 0591 0592 0593 0594 0595 0596 0597 0599 0600 0601
0602 0603 0604 0605 0606 0607 0608 0609 0610 0611 0612 0613 0614 0615

Hemolutic Disease of the Newborn/Pediatric Transfusions
0640 0641 0642 0643 0644 0645 0646 0647 0648 0649 0650 0651 0652 0653 0654
0655 0656 0657 0658 0659 0660 0661

Virus Inactivation of Blood and Plasma
0721 0722 0723 0724 0725 0726 0727 0728 0729 0730 0731 0732 0733 0734

Donors
0735 0736 0738 0739 0740 0741 0742 0743 0744 0745 0746 0747 0748 0749

Developing Countries/Miscellaneous
0750 0751 0752 0753 0754 0755 0756 0757 0759 0761 0762 0763 0764 0765 0766
0767 0768 0769 0770